This book is dedicated to the military medical professional in a land far from home, standing at the bedside of a critically ill child.

Dosage Selection:

The authors and publisher have made every effort to ensure the accuracy of dosages cited herein. However, it is the responsibility of every practitioner to consult appropriate information sources to ascertain correct dosages for each clinical situation, especially for new or unfamiliar drugs and procedures. The authors, editors, publisher, and the Department of Defense cannot be held responsible for any errors found in this book.

Use of Trade or Brand Names:

Use of trade or brand names in this publication is for illustrative purposes only and does not imply endorsement by the Department of Defense.

Neutral Language:

Unless this publication states otherwise, masculine nouns and pronouns do not refer exclusively to men.

The opinions or assertions contained herein are the personal views of the authors and are not to be construed as doctrine of the Department of the Army or the Department of Defense. For comments or suggestions on additional contents in forthcoming editions, please contact the publisher (www.bordeninstitute.army.mil).

Published by the Office of The Surgeon General
Borden Institute
Fort Detrick, Maryland, and Fort Sam Houston, Texas

Library of Congress Cataloging-in-Publication Data

Pediatric surgery and medicine for hostile environments / senior surgical editor, Michael M. Fuenfer ; senior medical and critical care editor, Kevin M. Creamer. -- Revised.
p. ; cm.
Includes bibliographical references and index.
I. Fuenfer, Michael M., editor of compilation. II. Creamer, Kevin M., editor of compilation. III. Borden Institute (U.S.), issuing body. IV. United States. Department of the Army. Office of the Surgeon General, issuing body. V. US Army Medical Department Center and School, issuing body. VI. Emergency war surgery. Third United States revision. 2004. Pediatric version of (work):
[DNLM: 1. Emergencies--Handbooks. 2. Wounds and Injuries--surgery--Handbooks. 3. Child. 4. Infant. 5. Military Medicine--Handbooks. WO 39]
RD151
617.9'9--dc23

2013003735

Printed in the United States of America
18, 17, 16, 15, 14, 13 5 4 3 2 1

Age / Weight	Chest Tube	Peripheral BP Cuff Size	IV Catheter	Central Line	Arterial Line	Nasogastric Tube	Foley Catheter
Premature infant (< 3 kg)	8–10 Fr	Premature infant–newborn 5 cm	24 g	5 Fr UVC or 5 Fr feeding tube	5 Fr UAC or 5 Fr feeding tube	5 Fr	5 Fr
Newborn (< 28 days; ≥ 3 kg)	10–12 Fr	Newborn 5 cm	24 g	5 Fr UVC	5 Fr UAC	5–8 Fr	6 Fr
Infant (1 m–1 y; 4–10 kg)	10–12 Fr	Newborn–infant 5 cm	22–24 g	3 or 4 Fr 5–8 cm or 20 g 12 cm pediatric IJ kit	2.5 Fr 2.5 cm (peripheral) or 24 g IV or 2.5 Fr 5 cm (central)	5–8 Fr	6–8 Fr
Toddler (1–2 y; 10–13 kg)	16–20 Fr	Infant–child 5–7 cm	22–24 g	4 Fr 8–12 cm or 20 g 12 cm pediatric IJ kit	2.5 Fr 2.5 cm (peripheral) or 22–24 g IV or 2.5 Fr 5 cm (central)	8 Fr	8 Fr
Preschool (3–5 y; 13–18 kg)	18–24 Fr	Child 7 cm	20–22 g	4–5 Fr 12 cm 8–12 cm	22 g IV catheter or 20 g pediatric IJ kit (central)	10 Fr	10 Fr
School age (6–12 y; 18–40 kg)	20–32 Fr	Child–small adult 7–9.5 cm	20 g	5 Fr–7 Fr 8–20 cm	22 g IV catheter	10–14 Fr	10–12 Fr
Adolescent (13–18 y; > 40 kg)	> 32 Fr	Small adult–adult > 9.5 cm	18–20 g	7 Fr adult triple lumen	22 g IV catheter	14–18 Fr	12–18 Fr

BVM: bag valve mask
IJ: internal jugular
IV: intravenous
UAC: umbilical arterial catheter
UVC: umbilical venous catheter

Pediatric Surgery and Medicine for Hostile Environments

Revised

Borden Institute
Walter Reed Army Medical Center
Washington, DC

Office of The Surgeon General
United States Army
Falls Church, Virginia

US Army Medical Department Center and School
Fort Sam Houston, Texas

The test of the morality of a society
is what it does for its children.

—Dietrich Bonhoeffer (1906–1945)

Contents

Pediatric Surgery and Medicine for Hostile Environments

Senior Surgical Editor

Michael M. Fuenfer, MD, FAAP, FACS

Colonel, Medical Corps, US Army Reserve
Pediatric Surgeon
Walter Reed Army Medical Center
6900 Georgia Avenue, NW, Washington, DC 20307;
National Naval Medical Center
8901 Rockville Pike, Bethesda, Maryland 20889;
Assitant Professor of Surgery and Pediatrics
Uniformed Services University of the Health Sciences
4301 Jones Bridge Road, Bethesda, Maryland 20814

Senior Medical and Critical Care Editor

Kevin M. Creamer, MD, FAAP

Colonel, Medical Corps, US Army
Chief, Pediatric Inpatient and Critical Care Services
Walter Reed Army Medical Center
6900 Georgia Avenue, NW, Washington, DC 20307;
Associate Professor of Pediatrics
Uniformed Services University of the Health Sciences
4301 Jones Bridge Road, Bethesda, Maryland 20814;
Pediatric Consultant to The Surgeon General
for Pediatric Subspecialties

Borden Institute Editorial Staff

Martha K. Lenhart, MD, PhD, FAAOS
Colonel, MC, US Army
Director and Editor in Chief

Ronda Lindsay
Volume Editor

Joan Redding
Managing Editor

Douglas Wise
Layout Editor

Marcia Metzgar
Technical Editor

Note to Revised Edition

This revision includes an expanded dental chapter and minor wording changes.

Editorial Board

Contributors

Karla Au Yeung, MAJ, MC, USA
Kenneth S. Azarow, COL, MC, USA (Ret)
Hans E. Bakken, MAJ, MC, USA
Randy S. Bell, LCDR, MC, USN
Paul L. Benfanti, COL, MC, USA
Richard H. Birdsong, COL, MC, USA
Scott E. Brietzke, LTC, MC, USA
Thomas R. Burklow, COL, MC, USA
Kathryn Camp, MS, RD, CSP
Wayne A. Cardoni, LCDR, MC, USN
Lisa Cartwright, LCDR, MC, USN
Debora S. Chan, PharmD, FASHP
Theodore J. Cieslak, COL, MC, USA
Bernard A. Cohen, MD
Annesley W. Copeland, COL, MC, USA (Ret)
James E. Cox, Jr., COL, MC, USAF (Ret)
Stephen J. Cozza, COL, MC, USA (Ret)
Kevin M. Creamer, COL, MC, USA
Arthur J. DeLorimier, COL, MC, USA
William C. DeVries, COL, MC, USAR
Robert L. Elwood, MAJ, MC, USAF
Nathan L. Frost, CPT, MC, USA
Charles J. Fox, LTC, MC, USA
Michael M. Fuenfer, COL, MC, USA
Satyen Gada, LCDR, MC, USN
Rebecca A. Garfinkle, MAJ, MC, USA
Curtis Goho, COL, DC, USA

Matthew D. Goldman, MAJ, MC, USAF
Gregory H. Gorman, LCDR, MC, USN
John Hanna, DDS
Patrick W. Hickey, MAJ, MC, USA
Alex Holston, LCDR, MC, USN
Nancy G. Hoover, LTC, MC, USA
Cheryl Issa, MS, RD, CSP, CNSD
David Jarrett, COL, MC, USA
Timothy K. Jones, COL, DC, USA (Ret)
Matthew Kelly, MAJ, MC, USA
Ryan J. Keneally, MAJ, MC, USA
Brent L. Lechner, LTC, MC, USA
Martha K. Lenhart, COL, MC, USA
Rebecca B. Luria, MAJ, MC, USA
Robert Mansman, MAJ, DC, USA
Chad Mao, LCDR, MC, USN
Jonathan E. Martin, MAJ, MC, USA
Donald R. McClellan, COL, MC, USA
Michael McCown, MAJ, MC, USA
Kathleen McHale, COL, MC, USA (Ret)
Margret E. Merino, LTC, MC, USA
Michael H. Mitchell, COL, MC, USA
Marisa G. Mize, DNP
Houman Motamen-Tavaf, LTC, MC, USA
Dawn D. Muench, MAJ, MC, USA
Harlan S. Patterson, COL, MC, USA
Philip L. Rogers, COL, MC, USA (Ret)
Shawn D. Safford, CDR, MC, USN
Erik P. Schobitz, MD
Cynthia H. Shields, COL, MC, USA
Elizabeth Shin, DDS
Steven E. Spencer, LTC, MC, USA
Phillip C. Spinella, MD
Robert Steelman, MD, DMD
Allen I. Stering, MAJ, MC, USAF
Frederick J. Stoddard Jr, MD
Carolyn A. Sullivan, COL, MC, USA
Deena Sutter, MAJ, MC, USAF
Sarah K. Taylor, MAJ, MC, USA
Martin E. Weisse, COL, MC, USA

Foreword

Throughout American history, military physicians have provided humanitarian care to civilians whenever possible. This was especially the case during the period of westward expansion in the 1800s, when, in many instances, Army doctors stationed at remote outposts represented the sole source of medical care for pioneering families. Today, officers and enlisted soldier–medics are deployed to over a hundred nations in all corners of the world. For much of the populace of these countries, especially children, these uniformed combat medics, nurses, physicians, and allied health professionals represent the only hope for modern and compassionate medical and surgical care.

Now, more than ever before, large numbers of indigenous children with a wide range of acute and chronic medical conditions are presenting for treatment at US military medical facilities. Family members travel for days over rugged terrain, sometimes carrying children on their backs, in order to reach a US military facility, knowing that their children will receive life-saving and compassionate treatment there. During my many visits to US military facilities in Iraq and Afghanistan, while participating in reviews of clinical research programs in Africa and Asia, or engaged in humanitarian missions in developing nations, I find few images are as heart rending as those of severely injured, ill, and wounded children. It is an unfortunate but irrefutable fact that the most innocent and vulnerable members of a society, its children, are often the first to suffer from the turmoil of an increasingly violent and unpredictable world.

Recognizing this state of affairs, my predecessor directed that the experience in pediatric care garnered by our deployed medical officers be incorporated into this book, *Pediatric Surgery and Medicine for Hostile Environments*. This manual will serve as a basic reference for military physicians and surgeons whose usual scope of practice entails limited exposure to childhood illness. To accomplish this objective, some of the most talented and experienced pediatricians and pediatric subspecialty surgeons throughout the active and retired ranks of the Medical Corps of the Army, Navy, and Air Force were enlisted as contributors. All are to be commended for an outstanding effort and remarkable final product. I feel this manual will contribute significantly to the success of the overall humanitarian mission of military medicine and will advance our collective efforts to mitigate the tragedy of violent conflict and, whenever possible, may prevent or arrest the spread of war.

Lieutenant General Eric B. Schoomaker, MD, PhD
The Surgeon General
US Army
Commanding General
US Army Medical Command

Washington, DC
May 2010

Prologue

Injuries to civilian populations are a tragic consequence of war. Unfortunately, the changing nature of warfare is resulting in a progressively higher proportion of civilian casualties. During World War I, civilians accounted for less than 20% of all deaths. In World War II, they made up 48% of all deaths. Civilians account for 80% of the war dead in more recent conflicts.[1] It is estimated that more than 2 million children perished as a result of war in the last decade of the 20th century, with over 6 million injured or permanently disabled.[2] The current US military conflicts, Operation Enduring Freedom (OEF) in Afghanistan and Operation Iraqi Freedom (OIF) in Iraq, have also resulted in a significant incidence of pediatric trauma.

The primary mission of the deployed military healthcare system is to "preserve the fighting strength" by caring for sick and injured US military and coalition forces. Another vital role is to provide humanitarian care for the civilian population. Local national admissions to level III facilities, such as combat support hospitals (CSHs), are supported by US military doctrine if the patient is suffering from an illness or injury that threatens life, limb, or eyesight. The Center for Army Strategic Studies reports pediatric patients comprise approximately 10% of all CSH admissions in Iraq and Afghanistan. Children comprised almost half of the humanitarian admissions in both theaters, and their length of hospital stay was roughly twice as long as that of all adult patients.[3] As of late 2009, it is estimated that between 5,000–6,000 children, many critically injured, have been admitted to deployed hospitals in Iraq and Afghanistan. Although nontraumatic and medical diagnoses were responsible for 25% of all pediatric admissions to CSHs, trauma injuries, of which 75% were penetrating, were the most common reasons for admission.[4] Traumatic injuries to children accounted for 12% of all occupied beds at CSHs, 11% of transfused and ventilated patients, and 13% of all combat hospital deaths.[5] Although the primary mechanisms of injury in children are gunshot wounds (39%), followed by explosive injuries (32%), there are distinct differences between theaters

(Tables 1 and 2, Figure 1).The length of hospital stay for these children averaged 7–15 days. On average, they each underwent more than two invasive or surgical procedures. The pediatric mortality rate has trended upward annually, and the overall mortality rate is 6.9% for children admitted to a CSH. This is significantly higher than for adults in both coalition and humanitarian emergency admissions, and more than double the reported pediatric civilian trauma mortality rate of 2.9%.[6]

Burns accounted for one third of inpatient deaths, followed by head injuries (75% of which were penetrating), at 25%. Infection and sepsis accounted for 10% of pediatric mortality, but when secondary infection was considered, it was evident that infections were a major factor in 30% of all pediatric CSH deaths. Head injuries resulted in the highest case fatality rates (20%), while pediatric burn injuries had a case fatality rate of 16% at the CSH. In contrast, the case fatality rate for all other diagnoses was 3.8%.

The scope of the pediatric mission is a compelling reason to refine predeployment and deployment education to improve

Table 1. Causes of Pediatric Injury by Theater

Known Cause of Injury (Pediatric Inpatients)	Percent of Total Injured in Afghanistan	Percent of Total Injured in Iraq
Gunshot wounds	21	56.6
Burns	14.6	5.8
Landmines	14.6	0.8
Motor vehicle crashes	12.5	6.8
Falls	12.3	1.5
Fragments	8.2	13.4
Blasts	7.4	8.7
Complications of previous injuries	4.8	4.7
Environmental (drowning, animal bites, cold, venomous bites/stings)	2.3	0.7
Poisoning	1.2	0.5
Stab wounds	1.1	0.3

Table 2. Principal Pediatric Traumatic Diagnosis by Theater*

Principal Diagnosis (Pediatric Inpatients)	Percent of Those Injured in Afghanistan	Percent of Those Injured in Iraq	Percent of Total Injured†
Burns	16.3	10.1	13.3
Abdominal wound with bowel/organ injury, penetrating	9.4	14.4	11.8
Lower extremity wound, fracture, open	6.4	12.3	9.2
Lower extremity wound, penetrating	5.3	8.5	6.9
Skull fracture, open	6.4	7.1	6.7
Upper extremity wound, fracture, open	3.8	5.5	4.6
Lower extremity wound, fracture, other	5.3	2.7	4.0
Skull fracture, other	5.7	2.1	4.0
Eye injury	5.8	1.6	3.8
Back/buttock/genitalia wound, penetrating	2.2	5.3	3.7
Lower extremity wound, traumatic amputation	5.5	1.7	3.6
Upper extremity wound, penetrating	2.8	4.0	3.4
Face/head/neck wound, penetrating	3.7	2.5	3.1
Upper extremity wound, traumatic amputation	4.1	2	3.1
Head injury/traumatic brain injury	3.0	3.1	3.1
Chest wound, penetrating	1.8	3.5	2.6
Upper extremity wound, fracture, other	2.7	1.5	2.1
Chest wound, pneumothorax	0.9	1.7	1.3
Vascular injury	0.9	1.6	1.2
Face/head/orbit fracture, open	0.8	1.7	1.2
Face/head/orbit fracture, other	1.7	0.5	1.1
Lower extremity wound, other	1.3	0.7	1.0
All others	4.4	5.9	5.1
Totals (average percent)	**51.20**	**48.80**	**100.00**

*Most common injuries grouped and sorted by theater.
†Total number injured in Afghanistan: 787; total number injured in Iraq: 750; total number injured overall: 1,537.

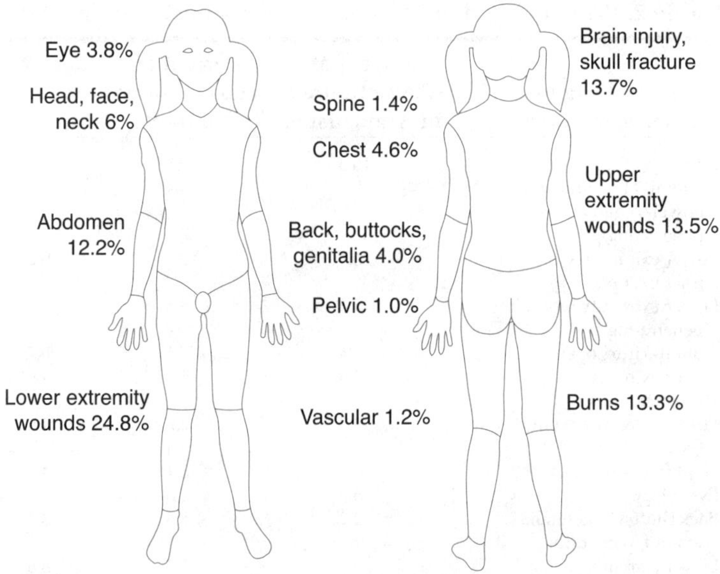

Figure 1. Distribution of injuries by anatomic region.

outcomes in this vulnerable population. This manual was created in recognition of the clear need for pediatric emergency and humanitarian care delivery by the US military healthcare system in Afghanistan and Iraq during OEF and OIF.

Our intention is to provide military physicians, often practicing in an austere environment, with a current and concise reference for the basic medical, surgical, and critical care of children. It should be used as a pragmatic reference but not as a substitute for published textbooks, current peer reviewed articles, or reasoned judgment. Operative procedures performed on children often entail significant risk even under ideal circumstances, and should not be attempted without a complete assessment of the available resources and equipment, experience of the operating room team, potential complications, nonoperative options, availability of follow-up care, and an honest overall assessment of the risk to the child from the procedure to be undertaken.

It is our ethical obligation to counsel the parent or guardian, if available, about the risks and benefits of a procedure, and to obtain their consent for nonemergent operations. Local custom and the family's desires must be respected in all cases, lest what was intended to be a humanitarian gesture results in unintended consequences that negatively impact the success of the overall military mission.

In many situations, the extent to which such aid can be rendered will be limited by operational considerations, lack of age-appropriate equipment and supplies, and limitation of other resources.

References

1. Aboutanos, MB, Baker SP. Wartime civilian injuries: epidemiology and intervention strategies. *J Trauma*. 1997;43:719–726.
2. Ursano RJ, Shaw JA. Children of war and opportunities for peace. *JAMA*. 2007;298:567–568.
3. Hassell LR, Wojcik BE, Stein CR. Overview of CASS studies and analysis. Paper presented at: Center for AMEDD Strategic Studies; June 7, 2007 (updated September 10, 2007); Ft Sam Houston, Tex.
4. Creamer KM, Edwards MJ, Shields CH, Thompson MW, Yu CE, Adelman W. Pediatric wartime admissions to US military combat support hospitals in Afghanistan and Iraq: learning from the first 2,000 admissions. *J Trauma*. 2009;67;762–768.
5. Borgman M, Spinella PC. Profile of pediatric patients at US Army combat support hospitals in Afghanistan and Iraq. *Crit Care Med*. 2007;35:12s, A158.
6. Burd RS, Jang TS, Nair SS. Evaluation of the relationship between mechanism of injury and outcome in pediatric trauma. *J Trauma*. 2007;62:1004–1014.

Introduction

Caring for Children in War: Military Humanitarianism and Fourth-Dimension Warfare

Caring for children injured in combat or stricken ill by the consequences of war has long been a priority for American military medical forces. But the potential impact of "military humanitarianism" on the outcome of war is only now being recognized as a key component of the National Military Strategy, which encourages American military forces to promote peace and stability worldwide to "shape the world, not merely to be shaped by it."[1]

Experts on modern warfare say that it has entered a "fourth" dimension. The first two dimensions encompassed war's breadth and depth, but were limited by time and space. The third dimension began with the advent of airpower, which reached across the boundaries of distance and represented one of the major revolutions in warfare. Technology and the digital transformation have been referred to as warfare's fourth dimension because the speed of information exchange allows for one warring faction to interrupt its enemy's information–decision–action (IDA) cycle.[2] However, this view of warfare's fourth dimension is too shortsighted.

The ancient Greeks had different concepts of time. The idea of time as "chronos" defines physical time measured in a linear fashion, in which each moment is like the next. "Kairos" reflects the perfect season or quintessential moment that must be seized and acted upon to achieve a desired result. Physicians caring for children in austere or hostile environments are able to interrupt the enemy's IDA cycle by affecting kairos time in the families and communities for which they provide care. They can be with the family at the exact moment of need, and can affect the family's perspective for a lifetime. This is how military humanitarianism, particularly the care of children in wartime and in complex humanitarian disasters, embodies the fourth dimension of warfare.

The impact of humanitarianism at these quintessential kairos moments can be seen throughout our history. The Lewis and Clark expedition, commissioned by President Jefferson, was the longest infantry patrol in US history. It traveled 8,000 miles in 28 months, and military humanitarianism was one of the key goals of the mission.[3] Lewis and Clark acknowledged their mission's success was in a large part due to the skill and leadership of their pregnant Shoshone guide, Sacagawea. Her knowledge of the geography and the languages and cultures of the tribes she encountered saved them on many occasions. When Sacagawea's labor failed to progress, Lewis cared for her and administered two rings of a rattlesnake rattle, according to a local American Indian folk medicine tradition. Sacagawea's child fell ill when he was 15 months old. On May 22, 1806, Lewis wrote, "The child . . . is very ill this evening . . . he was attacked with a high fever . . . and his neck and his throat are much swollen." After treatment with cream of tartar and repeated application of poultice of onions, the fever broke.[4] The attentive care with which Lewis and Clark ministered to Sacagawea during her labor and to her son during his life-threatening illness was the kairos that won them her heart and her loyalty.[5]

After the United States dropped a nuclear bomb on Hiroshima in 1945, a Japanese physician, Dr Hachiya Michihiko, was positively affected by US military doctors who helped him treat Japanese civilians wounded and sickened by the bomb. He wrote,

> They gave us great help, materially and spiritually, in the reconstruction of our hospital. Two doctors removed fear and hostility from our hearts and left us with a bright, new hope. The harsh winter that followed the autumn was less harsh for their having come.[6]

Military humanitarianism has also played a critical role in current conflicts. US Special Forces, focusing on engineering projects and delivering healthcare, helped radically improve the security on Basilan Island, Philippines. Over 4 years, this "volatile, uncertain, complex and ambiguous" situation was made more secure by allowing the Philippine military to reduce its presence from 15 battalions to 2.[7,8] The impact medical care had on young mothers and children—and, by association, future security—there remains to be seen.

In Afghanistan, humanitarian efforts may play an even greater role. In 2004, one in four children died before age 5, and one in twelve women died in childbirth. Afghanistan had been a training ground for enemies of the United States, and was far from becoming a developed nation. While talk in Iraq was about rebuilding, in Afghanistan, our efforts continue to be building from the ground up, and military physicians are deeply involved in this process. Caring for children is at the forefront of these efforts in military hospitals and in building host-nation capabilities.[9–11]

Although the nuances of fourth-dimension warfare are complex, the realities for doctors and nurses are much simpler. Service members caring for children in Iraq, Afghanistan, the Horn of Africa, the Philippines, Somalia, East Timor, and many other places around the globe focus their energies on building up nations' healthcare systems so that infants there have the same chance at survival as infants born in the United States. If our enemies are indeed finite, it is possible to diminish their number by taking away their ability to recruit from the children of the next generation. For example, consider a child whose first memories of Americans are the faces of the doctors and nurses in uniform who struggle to save her after she stepped on a mine. What will this child and her parents think of the Americans they have met? Will their memories make them less likely to become our enemies? This is fourth-generation kairos warfare.[12]

In his address to the House of Commons on June 8, 1982, President Ronald Reagan said, "The ultimate determinant in the struggle that's now going on in the world will not be bombs and rockets, but a test of wills and ideas, a trial of spiritual resolve, the values we hold, the beliefs we cherish, the ideas to which we are dedicated."[13] This book is directed at those engaged in this fight, and dedicated to everyone standing at the bedside of a critically ill child in a land far from home.

Colonel Chuck Callahan
DeWitt Health Care Network
Fort Belvoir, Virginia

Colonel Kevin M. Creamer
Walter Reed Army Medical Center
Washington, DC

Colonel Michael M. Fuenfer
Walter Reed Army Medical Center
Washington, DC

References

1. US Department of Defense. National Security Strategy 2008. US Department of Defense Defense Link Web site. http://www.defenselink.mil/news/2008%20National%20Defense%20Strategy.pdf. Accessed October 10, 2009.
2. Singh A. Time: the New Dimension in War. *Joint Forces Quarterly*. 1995/1996;10:56–61.
3. Ambrose S. *Undaunted Courage*. New York, NY: Touchstone Books; 1996.
4. Chuinard EG. *Only One Man Died: The Medical Aspects of the Lewis and Clark Expedition*. Glendale, Calif: The Arthur H. Clark Co; 1980: 405.
5. Callahan C. The roots of military medical humanitarianism. *US Army Med Dep J*. 2001;PB 8-01-7/8/9:39.
6. Michihiko H. *Hiroshima Diary*. Wells W, trans. New York, NY: Avon Publications; 1955: 220.
7. McAvoy A. U.S. forces find model for beating terror. *Washington Post*. May 31, 2006. http://www.washingtonpost.com/wp-dyn/content/article/2006/05/31/AR2006053100347.html.
8. Shambach SA. *Strategic Leadership Primer*. Carlisle Barracks, Pa: US Army War College; 2004.

9. Creamer K, Edwards MJ, Shields C, Thompson M, Yu CE, Adelman W. Pediatric wartime admissions to US combat support hospitals in Afghanistan and Iraq: learning from the first 2,000 admissions. *J Trauma*. 2009;67:762–768.
10. Burnett M, Spinella, P, Azarow K, Callahan C. Pediatric care as a part of the U.S. Army medical mission in the Global War on Terrorism: Afghanistan and Iraq, December 2001 to December 2004. *Pediatrics*. 2008;121:261–265.
11. Matos R, Spinella P, Holcomb J, Callahan C. Increased mortality of young children with traumatic injuries at a U.S. Army hospital. *Pediatrics*. 2008;122:e959–e966.
12. Callahan C. Editorial. *Honolulu Advertiser*. October 20, 2004.
13. Reagan R. Address to the House of Commons, June 8, 1982. Constitutional Concepts Foundation Web site. http://www.constitutionalconcepts.org/reaganspeech.htm. Accessed October 10, 2009.

Resuscitation and Critical Care

Chapter 1

Basic Approach to Pediatric Trauma

Approximately 75% of children admitted to deployed level-three facilities since 2001 have been victims of trauma, and 75% of that trauma was penetrating, caused by myriad mechanisms.[1] Although extremity wounds, including traumatic amputations, were the most frequent injuries reported, major sources of mortality in the resuscitation phase were head injury, penetrating thoracic wounds, and burns. Previous epidemiologic reviews have found significantly higher mortality rates for infants, younger children, and females (see Further Reading). Independent predictors of mortality include pH less than 7.1, Glasgow Coma Scale (GCS) score less than 4 on presentation, or the need for more than one unit of packed red blood cells or fresh frozen plasma.

Triage for children is similar to that for adults; it is a system used to prioritize treatment, taking into account the extent of the trauma (ie, polytrauma or a single injury), type of trauma (ie, blunt or penetrating), and the severity of the illness or injury. The goal is the same for children as for adults: to save as many patients as possible with the resources available.

Anatomical and Physiological Considerations

- General differences
  - Abnormal general appearance is indicative of a serious illness or injury
  - Normal responses differ by age (ie, developmental stages)
  - Vital signs are based on age
  - Bradypnea and bradycardia are both ominous
  - Children have a larger relative surface area for a given weight than adults
    - This puts them at higher risk for hypothermia
      - Hypothermia can increase oxygen requirements
      - Obtain rectal temperature; monitor and maintain temperature at 36.5°C–37.5°C

    - Hypothermia is associated with apnea and bradycardia
    - The head is a major source of heat loss; mitigate heat loss by covering the head with a hat or cap
  - Because of their larger surface-area-to-weight ratio, children also sustain greater insensible water loss and have different fluid requirements than adults (see Chapter 22, Basic Fluid and Electrolytes)
- Children have a conical airway; the cricoid is the narrowest portion of the airway
- The pediatric skull has expandable sutures until 18–24 months of age
- Children's short, fat necks make assessing for tracheal deviation or jugular venous distention more difficult than in adults
- Cervical spine fractures are less common than ligamentous injury
  - Injury is more likely to be at a higher cervical level in children than in adults
  - Spinal cord injury without radiographic abnormality can be seen in up to 50% of children with spinal cord injuries
- Children's pliable ribs make fractures less likely; transmitted energy is more likely to cause pulmonary contusion
- Tension pneumothorax is more likely in children than in adults due to the mobile contents of the mediastinum
- Solid abdominal organs are more susceptible to injury because of their anterior placement, children's less-developed abdominal walls, and subcutaneous fat
- Fractures of long bones with active growth plates can result in length discrepancies
- Medications are all dosed as milligrams per kilogram per dose. Use a Broselow tape for emergency medication dosing, and use a published reference to confirm all other pediatric drug doses (eg, *The Harriet Lane Handbook*; see also the comprehensive equipment table inside the front cover)
- Psychological impact
  - Very young children may regress in response to pain or

stress, or as perceived threats enter their environment
    - Involving a parent may help in calming the child and acquiring a history
- Neonates and young infants
  - This age group is at increased risk for sepsis due to decreased white blood cell function and count, decreased antibody synthesis, and decreased inflammatory response
  - Neonates are more sensitive to drugs because of their immature blood–brain barrier
  - Hypoglycemia is more common in this age group because of their smaller glycogen stores
  - Neonates' smaller functional residual capacity makes desaturation more common
  - Apnea and bradycardia occur in response to decreased partial pressure of oxygen and increased carbon dioxide in young infants
  - Hypocalcemia will result in hypotension; intravenous (IV) calcium is an inotrope in young infants

Assessment

- Life-threatening conditions should be treated as soon as they are identified
- Primary survey (should take no more than 5–10 min)
  - Start with a 30-second pediatric advanced life support (PALS) rapid cardiopulmonary assessment
  - **Airway** (the most common cause of cardiac arrest in children is respiratory failure; support the airway first)
    - Is the child's airway clear and maintainable, or does the patient require intubation?
    - Maintain and control open airway
    - The child's head should be placed in the sniffing position
      - Use jaw thrust if injury to the cervical spine is a concern
      - A child's relatively large tongue and prominent occiput cause the head to flex forward and potentially obstruct the pediatric airway
      - Position and suction the airway as necessary
        - The larynx is funnel shaped, cephalad, and ante-

rior in the neck
        - An infant's trachea is about 5 cm long; a toddler's is about 7 cm long
        - Unintentional right mainstem intubation is common in small children
    - Consider placing an oropharyngeal (in an unconscious patient) or nasopharyngeal airway
    - Intubation is indicated for any of the following:
        - GCS score ≤ 8
        - No gag reflex
        - Prolonged transport
        - If bag-valve mask ventilation is ineffective
        - If sensorium is depressed and hypovolemia or hypotension are present
    - Cricothyroidotomy (needle or surgical) is an option for those unable to be bag-mask ventilated or intubated (**NOTE:** surgical cricothyroidotomy should not be performed in children < 12 years of age)
- Rapid sequence intubation
    - Preoxygenate with 100% oxygen by a nonrebreather mask for 2 minutes or 4 vital capacity breaths
    - Administer atropine sulfate (0.02 mg/kg IV) to dry oral secretions and prevent bradycardia from succinylcholine for children < 6 months old
    - Administer an induction agent (Table 1-1)
    - Apply cricoid pressure using the thumb and index finger (5–10 lb pressure on cricoid cartilage)
    - Administer a paralytic: succinylcholine chloride (2 mg/kg for children < 10 kg; 1 mg/kg for children > 10 kg) or rocuronium (0.6–1 mg/kg)
    - Intubate (see comprehensive equipment table inside the front cover)
    - Confirm tube position with capnography or qualitative carbon dioxide first; follow with clinical confirmation (eg, auscultation, chest rise, mist in tube)
    - Release cricoid pressure
    - Secure tube
    - Obtain secondary confirmation with chest radiograph, if available

Table 1-1. Induction Agents for Intubation

Induction Agent	Dose	Characteristics
Etomidate	0.2–0.3 mg/kg IV	Quick onset; ultrashort acting; PALS recommended for head-injured patients
Thiopental	3–5 mg/kg IV	ATLS recommended for normotensive patients
Midazolam	0.1–0.3 mg/kg IV	ATLS recommended for hypotensive patients
Propofol	1–2 mg/kg IV	Avoid using in hemodynamically unstable patients; can worsen hypotension
Ketamine	1–2 mg/kg IV	Limited effect on circulatory system; useful in patients with hemodynamic instability

ATLS: advanced trauma life support
IV: intravenous
PALS: pediatric advanced life support

- **Breathing**
  - Does the patient exhibit increased respiratory rate for age?
    - Infant: > 60 breaths per minute (bpm)
    - Child < 5 years old: > 40 bpm
    - Child > 5 years old through adolescent: > 30 bpm
  - Does the patient exhibit effective air movement (tidal volume)?
    - Decreased air entry is a sign of parenchymal lung disease or poor effort
    - Hypoventilation is common in pediatric trauma
    - Avoid hypercarbia
  - Signs of respiratory distress
    - Retractions (inspiratory)
    - Grunting (expiratory) indicates airway or alveolar collapse
    - Stridor upon inspiration indicates extrathoracic obstruction
    - Wheezing indicates intrathoracic obstruction

- Apply supplemental high-flow oxygen and positive-pressure, bag-valve mask ventilation as necessary
  - Deliver 1 breath every 2–3 seconds
  - Deliver enough volume to generate good chest rise
- Perform needle decompression then insert a chest tube for tension pneumothorax (diagnostic signs and symptoms include hypoxemia, hypotension, and absent breath sounds)

◦ **Circulation**

- Observe mental status; the child's level of reactivity and responsiveness is usually a reflection of cerebral perfusion
- Measure heart rate
- Feel pulse quality and compare central and peripheral pulses
- Is there a differential skin temperature? Is the skin cooler distally than it is proximally?
- Observe capillary refill time; normal is 2 seconds, more than 3 seconds can indicate shock
- Check pulse pressure
- Measure blood pressure early
  - A child can be in shock and still have a normal blood pressure
  - Low blood pressure for the child's age indicates decompensated shock
- Establish vascular access (intraosseous if necessary)
  - Treat shock and hypotension aggressively
  - The preferred isotonic fluid is Ringer's lactate, unless the patient has a head injury (in that case, the preferred fluid is normal saline); bolus volume for a child is 20 mL/kg (repeat once if necessary)
  - Consider early transfusion for hemorrhagic shock
    - Use a 10–15 mL/kg packed red blood cell bolus for blood replacement
    - See Chapter 5, Transfusion Medicine, for further guidance on transfusion therapy
  - Inadequate resuscitation is common; it is most important to control bleeding
  - Diagnose and treat pericardial tamponade (diag-

in Morison pouch, subphrenic space, right pleural space, and retroperitoneum
    - Free fluid forms spicules or triangulates to follow the path of least resistance
    - Morison pouch pools excess fluid from pelvis and perisplenic areas; use the coronal view and slide caudally until the inferior pole of the kidney is seen. This allows detection of supra- and inframesocolic fluid around the tip of the liver
    - Pleural fluid is accurately detected in 98% of patients
  - Perisplenic (left upper quadrant)
    - Use an intercostal technique; place probe between ribs 9 and 10 or 10 and 11. Technically difficult to get good visualization this way
    - The spleen is located dorsally, so the probe must be placed posteriorly
    - The ideal view contains the left hemidiaphragm, spleen, and left kidney
    - Splenic injury is more difficult to visualize with FAST than with CT scan
  - Pelvic
    - This area is best examined when the bladder is full
    - Perform a complete examination before inserting a Foley catheter
    - Observe both longitudinal and transverse views
    - Place probe just above the pubic symphysis, with the probe indicator pointed toward the patient's head
    - In females, fluid will be present in the pouch of Douglas posterior to the uterus
    - In males, fluid appears in the rectovesicular pouch or cephalad to the bladder
- The presence of fluid or blood is not necessarily an indication for operative intervention

Further Reading

1. Creamer K, Edwards MJ, Shields C, Thompson M, Yu CE, Adelman W. Pediatric wartime admissions to US combat

support hospitals in Afghanistan and Iraq: learning from the first 2,000 admissions. *J Trauma*. 2009;67:762–768.

2. Matos R, Spinella P, Holcomb J, Callahan C. Increased mortality of young children with traumatic injuries at a U.S. Army hospital. *Pediatrics*. 2008;122:e959–e966.
3. McGuigan R, Spinella PC, Beekley A, et al. Pediatric trauma: experience of a combat support hospital in Iraq. *J Pediatr Surg*. 2007;42:207–210.
4. Gausche-Hill M, Fuchs S, Yamamoto L, eds. *The Pediatric Emergency Medicine Resource*. Revised 4th ed. Sudbury, Mass: Jones & Bartlett; 2007.
5. Mejia R, ed. *Fundamentals of Pediatric Critical Care Support Course*. Mount Prospect, Ill: Society of Critical Care Medicine; 2008.
6. American College of Surgeons Committee on Trauma. *Advanced Trauma Life Support of Doctors*. Chicago, Ill: American College of Surgeons; 2008.
7. Custer JW, Rau RE, Lee CK, eds. *The Harriet Lane Handbook*. 18th ed. New York, NY: Mosby; 2008.

Chapter 2

Anesthesia

Pediatric trauma anesthesia varies significantly from adult trauma anesthesia because of the anatomical and physiological differences between adults and children (Table 2-1).

Table 2-1. Anatomical Considerations

Airway Anatomy	Implications
Infants have a large occiput, anterior airway	The traditional sniffing position, which flexes the head downward, is not helpful; place a rolled towel under the shoulders to facilitate intubation
Small airway means small ET tube	Tube can easily become plugged with blood or secretions
Cricoid is the narrowest part of the airway	Ensure leak at 20–25 cm water pressure to avoid edema*
Short trachea	Endobronchial intubation is common; extubation can be caused by small movements of the head or ET tube
Infants have increased airway reactivity	Bronchospasm is common, especially during light anesthesia or if ET tube is near the carina
Infants have an increased dead space/minute ventilation ratio	Increased risk of rebreathing carbon dioxide; avoid adding connectors between ET tube and circuit

ET: endotracheal

*It may be necessary to have a seal of a greater magnitude than 25-cm water pressure when ventilating patients who have significant pulmonary contusions or edema that is a greater immediate threat than the eventual risk of postintubation croup or subglottic stenosis. Ventilating pediatric patients is difficult with field anesthesia machines, which rely on older, manually adjusted bellows. Intensive-care-unit-grade ventilators are more effective at generating exact tidal volumes and can be used with intravenous anesthesia.

Physiological Considerations

Infants and small children are unable to increase their stroke volume, making them dependent on heart rate to maintain cardiac output. In infants < 6 months old, consider using atropine before induction or giving neuromuscular blockade to maintain heart rate during rapid sequence intubation (see Table 2-2 for normal vital signs by age group).

Table 2-2. Normal Vital Signs by Age Group

Age	Weight (kg)*	Respiratory Rate (breaths/min)	Heart Rate (beats/min)	Normal Systolic Blood Pressure (mmHg)†
Premature infant	< 3 kg	40–60	130–170	45–60
Term newborn (< 28 days)	3 kg	35–60	120–160	60–70
Infant (1 mo–1 y)	4–10	25–50	110–150	70–100
Toddler (1–2 y)	10–13	20–30	90–130	75–110
Young child (3–5 y)	13–18	20–30	80–120	80–110
Older child (6–12 y)	18–40	15–25	70–110	90–120
Adolescent (13–18 y)	> 40	12–20	55–100	100–120

*Weight norms based on US children. Expect lower weights in countries where malnutrition is more prevalent.

†For children 1–10 years old, use the following equation: 70 + 2(age) = lowest acceptable systolic pressure for age.

- **Hypoventilation** is the most common cause of cardiac arrest in children
- **Respiratory acidosis**, further exacerbating a metabolic acidosis, is a common occurrence in injured children
- **Hypotension** is a late sign of **hypovolemia** in pediatric patients
  - Blood pressure usually remains normal until > 25% blood volume is lost
  - Poor perfusion, evidenced by cool extremities, delayed capillary refill, and diminished distal pulses, is an early sign of hypovolemia
  - The most common cause of hypotension in pediatric patients is hypovolemia
  - If the patient is not responding to volume resuscitation, medications may be needed to increase blood pressure
    - Phenylephrine **should not** be a first-line choice for treating intraoperative hypotension in children
    - Small doses of epinephrine are a better first-line choice

        - ▹ Start with 1–4 μg and titrate to effect
        - ▹ At low doses, the β effects of epinephrine predominate, increasing heart rate and contractility
    - ▸ Consider a continuous infusion of inotropes or pressors if hypotension persists despite adequate fluid and blood product resuscitation
    - ▸ Dopamine and epinephrine are preferred for pediatric patients

Intubation

- Indications: altered level of consciousness, impending or actual upper airway obstruction, and hemodynamic instability
- Orotracheal intubation is the most reliable means of establishing an airway and ventilating a child
    - The risk of penetrating the cranial vault or injuring the nasopharyngeal soft tissue is a relative contraindication to the use of the nasotracheal route in patients ≤ 12 years old
- In head-injured or comatose patients, intubation should be performed with cervical spinal immobilization
- For chronically malnourished children, consider starting with a slightly smaller tube

Airway Formulas

- Ways to estimate the appropriate endotracheal (ET) tube size:
    - (Age + 16)/4
    - Height (cm)/20
    - Size of child's small finger (fifth digit on hand)
    - Premature infant: 2.5
    - Term infant: 3.0
- Ways to estimate appropriate depth of ET tube (cm):
    - Infant: 6 + weight (kg)
    - Child: 3 × size (inner diameter) of tube
- **NOTE:** These are only estimates; always evaluate clinically

Surgical Airway

In infants and small children, cricothyroidotomy may cause long-term damage to the larynx, so tracheostomy is preferred. Cricothyroidotomy can be safely performed in children ≥ 11 years old.

Initial Ventilator Settings

- Tidal volume: 7–10 mL/kg
- If using pressure control, peak inspiratory pressure (PIP): 20–25 cm H_2O
- Positive end-expiratory pressure (PEEP): 3–5 cm H_2O
- Age-appropriate respiratory rates:
  - Adolescents: 10–15 breaths per minute (bpm)
  - Children: 15–25 bpm
  - Infants: 25–30 bpm
- Fraction of inspired oxygen (FiO_2): 100% initially, then titrate to nontoxic levels as permissible

Pediatric Equipment Sizing

In an emergency, the preferred method of determining equipment size for pediatric patients is using the Broselow Pediatric Measuring Tape (if available). To use the tape, measure the patient from the top of the head to the heels and use the equipment and drug doses indicated on the tape. For central line sizes, refer to Chapter 3, Vascular Access. Otherwise, refer to the equipment table on the inside and front cover of this book.

Pediatric Trauma Resuscitation

Acidosis, hypothermia, and coagulopathy are a deadly triad for patients presenting with major exsanguinating trauma.

- **Hypothermia**
  - Pediatric patients are predisposed because of their large surface-area-to-weight ratio, thin skin, and paucity of subcutaneous fat
  - Worsens preexisting acidosis by causing a leftward shift in the oxyhemoglobin dissociation curve, leading to decreased oxygen delivery to the tissues
  - Can cause decreased drug metabolism and, in infants, can lead to apnea and hypoglycemia
  - Aggressive rewarming and normothermia maintenance must be initiated immediately upon arrival of the pediatric trauma patient. Strategies for increasing or maintaining body temperature include, but are not limited to:
    - Increasing the room temperature
    - Using forced-air warmers

    - Preparing and working on one body part at a time while leaving the rest of the child covered
    - Wrapping the child's body and head in plastic bags
  - Fluid-warming devices are helpful; however, the volume of fluid and blood products administered to the pediatric patient must be controlled. One way to do this is to use a syringe at the end of the warming line to administer warm intravenous (IV) fluids and blood products
- Fluid resuscitation
  - In cases where blood products are not the initial therapy of choice, fluid resuscitation should be initiated with a 20 mL/kg bolus of normal saline (NS) or Ringer's lactate
    - The patient should be reassessed after each bolus of NS to evaluate whether or not more fluid or a change to blood is required. If child remains hypotensive after three 20 mL/kg boluses, administer packed red blood cells
    - If IV access is not rapidly achieved (1–3 min), immediately proceed to intraosseous (IO) access
    - Resuscitate through the IO access and then obtain reliable IV access
  - For small IV catheters (22 gauge and 24 gauge), bolusing with a 10–20 mL syringe is the most efficient way to rapidly deliver fluids and blood products (see Table 2-3

Table 2-3. Maintenance Fluid Requirements

Weight (kg)	Amount of Normal Saline to Administer
Up to 10	4 mL/kg/h
10–20 kg	40 mL/h + 2 mL/kg/h for each kg > 10
> 20 kg	60 mL/h + 1 mL/kg/h > 20 kg

for maintenance fluid recommendations)
  - Small children (< 2 years old) can occasionally become hypoglycemic during long operative cases
    - The tendency toward hypoglycemia is usually counterbalanced by the stress response of surgery
    - If potential hypoglycemia is concerning, run a

maintenance-only infusion using an infusion pump of D_5 0.45% NS (do not include glucose in any of the resuscitation fluids or the patient will become hyperglycemic)

- Blood therapy
  - See Chapter 5, Transfusion Medicine, for guidance on routine and massive transfusion strategies
  - Hypocalcemia is associated with rapid infusion of colloids, including blood products (particularly fresh frozen plasma and fresh warm whole blood)
    - Severe cardiac depression and hypotension can result from ionized hypocalcemia (potent inhalational agents dramatically exacerbate hypotension)
    - Do not **routinely** transfuse at a rate faster than 1 mL/kg/min
    - Prevention includes limiting the rate of fresh frozen plasma transfusion to less than 1 mL/kg/min and administering calcium chloride (5 mg/kg) or calcium gluconate (15 mg/kg)
  - If a patient is at risk for massive transfusion, packed red blood cells, fresh frozen plasma, and platelet transfusion should be initiated in a 1:1:1 ratio
    - Helps avoid coagulopathy
    - Has been shown in adults to reduce mortality

Burns (see also Chapter 9, Burns)
In children with unrecognized inhalational injuries, severe airway swelling may occur after fluid resuscitation. If there is uncertainty about whether an inhalational injury has occurred, intubate early.

- In addition to maintenance fluids (see Table 2-3), use the Parkland formula for fluid resuscitation in the first 24 hours after a burn:

4 mL/kg Ringer's lactate × body surface area (BSA) burned

  - Give half in the first 8 hours, half over the next 16 hours
  - **This formula is an estimate only.** The goal is to give enough fluids to maintain urine output of 1 mL/kg/h
- To calculate daily maintenance after the first 24 hours (mL/24 h):

$$[(\%\ \text{total BSA burned} + 35) \times \text{BSA}\ (m^2) \times 24] + 1{,}500\ \text{mL/m}^2$$

[1,500 mL/m^2 = daily maintenance fluid required in a burn patient]

Calculating BSA using a Web-based BSA calculator is easier, but the Mosteller formula can also be used:

$$\text{BSA}\ (m^2) = (\text{height (cm)} \times \text{weight (kg)}/3{,}600)^{1/2}$$

- Consider pulmonary injury, carbon monoxide poisoning, and chemical exposure, particularly in closed-space burns
- Consider airway burns and edema when patient presents with discolored sputum
- Nutritional support is critical; start tube feedings as soon as possible postoperatively
- Blood loss during burn excision: 3% of blood volume for every 1% of BSA excised
- Blood loss during skin grafting: 2% of blood volume for every 1% of BSA grafted

Preoperative Sedation

Children who require repeated operations after sustaining initial trauma will benefit from preoperative sedation. In children for whom IV access has been established, dose-adjusted preoperative sedation regimens similar to those used in adults are appropriate. For children without IV access, the following are some of the available options:

- Oral: **midazolam** 0.5 mg/kg (maximum dose 10 mg) 20 minutes prior to the procedure
- Rectal: **methohexital** 25–30 mg/kg (indicated for children weighing < 15 kg)
    - Mix 500 mg methohexital with water to a volume of 5 mL
- Intramuscular: 0.2 mg/kg **midazolam** + 1.5–2.0 mg/kg **ketamine** + 5–10 μg/kg **glycopyrrolate** (use 5 mg/mL concentration of midazolam or the volume will be too large)

Postoperative Pain Management

- Use a continuous IV opioid infusion (Table 2-4) if unable to use patient-controlled analgesia (PCA; eg, if patient is < 6 years old or if there is a language barrier)

Table 2-4. Intravenous Narcotics: Continuous Infusion*

Drug	Loading Dose	Continuous Infusion
Morphine	0.05 mg/kg	0.01–0.06 mg/kg/h
Fentanyl	1 μg/kg	0.2–3 μg/kg/h
Hydromorphone	10 μg/kg	0.5–4 μg/kg/h

*Bolus to achieve analgesia and start infusion at a lower rate. If analgesia is inadequate, rebolus with half the first dose, and increase rate by 25%.

Table 2-5. Patient-Controlled Analgesia Dosing*

Drug	Dose	Basal Rate	Lock out
Morphine	10–30 μg/kg	5–30 μg/kg/h	6–12 min
Fentanyl	0.25–1.0 μg/kg	0.25–1.0 μg/kg/h	6–12 min
Hydromorphone	2–6 μg/kg	1–3 μg/kg/h	6–12 min

*Patient-controlled analgesia can be used in a normal cooperative child as young as 6 years old.

- PCA is usually suitable for children > 6 years old (Table 2-5)
  - Communication must be sufficient to ensure both patient and parent understand appropriate PCA use
  - Loading dose is the same as for continuous infusion
  - Basal rates are associated with overdoses in adults; monitor closely or avoid if possible
  - Prevent family from pushing PCA button
- Intermittent IV opioid dosing
  - **Morphine**: starting dose is 0.05–0.1 mg/kg IV
    - Repeat dosing every 5–10 minutes until effective analgesia is established
    - Use this as basis for IV q2–4h dosing schedule
  - **Fentanyl**: starting dose is 0.5–1 μg/kg IV
    - Repeat dosing every 5–10 minutes until effective analgesia is established
    - Use this as basis for IV q1–2h dosing schedule
- Oral opioids and other adjuvant medications
  - **Acetaminophen** has opioid-sparing effects
    - Oral load 30 mg/kg, then 10 mg/kg q4h

- Rectal load 40 mg/kg, then 20 mg/kg q4h
- Maximum dose is 90–110 mg/kg/day
- Administer ketorolac 0.5 mg/kg IV q6h for no more than 3 days
- **Tramadol** is a weak μ-agonist
  - Administer 1–2 mg/kg orally q6h
  - Do not exceed 400 mg/day
- **Acetaminophen with codeine** can also be used
  - Codeine dosing is 0.5–1.0 mg/kg/dose orally q4–6h (dose is limited by maximum daily dose of acetaminophen)
  - 25% of patients cannot convert codeine to its active formulation and it will not be effective in these patients
- Administer **oxycodone** 0.05–0.15 mg/kg/dose orally q4–6h (daily dose is limited by maximum dose of acetaminophen if in a combined form)

Regional Anesthesia

Regional anesthesia may be contraindicated by shock or sepsis at initial presentation, but can be effective after initial stabilization and is usually performed while the child is anesthetized (Tables 2-6–2-8).

Table 2-6. Pediatric Drug Dosing for Caudal or Epidural Blocks

Age	Bupivacaine	Ropivacaine	Clonidine	Fentanyl
Single Injection				
< 1 y	0.25%, 1 mL/kg	0.2%, 1.2 mL/kg	1.0–1.5 μg/kg	2 μg/mL
> 1 y	0.25%, 1 mL/kg, max 20 mL	0.2–0.5%, max 20 mL or 3.5 mg/kg	1.0–1.5 μg/kg	2 μg/mL
Continuous Injection				
< 3 mo	0.0625%–0.125%, 0.2 mg/kg/h	0.1%–0.2%, 0.2 mg/kg/h	0.12–0.2 μg/kg/h	1–2 μg/mL
< 1 y	0.125%, 0.3 mg/kg/h	0.1-0.2%, 0.3 mg/kg/h	0.12–0.2 μg/kg/h	1–2 μg/mL
> 1 y	0.125%, 0.3–0.4 mg/kg/h	0.1%–0.2%, 0.4 mg/kg/h	0.12–0.2 μg/kg/h	1–2 μg/mL

Reproduced from: Buckenmaier C, Bleckner L. *Military Advanced Regional Anesthesia and Analgesia Handbook*. Washington, DC: Borden Institute; 2009: Table 30-2.

Table 2-7. Pediatric Spinal Dosing

Age	Bupivacaine (mg/kg)	Tetracaine* (mg/kg)	Ropivacaine (mg/kg)
Infants	0.5–1.0	0.5–1.0	0.5–1.0
1–7 y†	0.3–0.5	0.3–0.5	0.5
> 7 y†	0.2–0.3	0.3	0.3–0.4

*With tetracaine, use epinephrine wash (epinephrine aspirated from vial and then fully expelled from the syringe prior to drawing up local anesthetic) to increase duration up to 120 minutes.

†Additives: clonidine 1–2 μg / kg for children > 1 year of age.

Reproduced from: Buckenmaier C, Bleckner L. *Military Advanced Regional Anesthesia and Analgesia Handbook.* Washington, DC: Borden Institute; 2009: Table 30-3.

Table 2-8. Drug Dosing for Pediactric Single-Injection Peripheral Nerve Block*

Block	Dose Range (mL/kg)	Midrange Dose (mL/kg)	Maximum Volume (mL)
Parascalene	0.2–1.0	0.5	20
Infraclavicular	0.2–1.0	0.5	20
Axillary	0.2–0.5	0.3	20
Paravertebral	0.5–1.0	0.7	5
Femoral	0.2–0.6	0.4	17
Proximal sciatic	0.3–1.0	0.5	20
Popliteal	0.2–0.4	0.3	15
Lumbar plexus	0.3–1.0	0.5	20

*Children < 8 y: 0.2% ropivacaine or 0.25% bupivacaine. Children > 8 y: 0.5% ropivacaine or 0.5% bupivacaine. **Do not exceed maximum recommended doses of local anesthetic.**

Reproduced from: Buckenmaier C, Bleckner L. *Military Advanced Regional Anesthesia and Analgesia Handbook.* Washington, DC: Borden Institute; 2009: Table 30-4.

Further Reading

1. American College of Surgeons. *Advanced Trauma Life Support (ATLS) Course Manual*. 8th ed. Chicago, Ill: ACS; 2008.

2. US Department of Defense. *Emergency War Surgery, Third United States Revision*. Washington, DC: DoD; 2004.

3. Mattei P. *Pediatric Surgery: Surgical Directives*. 1st ed. Philadelphia, Pa: Lippincott Williams & Wilkins; 2003.

4. O'Neill JA Jr, Grosfeld JL, Fonkalsrud EW, Coran AG, Caldamone AA. *Principles of Pediatric Surgery*. 2nd ed. St. Louis, Mo: Mosby; 2003.

5. Motoyama EK, Davis PJ. *Smith's Anesthesia for Infants and Children*. 7th ed. Philadelphia, Pa: Mosby Elsevier; 2006.

6. Barcelona SL, Coté CJ. Pediatric resuscitation in the operating room. *Anesthesiol Clin North America*. 2001;19(2):339–365.

7. Smith HM, Farrow SJ, Ackerman JD, Stubbs JR, Sprung J. Cardiac arrests associated with hyperkalemia during red blood cell transfusion: a case series. *Anesth Analg*. 2008; 106:1062–1069.

8. Duchesne JC, Hunt JP, Wahl G, et al. Review of current blood transfusions strategies in a mature level 1 trauma center: were we wrong for the last 60 years? *J Trauma*. 2008;65:272–276.

9. González EA, Moore FA, Holcomb JB, et al. Fresh frozen plasma should be given earlier to patients requiring massive transfusion. *J Trauma*. 2007;62:112–119.

10. Al-Said K, Anderson R, Wong A, Le D. Recombinant factor VIIa for intraoperative bleeding in a child with hepatoblastoma and a review of recombinant activated factor VIIa use in children undergoing surgery. *J Pediatr Surg*. 2008;43:e15–e19.

11. Perkins JG, Schreiber MA, Wade CE, Holcomb JB. Early versus late recombinant factor VIIa in combat trauma patients requiring massive transfusion. *J Trauma*. 2007;62:1095–1101.

12. Spinella PC. Warm fresh whole blood transfusion for severe hemorrhage: US military and potential civilian applications. *Crit Care Med*. 2008;36:S340–S345.

Chapter 3

Vascular Access

Introduction

Obtaining vascular access in infants and children can be difficult even under optimal conditions. Attempting emergent access in a hypotensive, struggling infant is even more challenging.

Routine Access

Careful consideration should be given to the routine sites for peripheral intravenous (IV) access before more emergent techniques are employed. Often access can be obtained via peripheral veins on the back of the hand, in the antecubital space, or in the greater saphenous vein at the ankle. Common pitfalls in pediatric IV placement include attempting placement without sufficient assistance to restrain the child, especially the involved extremity, and an inexperienced provider using a catheter that is too small. Infants can tolerate 22- and 24-gauge IV catheters, while toddlers' and young children's veins can accommodate 20- and 22-gauge catheters. As older children's size approaches adult size, they are more likely to tolerate 16- and 18-gauge catheters.

When timely attempts at routine peripheral access fail, consideration should be given to either external jugular vein cannulation or intraosseous (IO) needle placement. In an emergency, these alternatives, especially IO needle placement, should be considered within 2 minutes.

External Jugular Vein Cannulation

The external jugular vein is a large peripheral vein that is relatively easy to cannulate, and it offers quick access to central circulation. It lies superficially along the lateral aspect of the neck, extending from the angle of the mandible downward until it pierces the deep fascia of the neck, just above the middle of the clavicle, ending in the subclavian vein. Because it is a very superficial vein, it tends to "roll" and be positional. Slight movement of the head may affect the flow of fluid.

- **Technique**
  - Position the patient in the supine, head-down position and rotate the head to the opposite side
    - Infants can be positioned at the edge of an examination table and their heads lowered (this is a 3-person technique)
  - Prepare the skin aseptically
  - Apply digital pressure to the vein distally (just above the clavicle), which will distend the vein (applying slight traction with the thumb at the proximal portion of the vein may prevent the vein from rolling)
  - Insert an IV catheter with an empty syringe attached into the middle of the vein, remembering its superficial position
  - Aspirate with the syringe after puncturing the skin and, immediately upon seeing a flashback, thread the catheter; stop if you meet resistance
  - Secure well
  - Keeping the head in a neutral position seems to optimize IV flow
- **Complications**
  - Trauma patients with potential cervical spine injuries should be approached with caution
  - Reduce the risk of air embolism by using a syringe attached to the angiocatheter during insertion
  - Pneumothorax is a remote possibility

Intraosseous Needle Placement

IO needle placement can provide emergency vascular access on a child when peripheral access is unobtainable. This technique can be used on patients of all ages. The bone marrow, a noncollapsible structure with a rich network of arteries and veins, can provide a rapid and reliable route for administering crystalloids, blood products, vasopressors, and drugs into the central circulation. Although products specifically designed for IO access are ideal, a styletted needle used for bone marrow aspiration or a large adult spinal needle can be used in an emergency.

- Technique
  - Common insertion sites (Figure 3-1):
    - Tibial plateau: the flat medial surface of the proximal tibia 1–2 cm below the tibial tuberosity

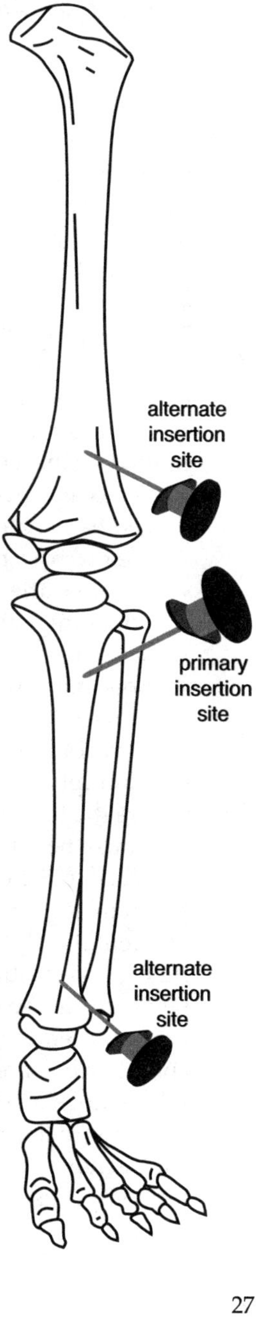

Figure 3-1. Preferred sites for intraosseous needle placement.

 - ▸ Distal femur: 3 cm above the superior aspect of the patella
 - ▸ Distal tibia, radius, and ulna; iliac crests; or sternum
- Apply rigid support to the posterior aspect of the insertion site (do not place your hand directly posterior to where needle will be driven)
- Using an aseptic technique, prepare the selected site with Chloraprep (Cardinal Health, Dublin, Ohio) or Betadine (Purdue Pharma LP, Stamford, Conn)
- In an awake patient, inject the skin with lidocaine for local anesthesia
- If using a product designed specifically for IO access, follow the manufacturer's directions
- If using a bone marrow aspiration needle, after penetrating the skin, direct the IO needle at a slight angle (10°–15°) caudad (in the femur, angle it cephalad) and apply pressure with a to-and-fro rotary motion
  - ▸ As the needle passes from the cortex of the bone into the marrow, resistance will diminish
  - ▸ Remove the stylet and check needle placement by attaching tubing connected to a saline-filled, 10-cc syringe
  - ▸ Bone marrow can be aspirated and fluid should be easily infused
- Observe for fluid infiltration of the calf; if this occurs, repeat the attempt in the opposite leg
- Secure the tubing to the leg with tape and gauze
- Minimize needle manipulation by attaching syringes or a stopcock to the tubing
- Maintain vigilant care and observation of the insertion site; accidental dislodgement of an IO needle will manifest as fluid extravasation into a swollen calf, or the needle will be mobile at the site
- Once the emergent condition is under control and the child has been resuscitated, attempt peripheral or central intravenous access, as IO lines are notoriously short lived (minutes to hours)

- **Complications**
  - Osteomyelitis
  - Fracture

- Necrosis of the epiphyseal plate
- Extravasation
- Compartment syndrome

Percutaneous Central Venous Lines
Percutaneous central venous lines are required when peripheral venous access is either unavailable or insufficient. Central venous lines last longer (days to weeks), allow for central venous pressure monitoring and phlebotomy, and can safely tolerate vasoactive medication drips and hyperosmoloar therapies. The preferred site for central vein access in children is the femoral vein. It is easier and safer to access than the internal jugular or subclavian veins, especially during resuscitation. Unlike in adults, there are no pediatric data suggesting a higher risk of infection at the femoral site. Lines placed under suboptimal conditions should be changed when the patient's condition warrants. Like adults, debilitated pediatric patients with indwelling central lines are at risk for catheter-related bloodstream infections and thrombosis. Fortunately, the risk of deep venous thrombosis is lower in children than in adults. The standard aseptic Seldinger technique is used for line placement. Rember the lateral to medial groin anatomy: NAVEL (nerve, artery, vein, empty space, lymphatics).

Arterial Lines
Arterial lines can be placed for minute-to-minute arterial blood pressure measurement, frequent arterial blood gas sampling, or continuous cerebral perfusion pressure measurement in cases of traumatic head injury (Table 3-1).

Table 3-1. Pediatric Central and Arterial Venous Line Sizes

Age/Size of Child	Central Line Sizes	Arterial Line Sizes
Infants < 5 kg	3 Fr 5–8 cm single lumen; 4 Fr 8 cm double lumen; **OR** 20-gauge 12 cm pediatric jugular vein kit	24-gauge IV catheter; 2.5 Fr 2.5 cm for peripheral (radial) access; 2.5 Fr 5 cm for central (femoral) access
Larger infants/ toddlers < 10 kg	4 Fr 8 cm double lumen; **OR** 20-gauge 12 cm pediatric jugular vein kit	22- or 24-gauge IV catheter 2.5 Fr 2.5 cm for peripheral (radial) access; 2.5 Fr 5 cm for central (femoral) access; **OR** 20-gauge 12 cm pediatric jugular vein kit for femoral access
Preschool children < 20–25 kg	5 Fr 8–12 cm double or triple lumen	20- or 22-gauge IV catheter
Older children	7 Fr adult triple lumen line	20- or 22-gauge IV catheter

Fr: french size
IV: intravenous

Chapter 4

Mechanical Ventilation

Equipment

When providing mechanical ventilation for pediatric casualties, it is important to select the appropriately sized bag-valve mask or endotracheal (ET) tube. The appropriately sized bag-valve mask will cover the child's mouth and nose and will sit below the eyes, across the bridge of the nose (Tables 4-1 and 4-2).

Table 4-1. Bag-Valve Mask Sizes

Age	Size
Infant	500 cc
1–3 y	1 L
>3 y	3 L

Table 4-2. Artificial Airways

Age	ET Tube Size	Tracheostomy Tube Size*
Newborn	3.0–3.5	3.0–3.5
6 mo	3.5	4.0
18 mo	3.5–4.0	4.0
24 mo	4.0–4.5	5.0
2–4 y	4.5–5.0	5.5
4–7 y	5.0–6.0	6.0
7–10 y	6.0–6.5	6–8
10–12 y	7.0	8

ET: endotracheal
*Tracheostomy tube should typically be a half size larger than the appropriately sized ET tube.

Safety

All ventilated patients should have an appropriately sized bag, mask, replacement ET tube, or tracheostomy tube available at the bedside. Wall suction and a Yankauer airway suction device should also be available at the bedside at all times.

Most modern ventilators are capable of safely, effectively, mechanically ventilating infants and small children. A knowledgeable respiratory therapist should be able to adjust for these patients' special needs during setup.

Settings for Getting Started

- Volume Ventilation Mode: Synchronized Intermittent Mechanical Ventilation/Volume Control
  - Fraction of inspired oxygen (FiO_2): 50%; if patient is hypoxemic, use 100%; wean rapidly to FiO_2 < 50% if possible
  - Inspiratory time ("I time") should be no less than 0.5 seconds, ranging up to 1 second in older children
  - Intermittent mandatory ventilation (IMV) rate should be appropriate for the patient's age (ie, 30 [for infants] down to 15 [for adult-sized patients]) to start
  - **Tidal volume** (Vt) should initially equal 10 mL/kg, rounding down
    - Look at chest rise, listen for breath sounds, and check peak inspiratory pressure (PIP)
    - **Decrease Vt** if examination reveals excessive chest rise, large air entry, and higher-than-expected PIPs (< 30–35 cm H_2O)
      - Elevated PIPs may result from right main stem ET tube placement, mucous plugging, excessive Vt, or poor lung compliance (ie, 1° pulmonary disease)
      - Goal Vt for patients with acute lung injury or acute respiratory distress syndrome (ARDS) should be around 6 mL/kg (as it is for adults)
      - Strongly consider switching to pressure-control (PC)–style ventilation for severe lung disease
    - **Increase Vt** if examination reveals poor chest rise, minimal air entry, and lower-than-expected PIPs (< 15 cm H_2O)
      - Adult-sized ventilator circuits may consume large amounts of volume each breath (2–3 cc for every centimeter H_2O pressure difference between PIP and positive end expiratory pressure [PEEP])
      - If this occurs, increase Vt or change to a PC-style breath

- **PEEP** should be 4 cm, or higher if functional residual capacity is compromised by atalectasis, abdominal distension, or severe lung disease
  - Increase in increments of 2 cm H_2O
  - Volume recruitment with PEEP takes hours but can be lost in minutes
- If available, start **pressure support** (PS) for spontaneously breathing patients at 10 cm H_2O
- Measure arterial blood gases to accurately access ventilation status
- Use chest radiographs to confirm the adequacy of the ET tube placement and chest expansion
- Use end-tidal carbon dioxide monitors if available

- Pressure Ventilation Mode: Synchronized Intermittent Mechanical Ventilation / Pressure Control
  - Same initial settings as volume control for FiO_2, I time, IMV rate, PEEP, and PS
  - Pressure-style ventilation offers advantages by allowing effective Vt at lower PIP and improves oxygenation for any given Vt
  - Strongly consider pressure ventilation (if available) for large air leaks due to small ET tube size, ineffective ventilation (eg, 2° adult ventilator circuit on infant or small child), or poor lung compliance
  - Set PC to give effective chest rise and adequate air entry
    - Expect PIPs between 18 and 22 cm H_2O in patients with healthy lungs, between 23 and 27 cm H_2O for those with moderate lung disease, and between 28 and 35 cm H_2O in those with more severe lung disease
  - Once PC is established, use machine-measured inspiratory and expiratory volumes as an estimate of the patient's lung compliance (volumes should be $\leq$ 10 mL / kg to avoid overstretch)

Problem Solving

- When a ventilated patient **acutely deteriorates**, don't be a **DOPE**

  Dislodged ET tube: check for equal breath sounds. Is end-tidal carbon dioxide waveform present?

Obstructed: suction mucous plug
Pneumothorax: check for equal breath sounds; use needle decompression or chest radiograph depending on relative urgency
Equipment failure: disconnect from circuit, hand bag, confirm 100% oxygen is flowing

- **Moderate to severe hypoxemia:** goal is to wean to FiO_2 < 50%
    - Minimize air leak by placing a larger ET tube, repositioning head, or changing to pressure mode
    - Increase PEEP in increments of 2 cm H_2O to increase functional residual capacity (aerated lung volume); consider paralytics for PEEP > 10
    - Increase I time to improve oxygenation by increasing mean airway pressure
    - Increase rate, especially if partial pressure of carbon dioxide (PCO_2) is also elevated and minute ventilation needs to be increased
    - Changing to PC will result in improved oxygenation for the same volume delivered
    - Once the appropriate Vt is established, avoid changing volumes; in ARDS, ventilator-induced lung injury is associated with Vt > 8–10 mL/kg
- **High peak pressures**: > 35 cm H_2O or **plateau pressure** > 30 cm H_2O
    - Suction ET tube
    - Check tube position with chest radiograph
    - Consider administering inhaled bronchodilators, especially if the patient exhibits wheezing, prolonged expiratory phase, or develops auto-PEEP
    - Changing to PC will result in lower peak pressure for the same Vt
    - Consider adopting a permissive hypercapnia strategy if lung compliance and oxygenation are poor in the face of high peak pressures
        - Limit delivered Vt to roughly 6 mL/kg of ideal body weight
        - Accept higher PCO_2 and lower saturations (85%)
        - Use higher PEEP and longer I time for recruitment and

oxygenation
  - Most pediatric patients will tolerate a pH of ≥ 7.2
  - Treat or minimize metabolic acidosis

Sedation Strategies for Ventilated Pediatric Patients

- **Postoperative short-term ventilation.** If the patient will be extubated in 6–12 hours, use:
  - Intermittent opioids, because pain will be the primary problem
  - Intermittent benzodiazepines as needed for sedation
  - A propofol drip can be considered for short-term sedation because it is titratable
  - Long-term propofol use in pediatrics is discouraged given the concern for fatal metabolic acidosis
- For **postoperative long-term ventilation,** use:
  - Continuous opioids to treat pain
  - Intermittent or continuous-drip benzodiazepines as needed for sedation
- For **medical short-term ventilation,** use:
  - Intermittent benzodiazepines because sedation is the primary requirement for ET tube tolerance
  - Intermittent opioids may be needed
- For **medical long-term ventilation,** use:
  - Continuous midazolam
  - Continuous or intermittent opioids if needed for pain

Remember, if the patient–ventilator synchrony is poor and adjustments to the ventilator are insufficient to make the patient comfortable, more sedation may be required.

Medications for Sedation

- **Midazolam:** starting dose is 0.05–0.1 mg/kg intravenous (IV); may repeat every 5–10 minutes until effective sedation is reached
  - Use this as basis for a dosing schedule of IV q1–2h
  - If effective intermittent regimen cannot be easily established, consider continuous drip at (0.05–0.1 mg/kg/h); watch for respiratory depression and hypotension
- **Lorazepam:** starting dose is 0.05–0.1 mg/kg IV
  - May repeat in 5–10 minutes until effective sedation is reached

- Use this as a basis for IV q2–4h dosing schedule
- **Morphine:** starting dose is 0.05–0.1 mg/kg IV
    - Repeat dosing every 5–10 minutes until effective analgesia established
    - Use this as basis for IV q2–4h dosing schedule
    - If effective intermittent regimen cannot be easily established, consider continuous drip
- **Fentanyl:** starting dose is 0.5–1 µg/kg IV
    - Repeat dosing every 5–10 minutes until effective analgesia is established
    - Use this as a basis for IV q1–2h dosing schedule (see Chapter 2, Anesthesia, Table 2-4)

Considerations for Extubation

- Has lung disease improved? Use **SOAP** memory aid:
  Secretions/sedation/spontaneous Vt (> 5 mL/kg): What is the minimal suction frequency? Is the patient awake enough to breathe and protect airway?
  Oxygenation: $FiO_2 < 35\%$
  Airway: If a child has been ventilated for more than 48 hours or has been intubated several times, there is a significant risk of airway edema that may compromise a successful extubation. The presence of an audible air leak around the ET tube can be reassuring. Otherwise, consider starting airway dosing of dexamethasone 0.5 mg/kg/dose, at least 12 hours prior to planned extubation and continue q6h for 4 doses
  Pressures: PIP < 25, PEEP < 5

Predictors of Extubation Failure

If a patient displays postextubation stridor, consider nebulized racemic epinephrine, heliox (if available), and steroids (Table 4-3).

Table 4-3. Predictors of Extubation Failure

Variable	Low Risk (< 10%)	High Risk (> 25%)
Vt (spontaneous)	> 6.5 mL/kg	< 3.5 mL/kg
FiO_2	< 0.30	> 0.40
PIP	< 25 cm H_2O	> 30 cm H_2O

FiO_2: fraction of inspired oxygen PIP: peak inspiratory pressure Vt: tidal volume

Chapter 5

Transfusion Medicine

Routine Transfusion Therapy

- Blood products should not be transfused on a unit basis in children
- Base the volume of transfusion products on weight to avoid over or under resuscitation
  - If only small-volume transfusions are needed, consider having the blood bank split a unit and save portions of it for later transfusion (24 h maximum); this will help avoid multiple donor exposures
  - Transfusing red blood cells (RBCs) that have been in storage for > 14 days has been associated with increased risk of organ failure in critically ill children; risk of immunologic, vasoregulation, and adverse hypercoagulation effects is also increased
- Estimated volume per unit of blood products is as follows:
  - Packed red blood cells (PRBCs): 300 mL / unit
  - Whole blood: 450–500 mL / unit
  - Fresh frozen plasma (FFP): 250–300 mL / unit
  - Platelets: 40–50 mL / unit
  - Cryoprecipitate: 10–12 mL / unit
- PRBCs
  - Initial volume of 10–15 mL / kg can be given quickly over minutes or over a 4-hour period, depending on the situation
  - The following equation can be used to determine the volume of PRBCs to transfuse; it requires the current hematocrit (HCT) level and the child's estimated blood volume (EBV; see Table 5-1 for average total blood volumes by age)

$$\frac{\text{desired HCT} - \text{present HCT}^{*} \times \text{EBV}}{\text{HCT of PRBC (avg 60\%–70\%)}}$$

*HCT of whole blood 40%–45%

Table 5-1. Blood Volume by Age

Age	Blood Volume (mL/kg)
Premature infant	100
Full-term neonate	85
Older infant	75
> 12 mo	70–75

- Transfusing a pediatric patient with 4 cc/kg will increase hemoglobin by 1 g/dL
- Transfusing 1 unit in an adult patient will raise hemoglobin by 1 g/dL (or HCT by 3%)

- FFP
  - Transfuse FFP 10–15 mL/kg
  - If close, round up or down to the closest unit
  - Routine FFP transfusion rates should not exceed 1 mL/kg/min because of the risk of hypotension caused by low ionized calcium during the FFP infusion
    - This complication can be treated with 10 mg/kg CaCl or 100 mg/kg calcium gluconate IV over 5–10 minutes
  - For patients with massive bleeding who are at risk for death secondary to hemorrhage, give FFP as fast as possible, paying attention to ionized calcium levels because large volumes of plasma and red cells will decrease ionized calcium concentrations
  - For patients with known clotting factor deficiencies, 10–15 mL/kg of FFP will raise factors levels 15%–20%
- Platelets
  - Pheresed platelet units have a volume of 6–10 random donor units
  - Transfuse 0.1–0.2 units/kg or 1 unit/5 kg of body weight
    - Equivalent to about 5–10 mL/kg
    - Increases platelet count by approximately 50,000/mm^3
- Cryoprecipitate
  - An excellent source of fibrinogen and factor VIII, factor XIII, and Von Willebrand's factor
  - Administering 1–2 bags for every 5–10 kg will raise fibrinogen levels 60–100 mg/dL

Massive Transfusion Therapy for Severe Hemorrhagic Shock

- The principles of damage-control resuscitation developed for adults are generally applicable in massively bleeding children
  - Current policies regarding hemorrhagic-shock resuscitation, regarding the use of whole blood and recombinant factor VIIa, are appropriate to guide therapy for children with severe injuries
- A "massive transfusion" in a child is when approximately one circulating blood volume is replaced within 24 hours
  - Consider using massive transfusion strategies when a child is anticipated to need more than two traditional 15 mL/kg transfusions of PRBCs during one resuscitation (equivalent to about > 6–8 PRBC units for an adult)
- Some clinical parameters may predict the need for a massive transfusion during active bleeding
  - Severe tachycardia or hypotension for age
  - Base deficit ≥ 6
  - Lactate ≥ 4 mmol/L
  - International normalized ratio ≥ 1.5
  - Hemoglobin ≤ 9 g/dL upon admission
- When transfusing through small IV catheters (22 gauge and 24 gauge), bolusing with a 10–20 mL syringe may be the most efficient way to deliver fluids and blood products rapidly
- If a patient is at risk for massive transfusion, PRBCs, FFP, and platelet transfusion should be initiated in a 1:1:1 ratio
  - Helps avoid coagulopathy and is associated with reduced mortality from hemorrhage in adults
  - Use of blood products in this ratio should continue until the life-threatening bleeding has stopped; at this point use more restrictive transfusion criteria. Formulas for calculating volumes of each product should be used
- Fresh warm whole blood (FWWB)
  - If FWWB is available, consider using it as a substitute for PRBCs, FFP, and platelets
  - FWWB can be beneficial in the massively transfused patient
    - Decreases the likelihood of hypothermia
    - Avoids the deleterious effects of large volumes of old stored RBCs and the accompanying anticoagulants

and preservatives
  - FWWB is particularly helpful when platelets or other component therapy is unavailable
  - Risk of transmitting infection and minor blood group incompatibilities is increased
  - Transfuse 15–20 mL/kg; repeat as necessary
  - Watch for hypocalcemia and hyperkalemia
- Factor VIIa has been used to reduce blood loss and restore hemostasis in combat casualties with coagulopathy associated with hemorrhagic shock
  - Works best with a pH > 7.1, a platelet count > 50,000/mm^3, and a fibrinogen level > 100 g/L
  - Has been used successfully in pediatric trauma for patients requiring massive transfusion
  - Dose is 90 μg/kg and may be repeated if persistent bleeding occurs secondary to coagulopathy within 1–3 hours

Risks Associated with Pediatric Transfusions

- Hyperkalemia
  - Potassium escapes from RBCs as they age; therefore, older units of PRBCs may contain high levels of potassium
  - Pediatric patients have small blood volume, so a potassium load results in a higher risk of hyperkalemia
  - Transfusion-associated hyperkalemic cardiac arrest is almost always associated with a low cardiac output state, acidosis, hyperglycemia, hypocalcemia, and hypothermia; all conditions commonly found in patients requiring massive transfusion
  - Avoiding older blood products and closely monitoring electrocardiogram (ECG) morphology and serum potassium can help avoid hyperkalemic cardiac arrest
- Hypocalcemia
  - Children are particularly prone to hypocalcemia secondary to citrate-containing blood products
  - Transfusion-related hypocalcemia is most likely to be caused by FFP and whole blood because these products contain the most citrate per unit volume
    - Monitor for hypocalcemia if FFP is transfused > 1 mL/kg/min

- Ca^{2+} is a potent inotrope in infants and children; severe cardiac depression and hypotension can result from ionized hypocalcemia
    - Potent inhalational agents dramatically exacerbate this hypotension
- Prevention includes limiting the rate of FFP transfusion to < 1 mL/kg/min if feasible and administering calcium chloride (5 mg/kg) or calcium gluconate (15 mg/kg)

- Hypothermia
    - This is a significant risk given pediatric surface-area-to-weight ratios
    - Consider using blood warmer, especially if large volumes will be transfused
- The risks of bacterial and viral contamination are the same as in adults
- Fluid overload
    - Patients with chronic anemias (eg, sickle cell anemia) undergoing transfusion are at risk for fluid overload and congestive heart failure
    - Use slow transfusions (1 cc/kg/h)
    - Consider administering furosemide (0.25–0.5 mg/kg) midtransfusion or after transfusion

Special Preparations (consider if available)

- Leukocyte-reduced blood products
    - Used to prevent febrile, nonhemolytic transfusion reactions
    - Microaggregate filters prevent febrile transfusion reactions and are useful in patients who have received blood frequently in the past
    - Leukopore filters are needed to decrease risk of cytomegalovirus transmission and human leukocyte antigen alloimmunization
    - White blood cell filters will dramatically slow the rate of a transfusion (may not be appropriate during a transfusion for hemorrhagic shock because of active bleeding)

Further Reading

1. Smith HM, Farrow SJ, Ackerman JD, Stubbs JR, Sprung

J. Cardiac arrests associated with hyperkalemia during red blood cell transfusion: a case series. *Anesth Analg*. 2008;106:1062–1069.

2. Duchesne JC, Hunt JP, Wahl G, et al. Review of current blood transfusions strategies in a mature level 1 trauma center: were we wrong for the last 60 years? *J Trauma*. 2008:65;272–276.
3. González EA, Moore FA, Holcomb JB, et al. Fresh frozen plasma should be given earlier to patients requiring massive transfusion. *J Trauma*. 2007;62:112–119.
4. Al-Said K, Anderson R, Wong A, Le D. Recombinant factor VIIa for intraoperative bleeding in a child with hepatoblastoma and a review of recombinant activated factor VIIa use in children undergoing surgery. *J Pediatr Surg*. 2008;43:e15–e19.
5. Perkins JG, Schreiber MA, Wade CE, Holcomb JB. Early versus late recombinant factor VIIa in combat trauma patients requiring massive transfusion. *J Trauma*. 2007;62:1095–1101.
6. Spinella PC. Warm fresh whole blood transfusion for severe hemorrhage: US military and potential civilian applications. *Crit Care Med*. 2008;36:S340–S345.

Chapter 6

Hemodynamics and Shock

Caregivers must have a basic understanding of pediatric vital signs to accurately perform hemodynamic monitoring and assess for shock (see Chapter 2, Anesthesia, Table 2-2). Cardiac output can be assessed by observing heart rate (HR) and capillary refill time, mental status changes, and urine output. Falling blood pressure (BP) is a late ominous sign. Preload can be assessed by observing changes in liver span or by viewing heart size with a chest radiograph. Systemic vascular resistance can be assessed by capillary refill time, pulse pressure, and differential temperatures peripheral to central (Table 6-1).

Table 6-1. Distinguishing Features of Clinical Shock States

	Physical				Monitoring		
Scenario	**WOB**	**CRT**	**Liver**	**Skin**	**CVP***	**SVR**	**CI**
Hypovolemic	nl	>2	nl	Cool	↓	↑	↓
Cardiogenic	+++	>2	+++	Cool	↑	↑	↓
Distributive	+/++	+/−	nl	+/−	↓	↓↑	↓↑

*Normal CVP for infants and children is 5–8 mmHg.
CI: cardiac index
CRT: capillary refill time
CVP: central venous pressure
nl: normal
SVR: systemic vascular resistance
WOB: work of breathing

Recognizing Shock

- Patient's history may include trauma, infection, heart murmur, or congenital heart disease
- Patient may exhibit poor perfusion manifested by capillary refill taking more than 3 seconds on the extremities or more than 2 seconds on the trunk
- Other signs and symptoms include tachycardia, hypotension (late finding), decreased peripheral pulses, decreased level of

consciousness, and decreased urinary output (normal goal ≥ 1 cc/kg/h), and may be associated with metabolic acidosis, tachypnea, and respiratory failure

- **Hypotension** is defined as a systolic BP of:
  - Infants 0–1 month old: < 60 mmHg
  - Infants 1–12 months old: < 70 mmHg
  - Children 1–10 years old: < 70 mmHg + 2(age [in years])

Types of Shock

- **Hypovolemic** shock results from blood loss or loss of other body fluids (Table 6-2)

Table 6-2. Assessing the Severity of Hypovolemic Shock*

Level	Weight Lost (infant)	Weight Lost (child)	Signs and Symptoms
Mild	5%	3%	Decreased urinary output, mild tachycardia, dry mucous membranes, decreased tearing
Moderate	10%	6%	Oliguria, tachycardia, dry membranes and tongue, sunken eyes and fontanelle, poor skin turgor, borderline to poor perfusion, mild to moderate tachypnea
Severe	15%	9%	Oliguria or anuria, possible shock, poor perfusion, decreased LOC, tachypnea, marked metabolic acidosis

*Percentages indicate actual weight loss from water loss or deficit.
LOC: level of consciousness

- **Cardiogenic** shock may be secondary to congenital heart disease
- **Distributive** shock includes septic shock and anaphylactic shock
- Other conditions that can cause shock include gastroenteritis, burns, trauma, hemorrhage, prolonged illness associated with poor oral intake, bowel obstruction, pneumonia, diabetic ketoacidosis, diabetes insipidus, neglect, cystic fibrosis, and inborn errors of metabolism

Treatment

- Stabilize airway, breathing, and circulation (ABCs); early mechanical ventilation may be indicated, particularly in septic shock
- Establish intravenous (IV) access (ideally in two locations)
- Administer rapid volume expansion with normal saline (NS) or Ringer's lactate bolus of 20 cc/kg in < 5–10 minutes, then reassess
  - Reassessment includes evaluating clinical appearance, chest auscultation, capillary refill, HR, BP, and, when possible, chest radiograph
  - If there is no improvement, repeat bolus as indicated by assessment; as intravascular volume is restored, the liver will expand and be palpable below the right costal margin
- Once perfusion has been normalized, continue to treat **hypovolemic** shock by calculating replacement fluids based on the estimated deficit (percent dehydration, see Table 6-2), ongoing losses, maintenance needs, and special situations (eg, hypernatremia or hyponatremia)
- Deficit replacement can be calculated using the following formula:

  $$\% \text{ deficit} \times \text{weight (grams)} = \text{fluid deficit in cc}$$

  For example, 10% dehydration of a 7-kg infant would be calculated as follows:

  $$10\% \times 7{,}000 \text{ g} = 700 \text{ g or } 700 \text{ cc}$$

  Add deficit to maintenance fluids of 700 cc to give 1,400 cc for the day
- Resuscitation of septic shock must be aggressive and timely
  - Signs of sepsis may be subtle but can include tachycardia, tachypnea for age along with high or low white blood cell count, fever, and hypothermia
  - Diagnosis: perfusional abnormalities accompanying suspected infection, and hypotension refractory to fluid resuscitation
  - Begin management by assessing ABCs and providing fluid resuscitation with isotonic crystalloid

Table 6-3. Vasoactive Support

Drug/Indication	Dosing	Effects	Action	Comments
Dopamine Septic shock Cardiogenic shock	Start at 5 μg/kg/min; range 2–20 μg/kg/min	β 5–10 μg/kg/min α > 15 μg/kg/min	Acts indirectly via NE release; inotrope, chronotrope, vasopressor	Give centrally if possible; not as effective in neonates who have limited NE stores
Dobutamine Cardiogenic shock	Start at 5 μg/kg/min; range 2–20 μg/kg/min	β	Direct-acting pure inotrope, lusitrope (diastolic relaxation)	May result in peripheral vasorelaxation and tachycardia
Epinephrine Postarrest shock Cold "septic" shock after dopamine	Start at 0.1 μg/kg/min; range 0.05–1.0 μg/kg/min	β at low doses α at higher doses	Direct-acting inotrope, chronotrope, and potent vasopressor	Give centrally if possible; may cause organ ischemia at high doses
Norepinephrine Warm septic shock refractory to dopamine	0.05–? μg/kg/min	α:β 3:1	Direct-acting potent vasopressor	Give centrally if possible; may cause organ ischemia
Phenylephrine Spinal shock Septic shock	0.05–? μg/kg/min	Pure α	Direct-acting potent vasopressor	Give centrally (burns)
Milrinone ↑ PVR or SVR with cardiac dysfunction	0.2–1 μg/kg/min; load 50 μg/kg	Phosphodiesterase inhibition (↑ cAMP)	Inotrope and vasodilator, lusitrope (diastolic relaxation)	Thrombocytopenia, T ½ h vs min
Nitroprusside Hypertension or ↑ SVR states	0.5–5 μg/kg/min	Exogenous NO donor	Potent arteriolar vasodilator	Need A-line to watch BP; cyanide toxicity

BP: blood pressure cAMP: cyclic adenosine monophosphate NE: norepinephrine NO: nitric oxide PVR: pulmonary vascular resistance
SVR: systemic vascular resistance

  - Pediatric patients in septic shock may need more than 60 mL/kg in the first hour
  - Consider transfusing packed red blood cells to reach goal hemoglobin of 10 g/dL
- Add vasoactive support in the first hour if fluid resuscitation fails to reverse septic shock (Table 6-3)
  - Initiate dopamine or epinephrine first
  - 80% of children will need inotrope before vasopressor
  - If shock persists despite fluids and dopamine is titrated up to 10 μg/kg/min:
    - Add epinephrine for cold shock (myocardial depression, leaky capillaries, metabolic acidosis, cool and mottled extremities)

      OR
    - Add norepinephrine for warm shock (increased carbon monoxide, bounding pulses, decreased systemic vascular resistance, warm extremities, normal or extremely fast capillary refill time, wide pulse pressures)
- Correct metabolic and electrolyte disturbances
  - Check and correct glucose and calcium levels
- When sepsis is suspected, administer broad-spectrum antibiotics within an hour
- Therapeutic goals include:
  - Normalized mental status
  - Central pulses equal to peripheral pulses
  - Urinary output > 1 mL/kg/h
  - Mean arterial pressure minus central venous pressure (if available):
    - > 60 mmHg in infants
    - > 65 mmHg for older children
  - Central venous oxygen saturation > 70% (if available)

Chapter 7

Managing Intracranial Pressure

Signs of Increased Intracranial Pressure

- Decreased level of consciousness
- Papilledema
- Tachycardia
- Hypotension
- Vomiting
- Irritability
- Photophobia
- Bulging fontanelle
- Split sutures
- Sunset eyes (chronic)
- Irregular respirations or apnea
- Widened pulse pressures
- **Cushing's triad (hypertension, bradycardia, abnormal respirations) is a preterminal event!**

Etiologies of Increased Intracranial Pressure

- Meningitis
- Encephalitis
- Head trauma
- Intracranial mass lesions
- Child abuse (eg, shaken baby)
- Status epilepticus
- Shock leading to hypoxic-ischemic encephalopathy

Treatment

- Assess and maintain airway, breathing, and circulation (ABCs)
    - Rapid sequence induction/intubation therapy may be necessary if airway protection is needed (eg, Glasgow Coma Scale score ≤ 8)
- Maintain **cerebral perfusion pressure (CPP) = mean arterial pressure – intracranial pressure (ICP)**

$$\text{mean arterial pressure (MAP)} = \frac{\text{systolic} + 2(\text{diastolic})}{3}$$

$$\text{Normal ICP} = < 20 \text{ mmHg}$$

Appropriate CPP is age dependent, as follows:
- **< 2 years**: 50 mmHg
- **2–6 years**: 55 mmHg
- **7–10 years**: 65 mmHg
- **11–16 years**: 70 mmHg
- **> 16 years**: 70–90 mmHg

  - If ICP monitoring is unavailable, use goal CPP as the minimally acceptable value for mean arterial pressure
- Avoid hypercarbia
  - Keep partial pressure of carbon dioxide (PCO_2) between 30 and 35 mmHg
  - Hyperventilation to PCO_2 below mid-30s mmHg should be reserved for temporary treatment of major ICP spikes
- Keep the partial pressure of oxygen in arterial blood (PaO_2) at 100 mmHg, or saturations at 97%–100%
- Keep patient's head midline and elevated to 30°
- Avoid free water; use isotonic fluid (normal saline) as the base solution for intravenous (IV) hydration
- Anticipate norepinephrine, dopamine, or epinephrine needs to maintain CPP once patient is euvolemic
- If patient is anxious and agitated while intubated, sedate with midazolam and fentanyl
  - Use paralysis if patient is persistently agitated
  - Sedation will alter neurological examination
- Avoid excess noise, vibration, light, and noxious stimulation that may increase ICP
  - Sedate with midazolam IV, fentanyl IV, or lidocaine IV, or via endotracheal tube before suctioning
- Treat seizures aggressively
  - Muscle relaxants will mask seizure activity
  - Consider prophylactic phenytoin for penetrating head injuries
- Keep patient cool and treat hyperthermia aggressively
  - Patient may need neuromuscular blockade to avoid shivering

- Monitor blood glucose
  - Add dextrose to IV fluids only after serum glucose ranges between 80 and 110 mmHg
- Place Foley catheter
- Monitor central venous pressure if available or indicated; maintain at 5–8 mmHg
- If increasing signs of ICP appear or if pupils suddenly dilate, administer hypertonic saline or mannitol (3% saline is preferred because it does not create an osmotic diuresis or result in hypovolemia)
  - **3% saline**: 2–4 mL/kg IV bolus for increased ICP
    - 10 mL/kg for herniation
    - 0.5 mL/kg/h for continuous infusion (range 0.1–1 mL/kg/h)
    - Patients will tolerate serum sodium rising to the 160 range, as long as the rise and eventual decline occurs gradually
  - **Mannitol**: 0.5–1 g/kg IV given over 20 minutes ; use in-line 5-μm filter for concentrations ≥ 20%
  - Consider **furosemide** 0.5–1 mg/kg IV slow push if patient is hypervolemic (maximum of 40 mg/dose)
  - Thiopental (3 mg/kg IV) may be given for continued evidence of increased ICP
    - Barbiturates are negative inotropes and vasodilators; watch for hypotension

Chapter 8

Aeromedical Evacuation

The Army utilizes dedicated rotary wing aircraft to support the air evacuation mission and provide medical air evacuation for all categories of patients and support to other services. In the Army, these assets are located in the medical company (air ambulance), which falls under the general support aviation battalion, combat aviation brigade. In addition, aircraft of opportunity (eg, USAF C-130 Hercules, C-17 Globemaster fixed-wing platforms, V-22 Osprey, UH-60 Blackhawk, and CH-47 Chinook rotary wing aircraft) may also be configured for patient transport. The evacuation and provision of en route medical care to combat wounded is the most recognized mission of medical evacuation assets. However, the essential and vital functions of medical evacuation resources encompass many additional missions and tasks that support the Military Health System, including transfer of patients between medical treatment facilities (MTFs) within the joint operations area and from MTFs to US Air Force aeromedical staging facilities, as well as emergency movement of class VIII medical supplies, blood and blood products, and medical personnel and equipment.

The United States Transportation Command (TRANSCOM) and the United States Air Force (USAF) Air Mobility Command operate a sophisticated worldwide air evacuation system capable of safely transporting critically ill patients of all ages. Crews are composed of flight nurses and technicians, augmented by Critical Care Air Transport Teams (CCATTs) when medically indicated. These expert teams are composed of a specially trained physician, nurse, and respiratory therapist. They have the expertise and equipment to provide in-flight intensive medical care.

Because pediatric patients are more vulnerable than adults to the stressors of flight, evacuating "stabilized" children and neonates by air presents unique challenges. Urgent treatment focused on life-threatening or organ-threatening problems must precede a definitive diagnosis. The impact of flight physiology and the need for specialized transport teams, or at least special consideration, should be factored into mission planning.

Stressors of Flight

- Hypoxia
  - Routine cruising altitude for strategic air evacuation flights is about 40,000 feet mean sea level (MSL)
  - A cabin altitude of approximately 8,000 feet MSL can be maintained by pressurization of the aircraft
  - In a child without cardiopulmonary disease, this results in a corresponding decrease in the oxygen saturation from near 100% at sea level to 90% at altitude (Dalton's Law)
  - Administering 2 L/m oxygen by nasal cannula increases the oxygen saturation to approximately 100%
    - In patients with cardiopulmonary disease, anemia, or increased metabolic demands due to burns, sepsis, or recent operative procedures, a higher flow rate may be required to maintain tissue oxygenation
    - A pulse oximeter is a useful guide when administering supplemental oxygen
- Decreased cabin air pressure
  - With climb from sea level to 40,000 feet, the volume of a trapped gas increases as the ambient barometric pressure decreases, causing trapped gases within body cavities (pleura, skull, viscera, etc) to expand (Boyle's Law); at a cabin altitude of 8,000 feet, volume increase approaches 40%
  - Nasogastric tubes, gastrostomy tubes, and ostomy bags must be vented
  - The pressure in ballooned devices (eg, endotracheal tube cuffs, Foley catheters) should be adjusted during the climb and descent phases of flight
  - Strongly consider leaving drains (including chest tubes) in place for flight; patients who have had chest tubes removed generally must wait 48 hours before flight and must be cleared radiographically to confirm pneumothorax resolution
  - When gas in cavities is not readily accessible to decompress

(eg, pneumocephalus) and urgent aeromedical evacuation (AE) is required, a cabin altitude restriction (CAR) can be requested (see below)

- Thermal stress/humidity
  - Temperature fluctuations can adversely affect infants because of their high surface-area-to-body-mass ratio and immature thermoregulatory systems
  - Decreased cabin humidity (~ 1%) can contribute to dehydration
    - An incubator or other flight-approved isolette can provide a neutral thermal and humid environment for infants
    - At cruise altitude, increased fluid flux occurs into the extravascular space, and increased insensible fluid losses exacerbate dehydration
- Vibration, gravitational forces, subdued lighting (due to combat conditions), and noise (auscultation is almost impossible) are all additional stressors
  - This is a difficult environment in which to manage pediatric patients; the above factors cause patient disorientation and fatigue
  - These factors are significant in tactical evacuation missions using rotary wing aircraft, where space limitation severely impedes the ability of a medical crew to monitor and perform intervention maneuvers in flight; fortunately these flights are usually of shorter duration
  - All lines and tubes must be carefully secured prior to transfer to the aircraft to prevent dislodgment during the requisite multiple patient movements
  - Orthopaedic casts must be bivalved
  - Consider fasciotomy in patients at high risk of developing a compartment syndrome
  - Intubate patients at risk for airway loss or with borderline respiratory status; establishing an emergent airway may be difficult or impossible in a child while in flight
- Prolonged mission duration
  - Strategic AE between major command areas of responsibility can exceed 10 hours and entail unanticipated delays due to operational considerations, equipment failure, weather,

  and other factors
  - Ensure patients have sufficient medication, blood products (if indicated), and pediatric age-appropriate equipment available; this is especially important with infant and toddler transports because most AE supplies are sized for adults
- CAR
  - Patients with severe pulmonary disease and marginal oxygenation at high ventilator settings may require a CAR to maintain the cabin air pressure near that of the origination altitude
  - A lower cruising altitude will most likely increase the duration of the mission due to increased fuel consumption (possibly necessitating a fuel stop), and often entails flight through more turbulent air
  - A CAR may place the aircraft at risk in the combat environment
  - Other conditions warranting a CAR include penetrating eye injuries with intraocular air and trapped air that cannot be evacuated before flight (eg, pneumoencephalus)
- Noncertified equipment
  - Approved AE equipment has been extensively tested to ensure that it is safe to operate in flight and that it will not interfere with an aircraft's navigation and electrical systems
  - A waiver may be granted for noncertified or nonstandard medical equipment
- Special considerations
  - Neonatal/pediatric intensive care patients: air evacuations of intubated, pressor-supported, or otherwise unstable pediatric patients demand special care and planning
  - Every effort should be made to create a transport team with the prerequisite pediatric skills
    - Adding a physician or nurse anesthetist skilled in pediatric intubation, a respiratory therapist, or a pediatric-skilled registered nurse may have a huge impact on patient safety
    - Physiological deterioration is common during pediatric critical care transport and should be anticipated;

unrecognized asphyxia is the primary cause of deterioration
- The transport team must be prepared for emergencies such as airway-related events, hypotension, loss of crucial intravenous access, and cardiopulmonary arrest
- Although pediatric and neonatal CCATTs exist, they are unlikely to be quickly available in hostile environments
    - Neonatal teams typically transport patients from birth to 3 months of age
    - Pediatric teams generally transport critically ill patients ages 3 months to 14 years of age

- Requests are coordinated between the originating physician, the validating flight surgeon at the patient movement requirements center (PMRC), and the destination/accepting physician
    - Close coordination between the sending facility and the PMRC is necessary to consider factors as such as weight, transport isolette size, in-flight care requirements, acuity, and team composition

Humanitarian Transport Requests

- The process of arranging pediatric humanitarian evacuations out of theater can take between 6 and 12 months
- Appropriate patient selection is critical; ideally these patients have only a single, fixable, stable problem
- The lack of suitable host-nation care must be confirmed and documented; regional care is preferred over transport to the continental United States (CONUS)
- Individual cases for humanitarian evacuation out of theater are unlikely to be successful without a passionate advocate; personalizing the case with photos and compelling narrative is crucial for success
- These complex requests often require coordination with the local US embassy or State Department, host-nation medical officials, and transit nations' ministries of foreign affairs (or equivalent)
- Identify partners within the country of origin and within

international nongovernmental organizations (eg, using resources within the US consulate and Shriners International for a child who needs reconstructive plastic surgery long after a disfiguring burn)

- For Southwest Asia, military approvals are required from local command through Central Command
- All evacuated children must have an attendant; those needing military transport require "Secretary of Defense Designee" status
- Coordination also includes travel to a receiving medical center once in CONUS, obtaining diplomatic transit clearance during wait for ongoing flights, and return transport
- Contact servicing PMRC for guidance

Key Steps for AE Request

- Contact local flight surgeon and / or AE liaison to assist in en route care plan and timing / precedence of evacuation; a patient movement request (PMR) is generated
- Include equipment and support requirements, nonmedical attendants (parent, guardian), precedence, litter, ambulatory (or both), and services required at accepting facility
- The servicing PMRC receives the PMR through the TRANSCOM Regulating and Command and Control Evacuation System (TRAC2ES) via the Internet
  - Facsimile, telephone, and Secure Internet Protocol Router Network (SIPRNet) messages are acceptable if TRAC2ES is unavailable
- PMRC reviews the PMR, validates the request, and establishes an AE requirement
  - The validating flight surgeon, a senior physician assigned to the PMRC, is primarily responsible for this action
- Determine the need for a CCATT (see "special considerations," page 56)
- Patient clearance
  - Local flight surgeon, working with the referring physician, determines that the patient is medically stable for transport and has appropriate equipment and medication for transport, then clears patient for flight
  - For CCATT patients, the transporting CCATT physician makes the final determination, considering the patient's

ability to tolerate transport and operational issues

- Patient movement precedence
  - **Urgent**: Immediate to save life, limb, or eyesight (transport as soon as possible)
  - **Priority**: Prompt medical care required and not available locally; use when condition can deteriorate and patient cannot wait for routine evacuation (transport within 24 h)
  - **Routine**: Requires evacuation, but condition is not anticipated to deteriorate significantly (transport within 72 h)

PMRC Contact Information

Global Patient Movement Requirements Center (GPMRC)
Scott Air Force Base, Illinois
CONUS, US Southern Command
Commercial (COMM) Telephone: (618) 229-4200 or 4129 (staffed all hours, 365 days a year)
Defense Switched Network (DSN): (312) 779-6241
Fax (DSN): (312) 779-4768

Theater Patient Movement Requirements Center–Pacific (TPMRC-P)
Hickam Air Force Base, Hawaii
US Pacific Command, East Asia
COMM Telephone: (808) 448-1602
DSN: (315) 448-1602
Fax (DSN): (315) 448-1606
E-Mail: 13af.sg.tpmrc@hickam.af.mil
Web page: http://www2.hickam.af.mil/units/13thafsurgeongeneral/index.asp

Theater Patient Movement Requirements Center–Europe (TPMRC-E)
Ramstein Air Base, Germany
US European Command, US Central Command, US Africa Command
COMM Telephone: 011-49-6371-47-2264 or 8040
DSN: (314) 480-2264 or 8040
Fax (DSN): (314) 480-2345
E-Mail: tpmrceurope@ramstein.af.mil

Surgery

Chapter 9

Burns

Introduction

Natural childhood curiosity and lack of supervision frequently combine to make thermal injuries a major cause of morbidity and mortality in the pediatric patient. Whether accidental or intentional, the most frequent etiologies are flame and scalding. Many factors contribute to the significant differences in the pathophysiology and treatment of burn injuries in children, including diminished thickness of skin and subcutaneous tissue, immaturity of immune and organ systems, difficulty establishing and maintaining intravenous (IV) access, pain management, and the psychological ramifications of hospitalization, parental separation, physical disability, and disfigurement.

- General considerations
  - Most burns occur in the home
  - Scalding is the most common etiology
  - Flame burns cause the highest incidence of full-thickness injuries and are associated with the highest morbidity and mortality
  - Metabolic responses are as follows:
    - Increased protein catabolism
    - Gluconeogenesis and hyperglycemia
    - Decreased insulin responsiveness
    - Increased plasma catecholamines (especially norepinephrine)
    - Increased heat production (basal metabolic rate)
- Pathophysiological considerations
  - Children's increased surface-area-to-body-weight ratio results in increased evaporative water loss
  - Decreased skin thickness and decreased insulating fat results in increased heat loss
- Point-of-injury care
  - Key steps in the first aid of pediatric burn patients:

        - Fire: stop the burning process
        - Chemical: remove contaminated clothing; lavage with copious quantities of water
        - Electrical: remove the patient from contact with the electrical current
        - Ensure airway patency
        - Prevent hypothermia
            - Cover the patient with a clean, dry sheet or thermal blanket
            - Increase room temperature
            - Provide warm IV fluids
        - Establish IV or intraosseous access and begin fluid resuscitation with Ringer's lactate
    - Conduct primary survey ("ABCDE")
        - Airway
        - Breathing
        - Circulation
        - Disability
        - Exposure/environmental control
    - Conduct secondary survey to uncover other injuries
        - History ("AMPLE")
            - Allergies
            - Medications
            - Past illnesses
            - Last meal
            - Events/environment
    - Perform head-to-toe physical examination
    - Examine every orifice
    - Conduct a complete neurological examination
    - Run special diagnostic tests as needed
    - Reevaluate
- Initial treatment
    - Administer supplemental oxygen
    - Place nasogastric tubes in all patients with burns > 15% body surface area (BSA) due to the high incidence of intestinal ileus
    - Place a Foley catheter
    - Monitor with electrocardiogram and pulse oximeter
    - Check hourly vital signs, monitor fluid input and output

  - Obtain chest radiographs of all intubated patients and those with suspected inhalation injury
  - Initial laboratory tests include:
    - Complete blood count (CBC)
    - Electrolytes
    - Blood urea nitrogen (BUN) / creatinine
    - Blood glucose
    - Urinalysis
    - Blood type and screen
    - Consider checking arterial blood gases and carboxyhemoglobin (inhalation injury)
  - Keep the patient warm by infusing warm IV fluids, elevating room temperatures, and minimizing patient exposure
  - Administer tetanus immunization
  - Stress ulcer prophylaxis
  - Systemic antibiotics are not indicated except for treating proven infection
- Determining burn depth
  - First degree
    - Involves the epidermis only (eg, sunburn)
    - Erythematous, painful, no blisters
    - Not included in calculation of BSA
  - Second degree ("partial thickness")
    - Superficial partial thickness
      - Involves injury to the epidermis and superficial dermis
      - Erythematous, painful, and characterized by intact or ruptured blisters
      - Heals spontaneously within 1–2 weeks, usually with minimal scarring
    - Deep partial thickness
      - Involves injury to the epidermis and deeper layers of the dermis, but some viable dermis remains
      - Whiter and less erythematous as the depth into the dermis increases; may appear mottled
    - Epidermal appendages (hair follicles, sweat and sebaceous glands) serve as the source of regenerating epidermal cells following a burn, as well as a source of bacterial contamination

- Third degree ("full-thickness")
  - Involves epidermis and full thickness of the dermis; these burns always require skin grafting
  - Painless because the nerve endings are destroyed
  - Whitish-gray and waxy to black, leathery appearance, dermal elements (hair, capillaries, nerves) are destroyed
  - Distinguishing between deep partial-thickness burns and full-thickness burns may initially be difficult
    - Deep partial-thickness burns often require 3–4 weeks to heal
    - The degree of scarring is related to the length of time needed for reepithelialization; deep partial-thickness burns that take longer than 3 weeks to heal should be excised and grafted to mitigate against hypertrophic scarring and improve long-term cosmesis
- Fourth degree
  - Involves destruction of epidermis, full-thickness of the dermis, and subdermal structures (eg, muscle, bone, or tendon)
  - Typically associated with electrical burns

- Estimating burn surface area
  - The pediatric modification of the adult rule of nines takes into account that a child's head size is relatively larger, compared to the torso and extremities, than an adult's; the increased ratio of the surface area of the head to the total BSA decreases as age increases
  - The palm of a child's hand approximates 1% BSA; this estimation can be useful for calculating splotchy patterned burns
  - A modified Lund and Browder chart can be used for calculations in children < 10 years old (Figures 9-1 and 9-2)
- Inhalation injury
  - Always suspect inhalation injury when a burn occurs in a closed space
  - Physical findings
    - Singed nasal hair and eyebrows
    - Carbonaceous sputum
    - Increased carboxyhemoglobin

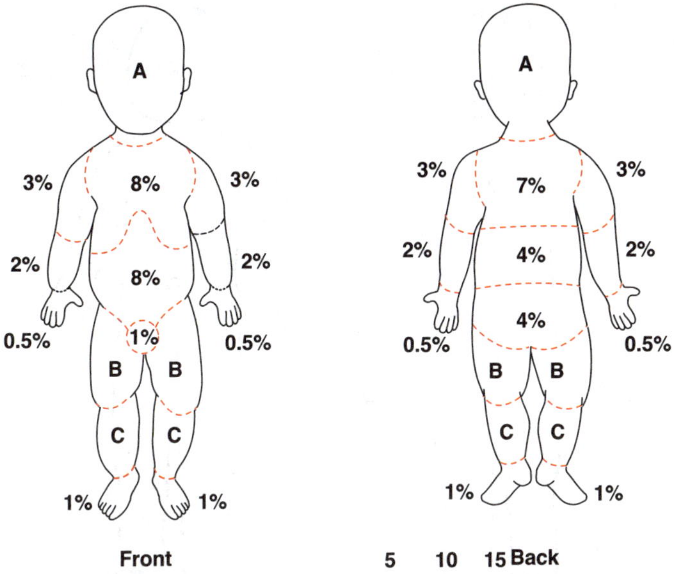

Area	Age 0	1y	5y	10y	15y	Adult
A = half of head	9 1/2	8 1/2	6 1/2	5 1/2	4 1/2	3 1/2
B = half of one thigh	2 3/4	4 1/4	4	4 1/2	4 1/2	4 3/4
C = half of one leg	2 1/2	2 1/2	2 3/4	3	3 1/4	3 1/2

Figure 9-1. Modified Lund and Browder chart for estimating burn severity in infants.

   - Hoarseness
   - Wheezing
   - Bronchorrhea
   - Altered mental status
- Diagnosis: bronchoscopy
- Indications for intubation
   - Compromised upper airway patency
   - Need for ventilatory support as manifested by poor gas exchange or increased work of breathing, or compromised mental status (Glasgow Coma Scale score ≤ 8)
- Carbon monoxide toxicity
   - Leading cause of death in patients with inhalation injury

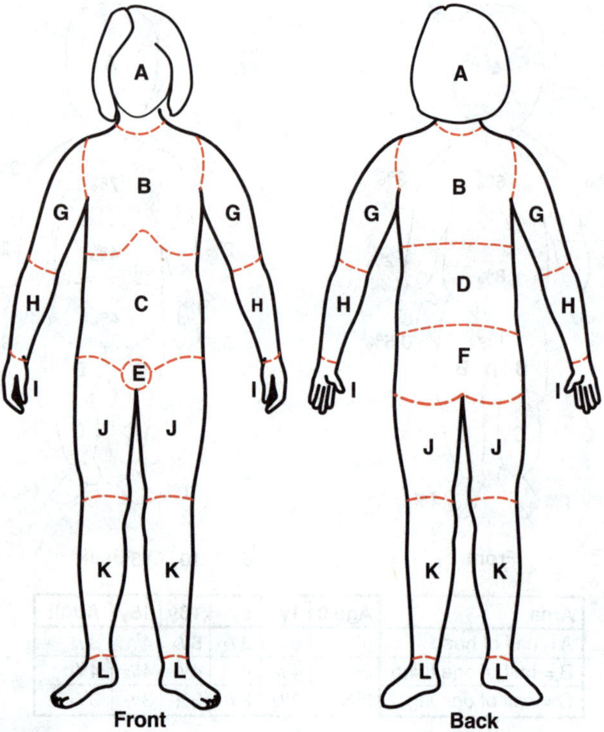

Area	Age 1y	5y	10y	15y
A = half of head and neck	8½	6½	5½	4½
B = half of chest	7	7	7	7
C = abdomen (front)	6	6	6	6
D = abdomen (back)	5	5	5	5
E = perineum	1	1	1	1
F = buttocks	5	5	5	5
G = half of arm	2½	2½	2½	2½
H = half of forearm	2	1½	2	2
I = half of hand	1½	2	1½	1½
J = half of thigh	3	4	4	4½
K = half of leg	2½	4	3	3
L = half of foot	1½	1½	1½	1½

Figure 9-2. Modified Lund and Browder chart for estimating burn severity in children.

- Carboxyhemoglobin levels:
  - < 20%: no symptoms
  - 20%–30%: headache, nausea
  - 30%–40%: altered mental status
  - 40%–60%: unconsciousness
  - > 60%: death
- Should be suspected with persistent metabolic acidosis, despite adequate volume resuscitation
- 100% oxygen should be administered via a high-flow, nonrebreathing mask to all patients suspected of having inhalation injury

- Guidelines for hospitalization or transfer
  - Second- or third-degree burns > 10% BSA in patients < 10 years old
  - Third-degree burns > 5% BSA
  - Full- or partial-thickness burns involving the face, eyes, ears, perineum, hands, or feet
  - Inhalation injuries
  - Electrical injuries
  - Chemical injuries (especially involving white phosphorus)
- Fluid resuscitation
  - Children with burns > 15% BSA require formal IV fluid resuscitation
  - An indwelling urinary catheter is required to accurately measure the adequacy of resuscitation
  - Avoid fluid boluses unless the patient presents with hypotension secondary to hypovolemia
  - Calculating resuscitation requirements:
    - First 24 hours (modified Parkland formula): total 24-hour volume = 3 cc/kg/%BSA burn Ringer lactate
      - Half of this volume is infused over the first 8 hours (calculated from the time of burning, not from when the patient actually arrives at the treatment facility)
      - The remaining half of the calculated 24-hour volume is infused over the next 16 hours
      - These calculations are only an initial estimate; the fluid rate is reassessed every hour and titrated as appropriate to achieve an hourly urine output of 1 cc/kg/h in toddlers, and 2 cc/kg/h in infants
      - Children < 30 kg should be administered D_5¼ normal

saline (NS) at a standard maintenance rate in addition to their calculated resuscitation requirement

- 24–48 hours after burn
    - At the 24th hour, discontinue Ringer lactate and infuse 5% dextrose in water (D_5W) at half the rate of the previous 16 hours
    - For burns > 30% BSA, infuse 5% albumin at a rate of 0.5 cc/kg/% BSA burn for 24 hours
- After 48 hours
    - Diuresis will usually commence at this time
    - Administer D_5W or D_5¼ NS at a maintenance rate
    - Estimate evaporative losses at 1–2 cc/kg/%BSA/day and replace with D_5W in addition to maintenance fluid to avoid hypernatremia
    - Monitor daily body weight, daily "ins and outs," urine-specific gravity, serum electrolytes, BUN/creatinine, and CBC
    - **NOTE**: it is critically important that BSA determination and resuscitation fluid calculations are accurate, and that ins and outs are recorded every 30–60 minutes on a burn resuscitation flow sheet

- Managing minor burns
    - The goals of treatment are to minimize the problems of pain, superficial infections, wound drainage, and prolonged convalescence
    - Small burns may initially be covered by a cloth cooled with saline solution
    - Ice should never be applied directly to a burn
    - Intact blisters should be left unbroken unless they are at flexion creases; ruptured vesicles should be debrided, and the area cleansed gently
    - Partial-thickness injuries may be treated with 1% silver sulfadiazine or by application of a fine-mesh gauze impregnated with petroleum jelly
    - Alternatively, second-degree burns may be covered with a biologic or synthetic dressing (polyurethane film or hydrocolloid semiopen dressing) without a topical antibiotic
    - Tetanus immunization should be given as indicated by immunization history

  - Nonsteroidal antiinflammatory agents may reduce pain
  - If the patient has evidence of group A streptococcal disease, give penicillin (50,000 units/kg/24h q6h oral or IV) to prevent colonization of the burn
- Burn wound care
  - Provide adequate IV (**not** intramuscular or subcutaneous) analgesics or conscious sedation for wound debridement and dressing changes
  - Devitalized skin, foreign bodies, and ruptured blisters should be debrided
  - Cleanse wounds with surgical soap
  - Apply topical agents bid
    - 1% silver sulfadiazine (may cause neutropenia)
    - 10% mafenide acetate (carbonic anhydrase inhibitor that may cause metabolic acidosis and compensatory hyperventilation)
    - 0.5% silver nitrate (may cause decreased serum sodium, resulting in seizures, methemoglobinemia, and indelible black staining)
  - Silver-impregnated dressings may be changed every 48 hours, rinsed, and reapplied on the same patient
  - Treat facial burns with antibiotic ointment to avoid ocular irritation
  - Treat burns to the external ear with mafenide cream
  - Artificial skin substitutes may be used to treat partial-thickness burns and have the advantage of eliminating the painful twice-daily dressing changes associated with standard dressings
  - Circumferential burns of extremities
    - The eschar of circumferential full-thickness and deep partial-thickness burns may result in vascular compromise as resuscitation proceeds
    - All extremities at risk should be monitored with hourly Doppler pulse checks
    - Extremity escharotomy is indicated for clinical symptoms of ischemia ("5-Ps": pain, pallor, paresthesias, paralysis, pulselessness)
    - Treatment: emergent escharotomy, preferably performed at the bedside using electrocautery

        - Because the nerve endings have been destroyed, no anesthesia is required
        - Incise the eschar longitudinally through the medial and lateral aspects of the extremity down to the subcutaneous fat, which should bulge into the wound if adequately incised
        - Arterial pulse should immediately return
    - Failure to adequately apply compartmental decompression will necessitate a fasciotomy
  - Circumferential chest wall burns
    - A child's respiratory efforts may become rapidly exhausted by the edema and restriction of a circumferential chest wall burn
    - Decreased compliance may impair oxygenation and ventilation, which are indications for chest wall escharotomy, performed by incising the chest along the anterior axillary lines bilaterally, extending onto the abdomen, with transverse bridging incisions across the chest
- Surgical treatment of burns
  - Early excision and grafting is effective in decreasing morbidity and improving the mortality rate of full-thickness burns
  - The goal should be to excise the wound within the first week following injury
  - Preoperatively, patients must be hemodynamically stable and be in optimal acid–base, fluid, and electrolyte balance
  - Adequate blood products must be available before excision and grafting can be considered
  - A prophylactic dose of a first-generation cephalosporin antibiotic may be used
  - It is extremely important to maintain the patient's body temperature at all times
    - Raising the temperature of the operating room is the most effective way to achieve this
    - On-table patient warming devices can also be used
  - Tangentially excise burn eschar down to viable tissue using a dermatome or freehand knife
  - Harvest meshed autografts from donor sites

        - Graft thickness varies in pediatric patients
            - Infant: 0.010–0.011 inch
            - Child: 0.012–0.013 inch
            - Teenager: up to 0.015 inch
    - Carefully apply appropriate wound dressings to prevent dislodgment of crucial skin grafts
    - Burn excision results in significant blood loss; the equivalent of 4 units of packed red blood cells (40 cc/kg) should be available for each 10% BSA excision
- Electrical burns
    - Low-voltage injuries result from sources of less than 1,000 volts and include oral injuries from biting electrical cords, outlet injuries from placing objects into wall sockets, and injuries from contacting live wires or indoor appliances
    - High-voltage injuries are caused by sources of more than 1,000 volts and result from contact with a live wire outdoors or from being struck by lightning
        - Children who have sustained high-voltage electrical injury require admission to the hospital with cardiac monitoring, serial electrocardiography, urinalysis, and determination of creatine kinase and urine myoglobin levels
        - If urine is dark, assume myoglobinuria and initiate treatment
            - Increase fluid administration to produce a urine output of 1–2 cc/kg/h
            - If pigment does not clear, administer 1 g/kg of mannitol IV, and add mannitol to IV fluids
            - Treat metabolic acidosis in a normovolemic patient with sodium bicarbonate to alkalize the urine and increase myoglobin solubility
    - Perform appropriate radiographic examinations to exclude concomitant long-bone and spine injuries
    - Myoglobinuria should be treated aggressively with IV hydration, osmotic diuretics, and alkalinization of the urine to avoid renal failure
    - Extremities must be monitored carefully for the development of compartment syndrome, which would necessitate fasciotomy

  - The definitive treatment of myoglobinuria is surgical debridement of dead muscle
- Chemical burns
  - The cornerstone of initial management is copious irrigation with water
  - Alkali burns may require several hours of lavage
  - Resuscitate and manage as a thermal burn
- Pain management
  - Pain and anxiety management are critical to the care of burned children
  - Succinylcholine should never be administered to a burn patient because of the risk of hyperkalemia
  - Initially, IV morphine should be used in small amounts and titrated to the child's physiological state
  - Analgesic agents are most effective when given on a regular schedule (rather than as needed)
  - Generous analgesia or conscious sedation should be used before dressing changes and wound debridement or other painful procedures
  - A bowel regimen, including both a stimulant and a stool softener, should be maintained as long as the child is being administered opioid-derived analgesics
  - Benzodiazepines alleviate the many psychological stresses impacting injured children
  - Use diphenhydramine to treat severe pruritis in children with healing second-degree burns
- Nutrition
  - Nutritional support should be started as soon as possible after injury, preferably via the enteral route
  - If patients cannot ingest adequate calories, a nasoduodenal feeding tube should be placed and isoosmolar feedings initiated
  - Estimated protein requirements are 3 g/kg/day
  - The daily caloric requirements of pediatric burn patients can be estimated using the Curreri formula:
    - Age 0–1 years: basic metabolic requirements + 15 kcal/%BSA burn
    - Age 1–3 years: basic metabolic requirements + 25

kcal/%BSA burn

  - Age 4–15 years: basic metabolic requirements + 40 kcal/%BSA burn

- Rehabilitation
  - Burns traversing joints must be treated with passive and active range-of-motion exercises during the healing process
  - Burned extremities should be splinted with the joints in the position of function at night
  - Attention to occupational and physical therapy is necessary to ensure optimal results
  - Burns requiring more than 2 weeks to heal, and all grafted burns, should ideally be treated for 1 year with compression garments that apply approximately 30 mmHg of pressure, which decreases the formation of hypertrophic scars

Chapter 10

Neurosurgery

Managing pediatric neurotrauma at medical treatment facilities (roles 1 to 3) requires a consolidated effort on the part of providers and administrators within the military healthcare system.

Mission Clarification

Pediatric neurotrauma patients require intensive resources. They may need prolonged mechanical ventilation and extensive rehabilitation, and few medical facilities in the developing world are capable of providing these services. Coalition healthcare providers are often unprepared for such limitations. It is essential to assess facility capabilities and address postresuscitation and posttreatment patient flow prior to the arrival of pediatric casualties; failure to make these assessments will result in poor patient outcomes, increased stress on healthcare providers, and potential erosion of relationships with local host-nation residents.

Head Injury in the Pediatric Patient

- Anatomical, physiological, cognitive, and social variances between adult and pediatric patients influence evaluation and treatment
  - Accurate neurological assessment is essential for appropriate patient triage and guides further management
    - Validity of the Glasgow Coma Scale (GCS; Table 10-1) is compromised in children due to the difficulty of accurately categorizing their verbal and motor responses
    - The Infant Face Scale (Table 10-2) is a validated clinical tool with a high degree of interrater reliability; it is a modified GCS for children
  - Triage decisions in pediatric patients in theater are difficult and can be emotionally charged
    - Although pediatric patients with neurological injuries are more likely to have favorable long-term outcomes than adults with similar injuries, their care is impacted

Table 10-1. Glasgow Coma Scale

Function	Score
Eye opening	
Spontaneous	4
Verbal stimulation	3
Painful stimulation	2
None	1
Motor	
Obeys commands	6
Localizes	5
Withdraws	4
Flexion	3
Extension	2
None	1
Verbal	
Oriented	5
Confused	4
Inappropriate	3
Incoherent	2
None	1

by limited resources in theater

- The decision between treatment and palliative care for an injured child is a sobering but necessary aspect of care in an austere environment
- Several factors can influence decisions on whether or not to proceed with treatment, such as:
  - A facility's capabilities
  - Options for later evacuation to military facilities with enhanced capabilities, or to a host-nation healthcare facility
  - Clinical factors
  - Physiological stability: abundant literature exists demonstrating poor neurological outcomes in patients following prolonged periods of hypotension and/or hypoxia; palliative care should be strongly considered for patients in these circumstances

- GCS and Infant Face Scale scores correlate well with neurological outcome
  - Accurate in normotensive, nonhypoxic patients with no

Table 10-2. Infant Face Scale Modifications to Glasgow Coma Scale

Function	Score
Best Motor Response	
Spontaneous, normal movements	6
Hypoactive movements	5
Nonspecific movement to deep pain	4
Abnormal, rhythmic, spontaneous movements	3
Extension, either spontaneous or to pain	2
Flexion	1
Best Verbal Response	
Cries spontaneously to handling or pain, alternating with quiet wakefulness	5
Cries spontaneously to handling or minor pain, alternating with sleep	4
Cries to deep pain only	3
Grimaces only to pain	2
No facial expression to pain	1

Data source: Durham SR, Clancy RR, Leuthardt E, et al. CHOP Infant Coma Scale ("Infant Face Scale"): a novel coma scale for children less than two years of age. *J Neurotrauma*. 2000;17(9):729–737.

pharmacologic agents compromising their examination

- After physiological stabilization, consider reversing sedation and neuromuscular blockade to facilitate a comprehensive neurological assessment
  - See Broselow tape for reversal-agent dosing
  - Muscle relaxation reversal should be confirmed with a peripheral nerve stimulator
  - A typical reversal regimen consists of **neostigmine** (50 μg/kg), **glycopyrrolate** (10 μg/kg), **naloxone** (10–20 μg), and **flumazenil** (10 μg/kg)
- Patients with GCS scores > 8 will often benefit from treatment; when resources are available, they should be treated aggressively
- Patients with GCS scores of 6–8 inhabit a "gray zone," and may proceed to treatment or palliative care, depending on additional clinical considerations and resource availability
- Patients with GCS scores ≤ 5 will rarely benefit from treatment in a forward environment and should be managed

expectantly

- Pupillary reactivity
  - Findings convey important information about the function of the eye and cranial nerves 2 and 3
  - Pupillary function can be impaired by several medications, including intravenous atropine (often used for resuscitation)
  - Pupillary function is not impaired by muscle relaxants
  - In the absence of penetrating injuries to the globe, bilateral mydriasis (large, nonreactive pupils) is a strong predictor of poor neurological outcome; treat patients with bilateral nonreactive pupils expectantly
  - Unilateral pupil dilation
    - May result from direct trauma to the globe, orbit, or cranial nerves
    - Can indicate impending herniation
    - Should be considered in concert with other clinical factors
- A computed tomography (CT) scan is important when determining the salvageability of neurological patients; the following two findings are the most likely to determine patient salvageability:
  - Midline shift: easily measured by dropping a line from the anterior and posterior insertion of the falx cerebri
    - Allows for quantification of intercompartmental shift
    - A shift exceeding 5 mm is worrisome; in excess of 1 cm, it portends a poor prognosis
  - Patency of basal cisterns (Figure 10-1): the basal cisterns, small-volume spinal fluid spaces at the base of the brain, are visible on nearly any CT scan of the head
    - Anteriorly, they are shaped like a pentagon, and posteriorly like a smile
    - When patent, they indicate low intracranial pressure (ICP) and increased likelihood of salvageability
    - When absent, the patient's prognosis is poor

Medical Management

- Avoiding hypoxia and hypotension are the most important goals
- Seizure prophylaxis is appropriate in the first week (Figure 10-2)
  - Minimizes the deleterious effects of increased cerebral blood flow (accompanying a generalized seizure) in pa-

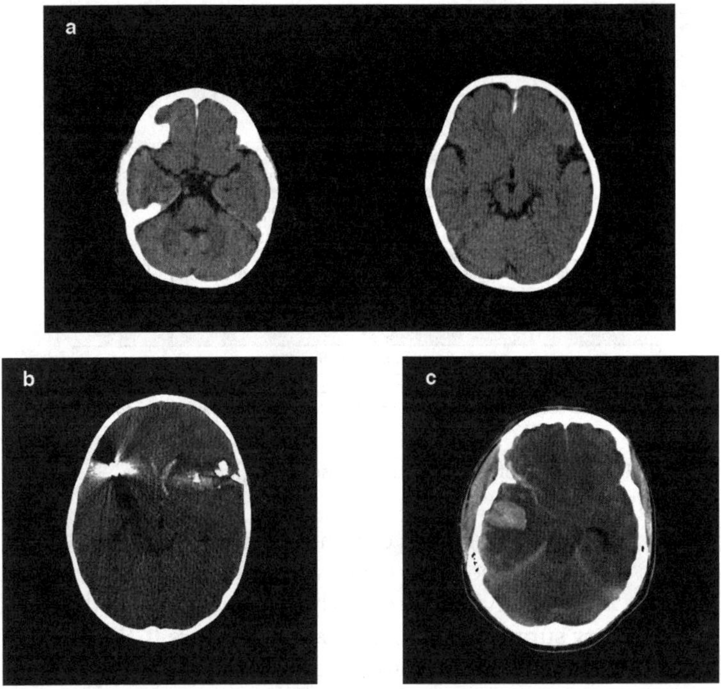

Figure 10-1. (**a**) Anterior and posterior basal cisterns on a normal computed tomography scan of the head. (**b**) Despite a fragment crossing the midline and ventricular system, no midline shift is present and the basal cisterns remain patent. The patient did well and was released from the hospital 4 days after admission. (**c**) Marked midline shift is present and the basal cisterns are effaced. Palliative care was elected, and the patient expired.

tients with impaired intracranial compliance

- Although phenytoin is an effective agent in adults, it is difficult to maintain therapeutic levels in infants and toddlers
- **Phenobarbital** is the preferred antiepileptic agent in patients < 2 years old
    - Loading dose: 20 mg/kg
    - Maintenance dose: 3–5 mg/kg/day divided bid

- ICP monitoring (when available) is indicated for all patients with GCS (including modified Infant Face Scale) score ≤ 8
    - This includes infants with a patent fontanelle

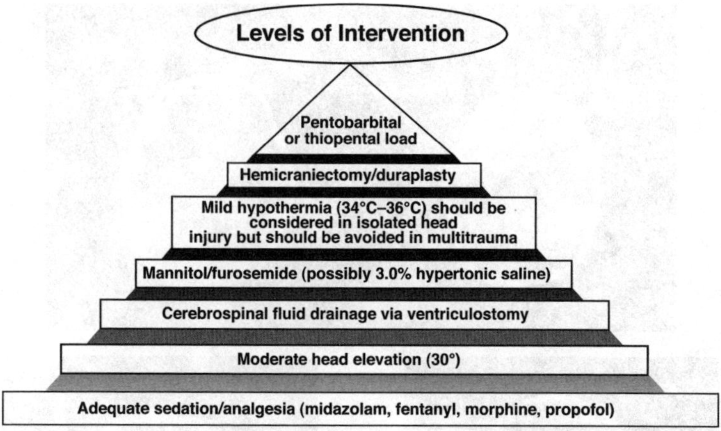

Figure 10-2. Levels of intervention in neurological injury.

- A patent fontanelle does not preclude elevated ICP
- There is no accurate, noninvasive means of estimating ICP
- Parenchymal monitors, which are available in the military supply system, accurately measure ICP
- Parenchymal monitors are easier to place and carry a lower infection risk, but provide no means of directly treating ICP
- Parenchymal monitors may be placed at a depth of 1–2 cm, regardless of patient's age

- Ventriculostomy catheters (Figure 10-3) are also accurate ICP measures available in military supply
  - Ventriculostomy catheters have the added advantage of allowing treatment of ICP elevations with spinal fluid drainage
  - Disadvantages include elevated risk of infection and potential difficulties with placement in patients with severe injury
  - Ventriculostomy catheters lie within the ventricle at a depth of:
    - 3–3.5 cm in infants
    - 4 cm in toddlers
    - 5 cm in older children and adults
  - Depth of insertion and cranial access in infants must be

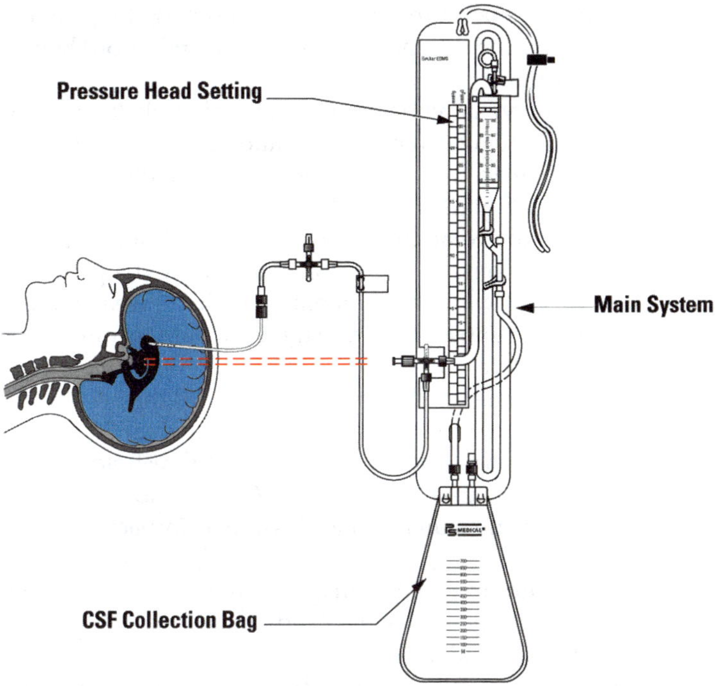

Figure 10-3. Schematic of ventriculostomy setup. Dashed red line represents the zero point of the system. Collection buretrol is set at desired height above the external auditory canal.
CSF: cerebrospinal fluid
Drawing courtesy of: Medtronic Neurosurgery, Goleta, California.

considered when placing ventriculostomy catheters in children

- For infants, the anterior fontanelle can be used instead of a craniostomy, provided the entry site is a minimum of 2 cm off the midline
- Drain setup is identical to that of any fluid-coupled system used in the intensive care unit, with the following exceptions:
  - Zero point for the system is the external auditory canal
  - The system should **never** be attached to a pressurized flush (such as that used for an arterial line)
  - When used for drainage purposes, one method is

to set the drain open at a certain height (eg, 10 cm above the external auditory canal) and record hourly output
      - To prevent hyponatremia and/or hypokalemia, each milliliter of cerebrospinal fluid (CSF) output should be replaced in infants and toddlers with a milliliter of 0.9% NaCl + 20 KCl
      - Rapidly wean the patient from CSF drainage if possible; do not place a CSF shunt while the patient is in a forward environment. Inability to wean patient from ventricular drainage is usually grounds for palliative care
- ICP and cerebral perfusion pressure (CPP) thresholds
   - ICP: treat sustained values of greater than 20 mmHg with the goal of reducing below this threshold
   - CPP (mean arterial pressure – ICP), due to age-related variance in mean arterial pressure, is impacted by patient age
      - Minimum of 40 mmHg for infants, and up to 65 mmHg for adolescents and adults
      - Medical adjuncts
- Propofol infusion is **contraindicated** for long-term sedation (> 24 h) in pediatric patients due to the risk of fatal metabolic acidosis (propofol infusion syndrome)
- 3% saline has replaced mannitol/furosemide as the preferred hyperosmolar or diuretic therapy
   - 3% saline: initial bolus of 2–3 mL/kg, followed by infusion, ranging from 0.1–1 mL/kg/h
   - Target serum sodium of 150–155 mEq/dL is an effective means of reducing ICP in most patients
      - Higher serum sodium targets have been reported, provided isovolemia is maintained without deleterious results
- Therapeutic hypothermia has not been validated for head injury in pediatric patients and is rarely practical in a deployed environment
   - Reduce cerebral metabolic rate by avoiding hyperthermia
- Barbiturate coma effectively manages refractory ICP in children, but is impractical in a deployed environment; do

not use routinely

- Surgical management
  - The spectrum of surgical management of pediatric head injury is broad. This chapter provides limited guidance for surgically managing head injuries; it is not a substitute for more conventional surgical education. Surgeons are advised to remain within their own skill set
  - Repair of scalp lacerations and low-velocity penetrating head injuries
    - Understanding the anatomy of the scalp and principles of scalp closure is essential (Figure 10-4)
    - Watertight repair of penetrating injuries to the scalp is necessary for stopping blood loss and preventing CSF efflux and the potential for meningitis from retrograde infection
    - The only surgical intervention required in the majority of head-injured patients with GCS score > 8 may be as simple as the following:
      - Fully exposing the wound by shaving the scalp
      - Conservatively debriding devitalized tissue
      - Performing layered closure of the galea, followed by the skin
    - Definitive treatment for many patients (particularly those with a GCS score ≥ 11) can be performed at facilities with limited surgical capabilities
  - **Craniotomy in the pediatric patient**
    - Positioning: a Mayfield headrest with pins is not appropriate for pediatric trauma patients in theater
      - A gel donut or cerebellar headrest (when available) helps avoid the potential for skull penetration in thinner pediatric skulls
      - A generous shoulder/hip roll can be used to maintain neutral positioning of the neck
    - Scalp incision: decreased absolute patient blood volume makes hemostasis imperative during scalp incision
      - Lidocaine (0.5% lidocaine with epinephrine 1:100,000) is a readily available, easy means of reducing blood loss at the time of skin incision
      - Lidocaine toxicity limits dosing to < 7.5 mg/kg

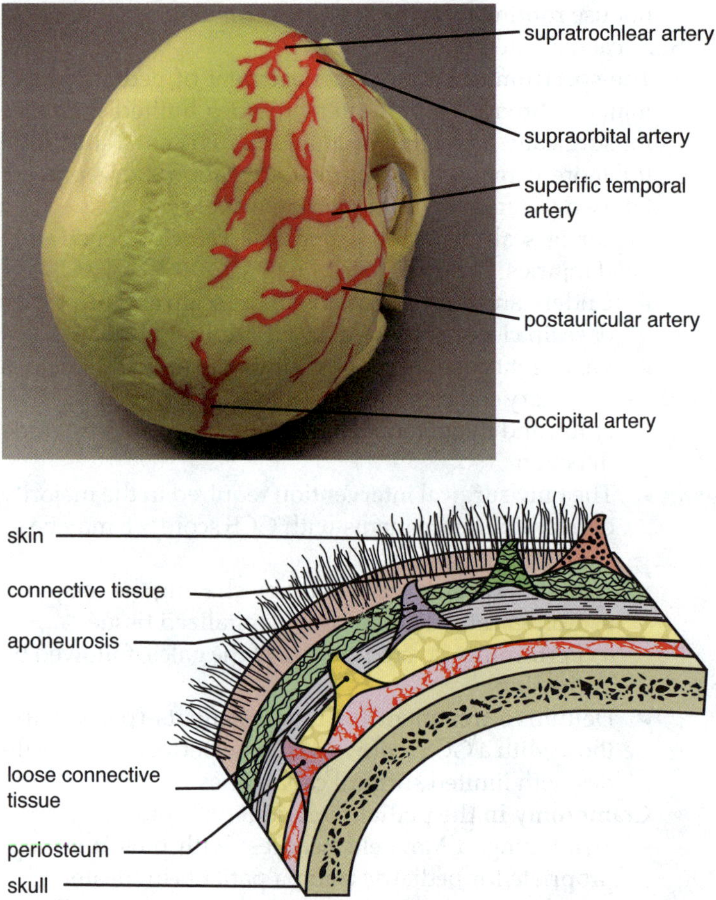

Figure 10-4. Scalp anatomy and blood supply.

- A **maximum** of 5 mg/kg of lidocaine or 7 mg/kg of lidocaine with epinephrine, injected intradermally, can be used in pediatric patients (1% lidocaine = 10 mg/mL)
- In children < 2 years old with decreased scalp thickness, Raney clips can be applied to achieve hemostasis
- Alternatively, apply hemostat to the galea during opening
- Consider extending the scalp incision through the

dermal appendages only, and complete the opening with monopolar cautery
    - A needle-tip bovie on settings of 7 cut/12 cauterize works well
  - Dural closure is rarely required, and often needlessly prolongs anesthesia for damage-control surgery
    - Onlay dural grafts are readily available and are the preferred tools in this setting for separating the brain from the scalp
    - Onlay repairs are effective in nearly all cases where the galea and scalp have been properly closed
  - Bone flap preservation: pediatric neurotrauma patients have limited options for reconstructive surgery following recovery in theater (Figure 10-5)
    - In acute injury, the bone flap is rarely replaced in the head at the time of surgery
    - Autologous "storage" of a flap that is not grossly contaminated is possible; at the time of cranial surgery, prepare the abdomen for subcutaneous bone-flap placement
    - The right lower quadrant is preferred to preserve the left upper quadrant for possible G-tube placement
    - The bone flap must occasionally be bisected and stacked to accommodate an expansive hemicraniectomy flap
    - The bone flap may become infected during the remainder of the patient's hospitalization and beyond
    - Bone flap replacement can be considered 3–6 months after injury

Spinal Injury in the Pediatric Patient

The pediatric spine, particularly the cervical spine, differs from the adult spine both anatomically and in its response to injury. Differences are most pronounced in patients ≤ 9 years old, after which anatomy and injury patterns tend to parallel those of adult patients.

- Anatomical and biomechanical differences between the pediatric and adult spine
  - Pediatric spine

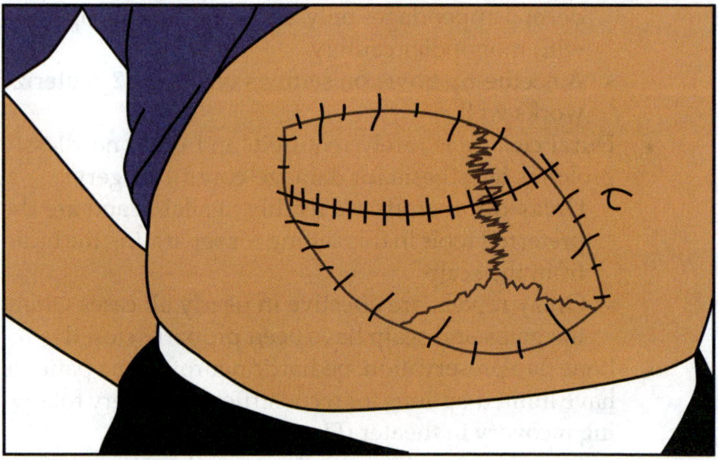

Figure 10-5. Subcutaneous abdominal placement of cranial bone flap.

- Contains more elastic ligaments
- Exhibits anterior wedging of vertebral bodies
- Facet joints are oriented more horizontally than in adults
- In cervical spine, absent uncinate processes decrease the stability of the spinal unit

- Children's proportionately larger heads increase the force applied to the upper cervical spine and cause neutral positioning differences when compared to adults
- The relative size of the spinal canal (which achieves near-adult cross-sectional area prior to the age of 9) presents a proportionately larger target for penetrating fragments in the thoracic and lumbar regions

- Pathophysiological differences between the pediatric and adult spine
  - The increased elasticity and proportionately larger head of a pediatric patient results in profound changes in observed injury patterns
  - Fractures are relatively uncommon in pediatric patients
  - The fulcrum of the cervical spine is shifted from C5–6 in adult patients to C2–3 in infants
    - Injuries most commonly occur between the occiput and

C3 levels

- Disruptions of unfused ossifications centers, such as the C2 synchondrosis, are common (as are ligamentous injuries at the craniocervical junction)
- Spinal cord injuries in the absence of plain radiographic findings are also more common in this age group

- Radiographic differences between the pediatric and adult spine
  - Radiographs and CT scans differ significantly between adult and pediatric patients
  - The large proportion of cartilage in the pediatric spine, coupled with primary and secondary ossification centers, are unfamiliar to most providers
  - Standard measurements, including the atlantodental interval and anterior soft tissue thickness at C2, are increased in pediatric patients in comparison to adults
  - Additional findings, such as C2–3 pseudosubluxation, also present challenges to the inexperienced provider
  - Providers likely to encounter pediatric patients in theater should familiarize themselves with these differences
- Transporting pediatric patients with suspected spinal injuries
  - A pediatric patient's proportionately large head size requires additional consideration at the time of transport
  - To maintain anatomical cervical lordosis and airway patency, the patient must be placed on a spine board with a bolster under the body at and distal to shoulder level, leveling the patient's face and allowing for proper spinal and airway positioning (Figure 10-6)
- Medical and surgical management of spinal injuries
  - Pediatric spinal injury management in current operational theaters is limited
    - Select US facilities in theater may have the prerequisite spinal instrumentation and intraoperative fluoroscopy
    - The majority of closed and penetrating injuries can be managed with resources available at facilities with less robust clinical and radiographic support
  - Closed injuries: management consists of restoring (near) normal anatomical alignment and immobilizing the patient

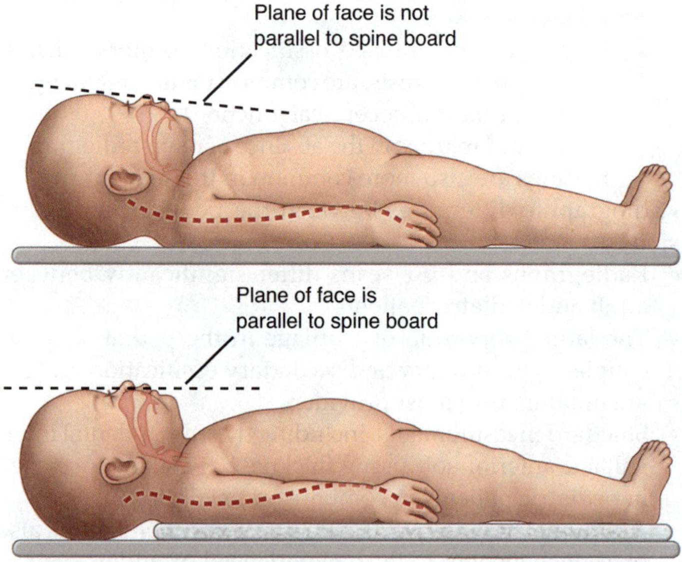

Figure 10-6. (**top**) Improper positioning of a child to maintain a patent airway. The disproportion between the size of a child's cranium and the midface leads to a propensity for the posterior pharynx to buckle anteriorly. The large occiput causes passive flexion of the cervical spine. (**bottom**) Proper positioning of a child to maintain a patent airway. Avoid passive flexion of the cervical spine by keeping the plane of the midface parallel to the spine board in a neutral position, rather than in the "sniffing position." Placement of a one-inch-thick layer of padding beneath a child's entire torso will preserve neutral alignment of the spinal column. Reproduced with permission from: American College of Surgeons. *Advanced Trauma and Life Support Student Course Manual*. 8th ed. Chicago, Ill: ACS; 2008: 230.

- Gardner-Wells tongs can be used for reduction in pediatric patients as they are in adults
  - Less weight is typically required to achieve reduction (2 lb per level in pediatric patients, as opposed to 5–10 lb per level in adults)
- Commercial cervical collars or expedient structural aluminum malleable (SAM) splints can be contoured to the patient to provide immobilization for cervical injuries

    - In the exceptional case that an appropriately sized halo vest is available, apply 6–8 pins at a force not to exceed 4 ft/lb of torque
    - Thoracolumbar fractures can be managed with 4–6 weeks of bed rest
    - Studies investigating the use of high-dose steroid therapy (methylprednisolone) in pediatric patients have not been performed; routine high-dose steroid therapy for pediatric spinal cord injuries **cannot be recommended**
- Penetrating injuries
    - Frequently encountered in theater
    - The absence of body armor and the proportionately large size of the spinal canal in children produce complex injuries, often traversing multiple body cavities in addition to the spinal canal
    - Antibiotic coverage is guided by the body cavities traversed and the relative cleanliness of the fragment and wound
    - Steroid therapy is inappropriate, based both on age and the penetrating mechanism
    - Spinal stability is rarely impacted by penetrating injuries
    - Most injuries are managed either with 6 weeks of bed rest for immobilization, or without positioning restrictions if upright radiographs demonstrate stability (in younger patients, sedation may be required to restrict activity)
    - CSF fistula presents one of the most serious challenges in these patients
        - If cutaneous CSF leakage is noted, or if clear fluid is noted at a high output from a chest tube following a transthoracic gunshot wound to the chest, a spinal fluid drain **must** be placed postoperatively, either under direct vision intraoperatively or percutaneously at the L4–5 interspace
        - Anesthesia providers are often qualified to assist with drain placement in the absence of neurosurgical support
        - Height-controlled drainage of 10–15 mL/h is usually

sufficient to stop drainage through the fistula

- ▹ 72 hours of drainage will often result in permanent closure of the fistula; clamp the drain for 24 hours to ensure successful resolution of the fistula prior to removal

Further Reading

1. Head injuries. In: *Emergency War Surgery, Third United States Revision*. Washington, DC: Department of the Army. Office of The Surgeon General, Borden Institute; 2004. Chap 15.
2. Wounds and injuries of the spinal column and cord. In: *Emergency War Surgery, Third United States Revision*. Washington, DC: Department of the Army. Office of The Surgeon General, Borden Institute; 2004. Chap 20.

Chapter 11

Ophthalmology

Portions of this chapter previously appeared as: Ocular Injuries. In: Emergency War Surgery, 3rd United States Revision. *Burris DG, Dougherty PJ, Elliot DC, et al, eds. Washington, DC: US Department of the Army, Borden Institute; 2004: Chap 14.*

The visual sensory system of a child less than 8–10 years old is developing and can be irreversibly damaged by a variety of conditions if they are not detected and treated early. In the US military, general ophthalmologists on active duty provide most pediatric eye care in many locations. At some facilities, optometrists may also provide nonsurgical refractive care and evaluate the eye health of pediatric patients, subsequently referring cases with more serious conditions to an ophthalmologist. Both general ophthalmologists and optometrists refer more complicated pediatric eye patients to subspecialty trained pediatric ophthalmologists, who, in the US Army, Air Force, and Navy, are generally located at larger facilities, such as regional medical centers and facilities with ophthalmology teaching programs. All facilities that have ophthalmology residency programs in the military have one or more pediatric ophthalmologists on staff.

- The pediatric eye examination
  - History
    - Obtain a history of the present condition
    - Gather information about birth history
      - Prematurity may be associated with retinopathy of prematurity (ROP), intraventricular hemorrhage with secondary hydrocephalus, and ventriculoperitoneal shunts; a failing shunt may be responsible for abducens palsy ("sun-setting eyes") or papilledema
      - Forceps delivery is associated with corneal clouding (edema of the cornea from Descemet's membrane tears)

    - Shoulder dystocia, difficult delivery, and neck traction may be associated with Horner's syndrome (ptosis, miosis, anhydrosis). Anisocoria is worse in the dark and there is mild ipsilateral ptosis
  - General medical history should include family history (especially of strabismus and heritable eye and systemic conditions) and surgical history (ie, prior eye surgery)
- Examination
  - Observe general appearance
  - Note head position
    - Observe for head tilts, face turns, and chin-up or chin-down posture
    - A goniometer is useful for quantifying abnormal head positions
  - Check facial symmetry (look for gross abnormalities and size or shape disparities)
  - Determine visual acuity (one of the vital signs of eye health); visual acuity evaluation and documentation is age dependent (Table 11-1)

Table 11-1. Normal Visual Acuity by Age

Age (years)	Vision
3–4	20/30
5	20/25
6–12	20/20
12–18	20/15

    - Premature infants and neonates (up to 2 mo old) should blink in response to a bright penlight
    - Infants (2–6 mo old) should fixate on and follow a target
    - In infants and toddlers (6 mo–2½ y old), vision should be central (eye appears properly aligned with target), steady (no nystagmus or searching movements), and maintained (eye can hold fixation for at least a few seconds when the other eye is covered and then uncovered; this is especially useful in the presence of strabismus)

  - Preschool (2½–5 y old) should be able to see pictograms at 20/20 (feet) or 6/6 (meters)
  - Children of school age and older should be able to see an alphabet at 20/20 (feet) or 6/6 (meters)
- Intraocular pressure (IOP; the other vital sign of eye health) is always measured indirectly (through the cornea or through the lids and cornea). IOP checks may be obtained while a child is sedated or at the onset of general anesthesia
  - Digital (finger) method: eyes are palpated through the closed lids; annotated as normal finger tension; this method is acceptable for the majority of patients
  - Instrument method: measured through the cornea. This method is more accurate, but more frightening to the patient; reserved for older children or for those in whom increased IOP is suspected
- Binocularity is a special vital sign of pediatric eye health. Binocular vision occurs in the cerebral cortex and involves integrating the sensory input from each eye to produce a single three-dimensional image
  - Stereo vision testing (often called "depth perception" testing) is commonly used to check binocularity
  - The Titmus (Titmus Optical Inc, Chester, VA) and Randot (Stereo Optical Company, Inc, Chicago, IL) stereoacuity tests use polarized glasses and slightly horizontally dissimilar photographs to create a three-dimensional illusion to detect the highest level of binocularity; these can be used on children as young as 2 years old
  - With the Worth 4 Dot Test (Richmond Products, Inc, Albuquerque, NM), glasses with red and green lenses are used to view red and green lights in an otherwise dark room; this test detects a lesser level of binocularity and is used on children around 5 years old and older
  - A base-out prism test calls for a low-power, clear prism (4–8 prism diopter power) to be brought over one eye, oriented apex toward the nose. The presence or absence of a corresponding fusional convergence

movement is noted. This test can be used on children as young as 6 months old

- Extraocular motility
  - Follow movement in lateral, medial, upward, downward, and diagonal directions of gaze. The examiner will need an assortment of fixation targets (eg, toys) to maintain the child's interest
  - Observe for over- or under-muscle action, baseline or induced nystagmus, or strabismus
- Examine pupils. Check size, shape, and location of the pupils, as well as direct and consensual response to light
  - Results are more reliable if the child's attention is diverted toward a distant target and away from the examiner's light source
  - A finding of afferent pupillary defect requires further evaluation, especially of the optic nerve. Magnetic resonance imaging (preferred) or a computed tomography (CT) scan may be indicated
- The examination for muscle balance is performed in primary position (face straight) at a distance and then near (14–16 inches), followed by other gaze positions as indicated (right, left, up, down, right tilt, and left tilt)
  - Cover–uncover test: one eye is covered by an occluder while the examiner observes the other eye; if movement is detected, strabismus is manifest
  - Alternate cover test: an occluder is moved back and forth from one eye to the other; movement represents latent or manifest strabismus
  - Simultaneous prism cover test: an occluder is placed over the fixing ("straight") eye while a correcting prism is placed over the nonfixing eye
  - Deviations in magnitude are measured with calibrated prisms. The endpoint is no movement on the alternate cover test or simultaneous prism cover test
- External examination
  - Check lid position (observe for unilateral or bilateral ptosis)
  - Epicanthal folds are frequently associated with pseudoesotropia

        - Increased tear lake, mucoid discharge, and epiphora may be signs of nasolacrimal duct obstruction
        - Look for lid masses and lesions (eg, dermoids, molluscum lesions)
        - Note telecanthus (increased distance between medial canthi)
        - Check for hypertelorism (increased distance between orbits; associated with midface abnormalities)
        - Examine the anterior segment (cornea, conjunctiva, anterior chamber, and iris)
    - Cycloplegic refraction is the most accurate method of determining a refractive state of the eye
        - Autorefraction is often unreliable in children; use only in adolescents
        - Manifest refraction (using phoropter) is unreliable in young children; it is easy to overestimate the power required ("over minus"); however, manual cycloplegic refraction with free-held lenses or devices (skioscopy bars) is helpful
    - Perform a retinoscopy (if the retinoscopic reflex is obscured, the visual axis is likely affected enough to produce amblyopia)
    - A dilated fundus examination is best performed with an indirect ophthalmoscope set set on the dim light setting
        - A posterior central fundus view is usually all that is required
        - The standard eight views of the periphery per eye is rarely indicated or tolerated by most younger children; evaluation under anesthesia or sedation may be required for periphery views

- Pediatric ophthalmic disease diagnosis and treatment
    - Nonstrabismic conditions
        - Orbital dermoid cyst
            - Most commonly located along the superior–temporal orbital rim; occasionally attached by a narrow transosseous isthmus to an intraorbital component
            - Slowly enlarges; may internally rupture and produce intense regional inflammation after minor local trauma

- Surgical removal is indicated after CT scan to rule out intraorbital portion
- Ptosis
  - Eyelid droop (usually unilateral). Urgent treatment is needed if the visual axis is obscured. Less urgent correction is indicated for chin-up head position (when children maintain a chin-up position, they are attempting to use the ptotic eye; when the lid droop is such that the child is not even trying to use the ptotic eye, the visual axis is usually blocked in that eye by the lid)
  - The most common form of ptosis includes poor levator muscle function (upper lid movement is limited), manifested by reversal of ptosis on down-gaze. Treat with a frontalis sling
  - If levator function is adequate (ie, upper lid has good movement), treat with levator resection
- Prominent epicanthal folds (skin fold over medial canthus gives the illusion of small-angle esotropia or crossed eyes); this is a normal variant and no treatment is needed
- Blepharitis (erythema of the lid margin)
  - Patient may have lash loss and scaling skin debris
  - Common in those with trisomy 21
  - May be a sign of immunologic deficiency in severe or chronic cases
  - Can be treated with proper lid hygiene and a mild topical antibiotic ointment before sleep
- Nasolacrimal duct obstruction
  - Common in neonates and infants
  - Usually unilateral, manifests as chronic mucopurulent discharge with excess tearing (epiphora)
  - May be mistaken for chronic or recurrent conjunctivitis; symptoms often improve while on antibiotic drops or ointment, only to recur when the medication is discontinued
  - Most cases resolve by 1 year of age
  - Massaging the nasolacrimal sac may assist resolution

- Nasolacrimal duct probing and irrigation is indicated for those cases persisting at 1 year old; if probing fails to resolve symptoms, temporary silicone-tube stinting may be required (see Figure 11-1)

- Conjunctivitis
  - Usually viral and self-limited
    - Acute purulent conjunctivitis is characterized by hyperemia, edema, mucopurulent exudates and ocular discomfort. The most frequent organisms are staphylococci, pneumococci, *Haemophilus influenzae*, and streptococci. Gram stain and culture are used to identify the specific organism, and infections usually respond to warm compresses and frequent instillation of topical antibiotic drops
    - Viral conjunctivitis is usually associated with adenovirus and manifested by a watery (as opposed to purulent) discharge. Usually self-limited, Gram stain and bacterial cultures are negative, and treatment with topical sulfonamides is sufficient
    - Chemical conjunctivitis may occur after prophylactic instillation of silver nitrate (1%), erythromycin ophthalmic ointment (0.5%), or azithromycin ophthalmic solution (1%) 12–24 hours after birth. No pathogens are identified and no treatment is necessary
  - Most cases are treated by the patient's primary physician, but severe, chronic, recurrent, or unusual cases are often referred to an ophthalmologist
  - Treat raised umbilicated lid lesions (molluscum contagiosum) by scraping
  - Recurrent and associated with epiphora; if it always occurs on the same side, suspect nasolacrimal duct obstruction and arrange for probing and irrigation. If probing fails to give long-term symptom relief, patient may need a stint
  - Epidemic keratoconjunctivitis: small, scattered, superficial corneal infiltrates that are self-limited

a

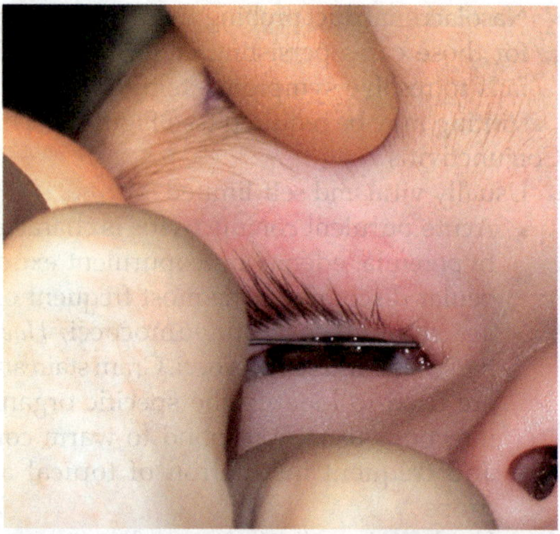

b

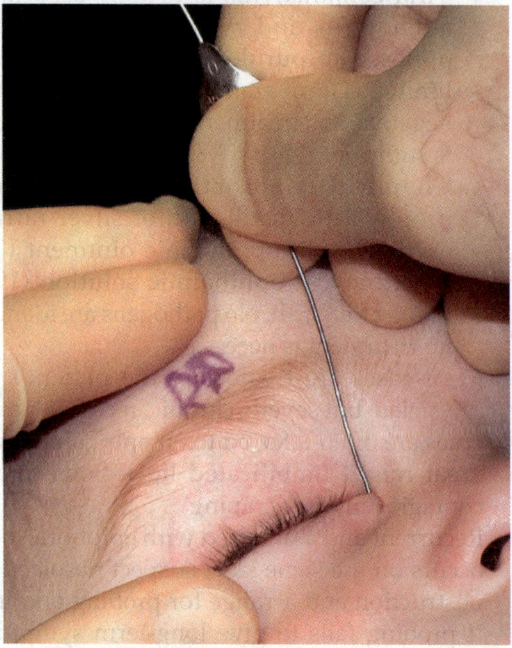

Figure 11-1. **(a)**"00" Bowman probe introduction into right superior puncta and canuliculus. **(b)** Medial and superior rotation of probe, then inferior advancement of probe to hard palate. (**Figure 11-1** *continues*)

c

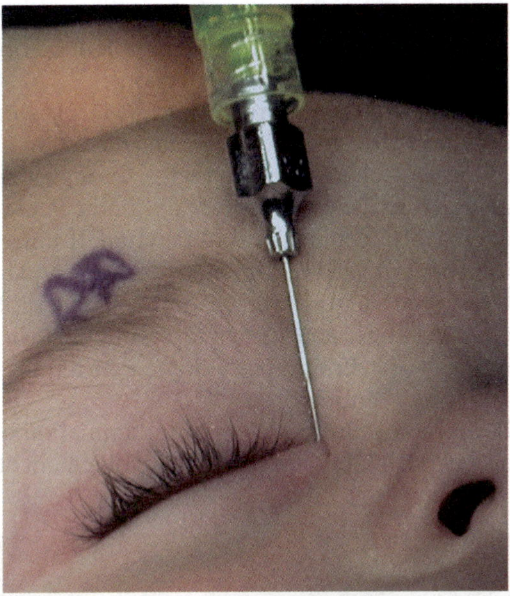

d

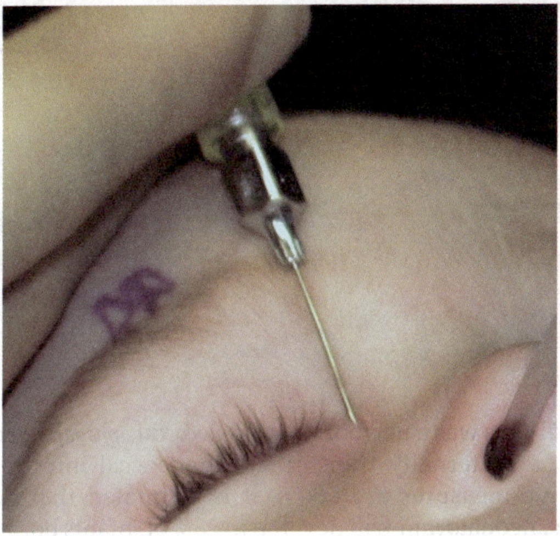

Figure 11-1 ***continued*****. (c)** Replacement of probe with a long, 23-gauge, blunt-tip canula, then, irrigation of a very small amount (< 1 cc or mL) of fluorescein-stained normal saline. **(d)** Recovery of fluorescein from ipsilateral nares with 8 Fr suction catheter confirms open nasolacrimal duct. Avoid airway compromise from excessive irrigation.

(may take 6–10 wk). Treat with supportive care and mild topical antibiotic ointment before sleep to prevent bacterial superinfection

- Ophthalmia neonatorum (Figure 11-2) is caused by infection due to *Neisseria gonorrhoeae* or *Chlamydia trachomatis* acquired by passage through the infected genital tract. There is profuse discharge, marked eyelid edema, and conjunctival hyperemia. If untreated, GC infection can lead to corneal perforation and blindness. Gram stain demonstrates Gram negative diplococci in GC infections, and intracytoplasmic inclusion bodies in *Chlamydia*. Both types of infections require systemic and topical antibiotics.
- Periorbital cellulitis refers to inflammation of the lids and periorbital tissues without involvement of the orbit

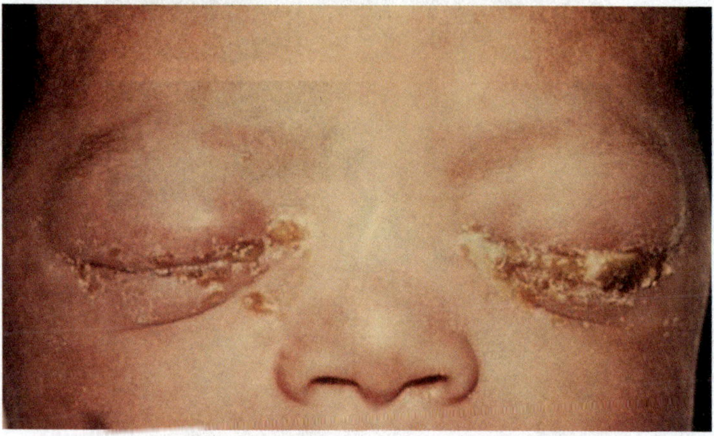

Figure 11-2. This was a newborn with *gonococcal ophthalmia neonatorum* caused by a maternally transmitted gonococcal infection. Unless preventative measures are taken, it is estimated that gonococcal ophthalmia neonatorum will develop in 28% of infants born to women with gonorrhea. It affects the corneal epithelium causing microbial keratitis, ulceration, and perforation.
Reproduced from: Centers for Disease Control and Prevention Public Health Image Library Web site. Photograph courtesy of J Pledger. http://phil.cdc.gov. Accessed September 9, 2010. Image 3766.

itself and may be associated with trauma, wound, or abscess of the lid or periorbital region. *Staphylococcus* and *Streptococcus* species are the most common organisms, and prompt treatment with systemic antibiotics is indicated to prevent development of an orbital abscess, cavernous sinus thrombosis, or meningitis.

- Anterior uveitis (iritis)
  - Uncommon in children; usually follows blunt ocular trauma
  - Symptoms may be photophobia and conjunctival injection (redness)
  - Associated with juvenile idiopathic arthritis
    - May be painless in these patients; perform a baseline examination and periodic screening on all patients
    - Treat with topical antiinflammatory steroids; systemic immune suppressive agents may also be required
  - Associated with sarcoidosis, especially in older children, children of African descent, and those with a positive family history
    - Treat sarcoidosis with intensive topical anti-inflammatory steroids, followed by a tapered dose
    - Patients may require higher doses of oral steroids for a time; severe cases may require long-term topical or oral steroids to prevent rebound inflammation
- Leukocoria (white pupil)
  - Retinoblastoma is a life-threatening malignancy that must be ruled out first in all leukocoria cases
    - May be bilateral
    - May be familial
    - CT scan shows intralesional calcification
  - A cataract is a lens opacity and is visually significant if the visual axis is blocked
    - May be unilateral or bilateral; all bilateral cases require evaluation for infectious, genetic, and metabolic causes
    - Congenital cataracts are present at birth; urgent

removal is indicated. If left untreated by 6–8 weeks of age, irreversible nystagmus and amblyopia may occur. Congenital cataracts are highly associated with subsequent glaucoma

- Infantile cataracts are present within the first year of life; urgent removal is indicated, but there is a lower association with glaucoma
- Acquired cataracts may be associated with trauma, steroid use, or less-common lens defects (posterior lentiglobus or lenticonus; Figure 11-3)
- Amblyopia management is required for many years after cataract removal (until age 8). Unilateral aphakia (absent lens) makes amblyopia more difficult to manage. Patching the better eye for 4–6 hours a day forces vision development in the aphakic eye, and refractive treatment with special aphakic lenses is preferred over unilateral aphakic glasses for better binocularity development. Bilateral aphakia makes amblyopia management less difficult. Aphakic contact lenses or aphakic glasses may be used. Patching is only needed if a disparity in visual acuity is noted

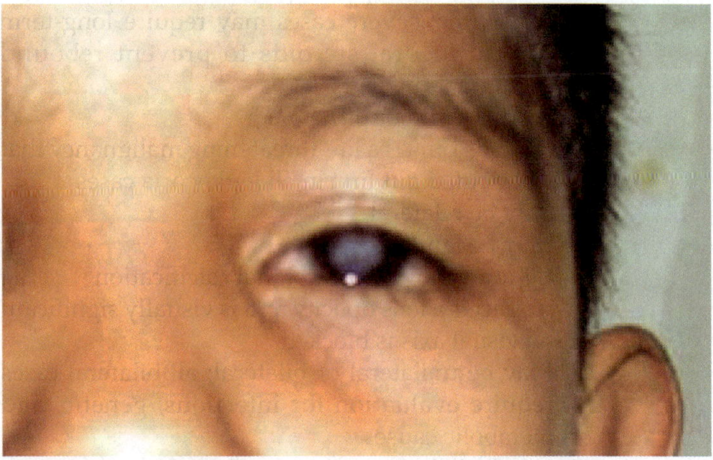

Figure 11-3. Acute traumatic cataract left eye.

      - Following cataract removal, up to a third of all eyes may develop glaucoma by adulthood
      - Pediatric cataracts are best managed by those experienced in their evaluation and treatment
    - Toxocara granuloma (from dog hookworm larvae) is an ocular form of visceral larva migrans characterized by severe local granulomatous inflammation to dead worm larvae
- Retinal disorders
    - ROP: abnormal blood vessel growth with a risk of tractional retinal detachment
      - Associated with prematurity (24–28 wk) and birth weight less than 1,300 g
      - These patients are screened while in the neonatal intensive care unit, and screening is continued until the ROP resolves or the treatment threshold is met
      - Treatment consists of laser photocoagulation of the peripheral avascular retina. Evaluation and treatment of ROP during the acute phases should be performed by ophthalmologists experienced in dealing with this condition
      - Long-term periodic follow-up is required to screen for early onset myopia
    - Nonaccidental trauma or shaken baby syndrome may cause multiple intraretinal and preretinal hemorrhages in the macula, extending to the mid periphery
      - When intraretinal hemorrhages are present, there is often also neurological depression, which may be life threatening
      - Screening examinations are usually requested by the pediatrics service associated with infants or toddlers presenting with injuries inconsistent with their history or with multiple injuries of various chronology
      - Social services and law enforcement officials are required to be notified in all suspected nonaccidental trauma cases. Photo documentation of the retinal findings is becoming the medical–

legal standard for prosecuting the responsible individuals (though this is not usually available in a deployed environment)

- Optic nerve abnormalities
  - A large cup-to-disc ratio is an indicator of possible glaucoma in adults, but the majority of pediatric patients with large cup-to-disc ratios do not have glaucoma. Check the patient's IOP and central corneal thickness (pachymetry), then follow with baseline photos and ocular coherence tomography
  - Papilledema is a sign of increased intracranial pressure characterized by a blurred disc margin, elevated disc, obscuration of vessels, and hemorrhages. It may indicate an intracranial tumor. An immediate CT scan of the brain is indicated, and neurological or neurosurgical evaluation is required
  - Optic nerve coloboma (incomplete closure of embryologic fetal fissure) presents an increased lifetime risk of retinal detachment. Patients with this disorder may also have chorioretinal coloboma at the inferior nasal location. It may be associated with systemic abnormalities or syndromes and requires periodic observation and surgery for retinal detachment (as needed)
- Refractive error
  - Treat a high refractive error (like one of the following) with eyeglasses to prevent or treat amblyopia
    - Symmetric astigmatism > 3 diopters
    - Myopia > 7 diopters
    - Hyperopia > 6 diopters
  - Anisometropia > 1.50 diopters difference requires refractive treatment
  - Mild to moderate levels of myopia do not need treatment; however, school-aged children with this level of myopia will need to wear eyeglasses for good distance vision. Encourage children to remove their glasses for prolonged near tasks
  - Mild to moderate levels of hyperopia do not require

treatment unless there is intermittent esotropia (see strabismus section below); however, school-aged children with mild to moderate hyperopia may need glasses for prolonged near work

- Strabismus is defined as an eye misalignment of any type and is the most common reason for pediatric eye surgery
  - Comitant strabismus is an ocular misalignment in which there is a similar quantitative deviation in all directions of gaze
  - Congenital esotropia is the most common strabismus. There is usually a large angle of deviation, but not amblyopia because of cross-fixation (spontaneous alternation of eyes). Treat with strabismus surgery (bilateral medial rectus recessions) around 5–7 months of age, if possible
  - Accommodative esotropia is associated with hyperopia
    - Onset is around 1½–4 years of age and is usually initially intermittent
    - Child may have greater esodeviation on near sight and a high ratio of accommodative convergence to accommodation
    - Patient may develop amblyopia quickly in the nondominant (esodeviating) eye
    - Treat with "plus power" eyeglasses; initially give less than full cycloplegic refraction, but if esodeviation is not corrected, full cycloplegic refraction may need to be prescribed
    - Patients with a high ratio of accommodative convergence to accommodation require bifocals; the bifocal segment must be 1 mm below the visual axis. Surgery is reserved for patients with residual esodeviations while in full cycloplegic refraction. Use bilateral medial rectus recessions (preferred) or unilateral medial rectus recession and lateral rectus resection (recess-resect procedure)
  - Intermittent exotropia often manifests when an individual is inattentive, fatigued, or has taken substances that decrease state of alertness

    - Highly variable age of onset
    - Individuals typically have excellent control of ocular alignment at near distances, only exhibiting exophoria
    - Vision is usually normal in each eye
    - Stereopsis is usually normal
    - Up to a third of patients may improve with accommodative exercises, and daily alternate-eye patching may improve some cases
    - Patients not responding to the above measures may be treated with strabismus surgery (bilateral lateral rectus recessions)
  - Consecutive strabismus is a deviation that occurs months to years after strabismus surgery, usually in the opposite direction of the initial surgery (typically exotropia after surgery for esotropia). Treat with bilateral recessions of the lateral rectus muscles (for exotropia) or medial rectus muscles (for esotropia)
  - Noncomitant strabismus is a condition in which ocular misalignment varies according to the direction of the patient's gaze
  - Superior oblique, or trochlear, palsy (cranial nerve 6 palsy) usually presents with a head tilt away from the affected side. Longstanding cases often present with intermittent diplopia (rare in children). The patient may have facial asymmetry with contralateral facial hypoplasia. Treat with strabismus surgery. The most common procedure is to weaken the ipsilateral inferior oblique muscle either by recession or myectomy; the next most common is a tuck (shortening) of the affected superior oblique tendon
- Other conditions associated with strabismus
  - Duane syndrome
  - Brown's syndrome
  - Monocular elevation deficiency
- Ocular manifestations of systemic disease
  - Aniridia: Wilms tumor
  - Blue sclera: osteogenesis imperfecta
  - Kayser-Fleischer corneal ring: Wilson disease

        - Congenital cataracts: intrauterine infection
        - Leukocoria (white reflex in the pupil): retinoblastoma
        - Retinal hemorrhages with white centers (Roth spots): subacute bacterial endocarditis
        - Chorioretinitis: toxoplasmosis, histoplasmosis, cytomegalovirus, tuberculosis, syphilis

Eye Injuries

- General guidance for pediatric eye injuries
    - The examiner must have high index of suspicion; patients may not self-report because they are too young or fear reprisal for having participated in unapproved behavior that resulted in the injury. These injuries are not frequently witnessed by adults and may only be suspected after a delay
    - Physical symptoms
        - Reluctance to open an eye
        - Reported or observed redness of an eye
        - Photophobia
        - Excessive tear production
        - Pain
    - Vision examination
        - Carefully measure vision (patient's reaction to light, distance at which patient can count fingers, etc)
        - Use any printed material (books, medication labels, etc) if a vision-screening card is not available
        - Compare sight in the injured eye to that in the uninjured eye
        - Severe vision loss is a strong indicator of serious injury
        - If there is a lid laceration, suspect and carefully check for signs of possible underlying globe laceration; examine the eyes prior to lid repair
- Ruptures and lacerations (open globe)
    - These may result from penetrating or blunt eye trauma and may cause vision loss from either disruption of ocular structures or secondary infection (endophthalmitis)
    - Signs
        - Hemorrhagic chemosis (elevation of the conjunctiva from the sclera by dense bleeding)

        - Hyphema (blood in the anterior chamber); if complete, an "eight ball" hyphema is present (may also be present in severe blunt trauma)
        - Disrupted anterior chamber architecture
            - Irregular or teardrop pupil shape (peaked pupil)
            - Dark iris or uveal tissue protruding through cornea
        - If there are signs of fragmentation injury (by either primary or secondary missiles) to the head, neck, or face, intraocular foreign bodies may be present
        - Proptosis may indicate a retrobulbar hemorrhage; urgent lateral canthotomy and cantholysis may be indicated
        - Decreased motility of one eye may be a sign of an open globe; other causes of limited motility include muscle injury, orbital fracture, and orbital hemorrhage
    - Initial treatment of an open globe injury: in a casualty with severe vision loss, biplanar radiographs or a CT scan of the head may help identify a metallic intraocular fragment, a traumatic hyphema, a large subconjunctival hemorrhage, or other signs of an open globe injury with an intraocular foreign body
    - Immediate treatment of an open globe injury
        - Tape a rigid eye shield (**not** a pressure patch) over the eye
        - Do not apply pressure to or manipulate the eye
        - Do not apply any topical medications
        - Start quinolone antibiotic (oral or intravenous [IV]; dose for patient weight)
        - Schedule an urgent (within 12–24 h) referral to an ophthalmologist
        - Administer tetanus toxoid, if indicated
        - Use antiemetics (dose for patient weight)
        - Patient can expect surgical exploration and globe repair under general anesthesia by the initial ophthalmologist; further procedures may be required later
- Subconjunctival hemorrhage (SCH)
    - Small SCHs may occur spontaneously or in association with blunt trauma; these lesions require no treatment and resolve in days to weeks

  - SCH may also occur in association with a rupture of the underlying sclera
  - Warning signs for an open globe include a large SCH with chemosis (conjunctiva bulging away from globe) in the setting of blunt trauma, or any SCH in the setting of penetrating injury. Casualties with blast injury and normal vision do not require special immediate ophthalmologic care, but should get a complete ophthalmic examination at the earliest opportunity. Suspected open globe patients should be treated as described above (see Ruptures and lacerations)
- Chemical injuries of the cornea
  - Initiate immediate copious irrigation (maintain for 30 min) with normal saline, lactated Ringer's, or balanced salt solution (nonsterile water may be used if it is the only liquid available); use topical anesthesia before irrigating, if available
  - Measure tear pH to ensure that irrigation continues until the pH returns to normal (7.35–7.45); **Do not use** alkaline solutions to neutralize acidity (or vice versa)
  - Remove any retained particles
  - Using fluorescein strips or drops, examine for epithelial defects
    - If none are found, treat mild chemical injuries or foreign bodies with artificial tears
    - If an epithelial defect is present, use a broad-spectrum antibiotic ophthalmic ointment (bacitracin / polymyxin, erythromycin, or bacitracin) 3–4 times per day (same dosing as for adults)
  - Apply a pressure patch between drops of ointment if a large epithelial defect is present
  - Monitor (via daily topical fluorescein evaluation) for a corneal epithelial defect until epithelial healing is complete (as determined by a negative fluorescein evaluation)
  - Noncaustic chemical injuries usually resolve without sequelae
  - Severe acid or alkali injuries of the eye (recognized by pronounced chemosis, limbal blanching, or corneal opacification) can lead to infection of the cornea,

glaucoma, and possible loss of the eye. Refer patient to an ophthalmologist within 24–48 hours. These more severe chemical injuries may also require treatment with prednisolone 1% drops 4–9 times per day, and scopolamine 0.25% drops 2–4 times per day (these should only be started on the direction of an ophthalmologist)

- Corneal abrasions
  - Be alert for the possibility of an associated open globe injury
  - The eye is usually symptomatic with pain, tearing, and photophobia; vision may be diminished from the abrasion itself or from the profuse tearing
  - Diagnose with topical fluorescein and cobalt blue light or Wood's lamp (if available)
  - A topical anesthetic may be used for diagnosis, but should **not** be used as an ongoing analgesic agent (this delays healing and may cause other severe complications)
  - Apply broad-spectrum antibiotic ointment (polymixin B, erythromycin, or bacitracin) 4 times a day
  - Pain relief options include:
    - Pressure patch (usually sufficient for most abrasions)
    - Diclofenac 0.1% drops 4 times a day
    - Larger abrasions may require a short-acting cycloplegic agent (1% tropicamide or 1% cyclopentolate) and a pressure patch
    - More severe discomfort can be treated with 0.25% scopolamine (1 drop bid), but this will result in pupil dilation and blurred vision for 5–6 days
  - Small abrasions usually heal well in 1–4 days without patching; if the eye is not patched, antibiotic drops (fluoroquinolone or aminoglycoside) may be used 4 times a day in lieu of ointment. Sunglasses are helpful in reducing photophobia
  - All corneal abrasions need to be checked once a day until healing is complete to ensure the abrasion has not been complicated by secondary infection (eg, corneal ulcer, bacterial keratitis)
- Thermal burns of the cornea are initially treated in the same manner as corneal abrasions

- Laser-induced injuries usually involve the retina, which is the tissue most vulnerable. Degree of injury will depend on the duration of exposure and amount of energy delivered. A reduction in visual acuity, tearing and pain are the main symptoms of laser injury. Nonpenetrating corneal injuries (anterior segment) should be treated as for corneal abrasions. Injury involving the posterior segment should be referred to an ophthalmologist as soon as possible
- Corneal ulcer and bacterial keratitis
  - Corneal ulcer and bacteria keratitis are serious conditions that may cause vision or eye loss
  - These conditions are associated with soft-contact lens wear, especially if contacts are not taken out prior to sleep
  - Symptoms include increasing pain and redness, decreasing vision, persistent or increasing epithelial defect (positive fluorescein test), and a white or gray spot on the cornea (seen on examination with penlight or direct ophthalmoscope)
  - Treatment includes quinolone drops (1 drop every 5 min for 5 doses initially, then 1 drop every 30 min for 6 h, then 1 drop hourly thereafter)
    - Scopolamine 0.25% (1 drop bid) may help relieve discomfort caused by pupillary spasm; patching and use of topical anesthetics for pain control are contraindicated
    - Expedite referral to an ophthalmologist (within 1–2 days)
- Conjunctival and corneal foreign bodies
  - These present with abrupt onset of discomfort or history of suspected foreign body
  - If an open globe injury is suspected, treat as discussed above
  - Definitive diagnosis requires visualization of the offending object, which may be difficult; a hand-held magnifying lens or pair of reading glasses will help
    - Stain the eye with fluorescein to check for a corneal abrasion
    - The patient may be able to indicate the perceived location of the foreign body prior to instillation of topical anesthesia

- Eyelid eversion with a cotton-tipped applicator helps the examiner identify foreign bodies located on the upper tarsal plate
- Treatment
  - Superficial conjunctival or corneal foreign bodies may be irrigated away or removed with a moistened sterile swab under topical anesthesia
  - Objects adhering to the cornea may be removed with a spud or the edge of a sterile 22-gauge hypodermic needle mounted on a tuberculin syringe (hold the needle tangential to the eye)
  - If no foreign body is visualized but the index of suspicion is high, the foreign body may be removed by vigorous irrigation with artificial tears or sweeps of the conjunctival fornices with a moistened, cotton-tipped applicator (after applying topical anesthesia)
  - If an epithelial defect is present after the foreign body is removed, treat as a corneal abrasion (see page 112)

- Hyphema (blood in the anterior chamber)
  - Treat to prevent vision loss from increased intraocular pressure or corneal blood-staining
  - Suspect a possible open globe and treat appropriately
  - A major goal of management is to avoid rebleeding
    - Avoid aspirin and nonsteroidal antiinflammatory drugs
    - Limit activity (require bed rest, with the patient only getting up to use the bathroom) for 7–10 days
  - Administer prednisolone 1% drops 4 times a day, and scopolamine 0.25% drops twice daily
  - Cover the eye with a protective shield
  - Elevate the head of the bed to promote settling of red blood cells in the anterior chamber (Figure 11-4)
  - Patient should be seen by an ophthalmologist within 24–48 hours to monitor for increased intraocular pressure (which may cause permanent injury to the optic nerve or corneal blood-staining and secondary deprivation amblyopia) and to evaluate for associated eye injuries. If evaluation by an ophthalmologist is delayed (> 24 h), treat with a topical β-blocker (timolol or levobunolol) twice a day

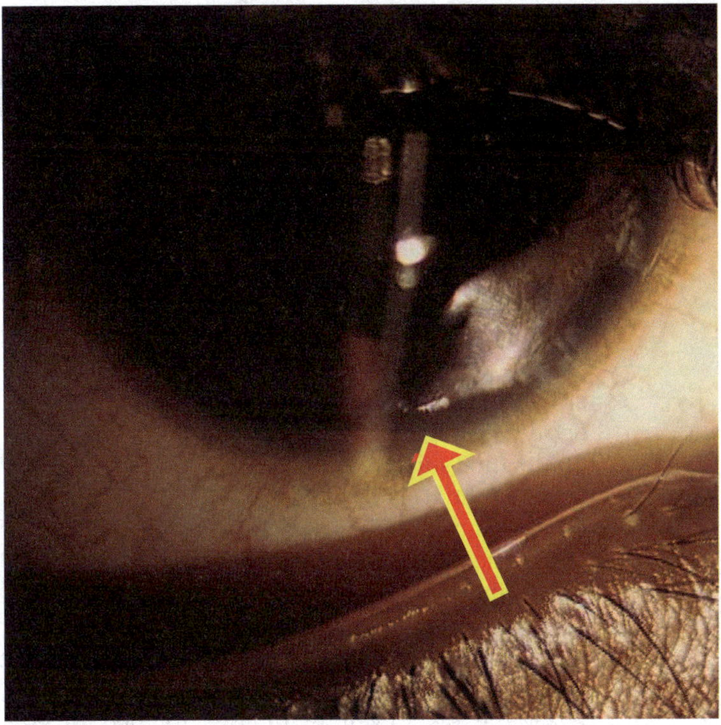

Figure 11-4. Blood aqueous level (arrow) indicates 5% hyphema.

to help prevent intraocular pressure elevation

- If intraocular pressure is found to be markedly elevated (above 30 mmHg) with a portable tonometry device, other options for lowering intraocular pressure include administering acetazolamide (oral or IV) or mannitol (IV), dosed for the patient's weight

- Retrobulbar (orbital) hemorrhage
  - Symptoms include severe eye pain, proptosis, vision loss, and decreased eye movement
  - Marked lid edema may make the proptosis difficult to recognize
  - Failure to recognize may result in blindness from increased ocular pressure
  - Treatment

- Perform an immediate lateral canthotomy and inferior cantholysis
- Provide an urgent referral to an ophthalmologist (within 6–12 h)
  - If evaluation by an ophthalmologist is delayed (> 24 h), treat with a topical β-blocker (timolol) twice a day to help lower intraocular pressure elevation
  - If intraocular pressure is found to be elevated (> 30 mmHg), follow first two steps under Treatment (see page 114)
- Lateral canthotomy and cantholysis
  - Do not perform these procedures if the eyeball structure has been violated; if the globe is open, apply a Fox shield for protection and seek immediate ophthalmic surgical support
  - Inject 2% lidocaine with 1:100,000 epinephrine into the lateral canthus
  - Crush the lateral canthus with a straight hemostat, advancing the jaws to the lateral fornix
  - Using straight scissors make a 1-cm long horizontal incision of the lateral canthal tendon, in the middle of the crush mark
  - Grasp the lower eyelid with large, toothed forceps, pulling the eyelid away from the face; this pulls the inferior crus (band of the lateral canthal tendon) tight so it can be easily cut loose from the orbital rim
  - Use blunt-tipped scissors to cut the inferior crus; keep the scissors parallel (flat) to the face with the tips pointing toward the chin
  - Place the inner blade just anterior to the conjunctiva, and the outer blade just deep to the skin; the eyelid should pull freely away from the face, releasing pressure on the globe
  - Cut residual lateral attachments of the lower eyelid if it does not move freely (cutting ½ cm of conjunctiva or skin is not cause for alarm)
  - Once the lower eyelid is cut, relieving orbital pressure, if the intact cornea is exposed, apply copious erythromycin ophthalmic ointment or ophthalmic lubricant ointment hourly to prevent devastating

corneal desiccation and infection. Orbital pressure relief must be followed by lubricating protection of the cornea and urgent ophthalmic surgical support. **Do not** apply absorbent gauze dressings to the exposed cornea

- Orbital floor (blowout) fractures
  - These fractures are usually the result of a blunt injury to the globe or orbital rim and may be associated with head and spine injuries
  - Blowout fractures may be suspected on the basis of enophthalmos, diplopia, decreased ocular motility, hypoesthesia of the V2 branch of the trigeminal nerve, associated subconjunctival hemorrhage, or hyphema
  - Immediate treatment includes administering broad-spectrum antibiotics for 7 days, applying ice packs, and instructing the casualty to avoid nose blowing
  - Definitive diagnosis requires a CT scan of the orbits with axial and coronal views
  - Indications for repair include severe enophthalmos and diplopia in the primary or reading-gaze positions. The surgery may be performed 1–2 weeks after the injury, but may have greater success in children if it is performed as soon as possible in trapdoor-style blowout fractures
  - Patients with an orbital floor (blow-out) fracture often have a limited (restricted) up gaze on the affected side and may also have a restricted down gaze on the affected side. Early surgical intervention may be indicated, especially if there is a trapdoor fracture that results in entrapment of the inferior rectus on the effected side. Strabismus surgery is reserved for patients with diplopia in the primary gaze (straight ahead) or in the reading position (moderate down gaze)
- Lid lacerations
  - Treatment for lid lacerations not involving the lid margin
    - Delayed primary closure is not necessary when there is adequate blood supply
    - Eyelid function (protecting the globe) is the primary consideration
    - Begin with irrigation and antisepsis (using any topical solution), and check for retained foreign bodies
    - Superficial lacerations of the eyelid that do not involve

the eyelid margin may be closed with running or interrupted 6-0 silk (preferred) or nylon sutures
- Horizontal lacerations should include the orbicularis muscle and skin in the repair
- If skin is missing, an advancement flap may be created to fill in the defect. For vertical or stellate lacerations, use traction sutures in the eyelid margin for 7–10 days
- Apply antibiotic ointments 4 times a day until sutures are removed
- Skin sutures may be removed in 5 days

- Treatment guidelines for lid lacerations involving the lid margin
  - Tissue loss greater than 25% will require a flap or graft
  - When repairing a marginal lower-eyelid laceration with less than 25% tissue loss, the irregular laceration edges may be freshened by creating a pentagonal wedge. Remove as little tissue as possible
  - Place a 4-0 silk or nylon suture in the eyelid margin (through the meibomian gland orifices, 2 mm from the wound edges and 2 mm deep) and tie it in a slipknot; symmetric suture placement is critical to obtaining post-operative eyelid margin alignment
  - Loosen the slipknot and place two or three absorbable 5-0 or 6-0 sutures internally to approximate the tarsal plate; the skin and conjunctiva should not be included in this internal closure
  - Place anterior and posterior marginal sutures (6-0 silk or nylon) in the eyelid margin just in front and behind the previously placed 4-0 suture
  - Leave the middle and posterior sutures long and tie them under the anterior suture; ensure that the wound edges are everted
  - Close the skin with 6-0 silk or nylon sutures and place the lid on traction for at least 5 days
  - Remove the skin sutures at 3–5 days, and the marginal sutures at 10–14 days
  - If there is orbital fat in the wound or if ptosis is noted in an upper lid laceration, damage to the orbital septum

and the levator aponeurosis should be suspected

- If the eyelid is avulsed, the missing tissue should be retrieved, wrapped in a moistened, nonadherent dressing, and preserved on ice. The tissue should be soaked in a dilute antibiotic solution prior to reattachment. If necrosis is present, minimal debridement should occur to prevent further tissue loss. The avulsed tissue should be secured in the anatomically correct position in the manner described for lid margin repair above
- Damage to the canalicular system can occur as a result of injuries to the medial aspect of the lid margins
  - Suspected canalicular injuries should be repaired by an ophthalmologist to prevent subsequent problems with tear drainage
  - This repair can be delayed for up to 24 hours

- Enucleation
  - A general surgeon in a forward unit should not remove a traumatized eye unless the globe is completely disorganized. Enucleation should only be considered if the patient has a very severe injury, exhibits no light perception when the provider uses the brightest light source available, and is not able to be evacuated to a facility with an ophthalmologist. Sympathetic ophthalmia is a condition that may result in loss of vision in the uninjured eye if a severely traumatized, blind eye is not removed, but it rarely develops prior to 14 days after an injury; thus, delaying the enucleation until the patient can see an ophthalmologist is relatively safe and advisable

Chapter 12

Dentistry

Caries

- Dental caries is a transmissible infectious disease
    - Transmitted vertically (caregiver to child)
    - The most prevalent chronic infectious disease of childhood
- Early childhood caries is defined as decay that occurs within the first 71 months of life
    - The American Academy of Pediatric Dentistry and the American Academy of Pediatrics recommend that a child's first dental visit occur upon eruption of the first tooth and no later than 12 months of age (Figure 12-1)

Upper Teeth	Primary Erupt	Permanent Erupt
Central incisor	8–12 mo	7–8 y
Lateral incisor	9–13 mo	8–9 y
Canine (cuspid)	16–22 mo	11–12 y
First premolar		10–11 y
Second premolar		10–12 y
First molar	13–19 mo	6–7 y
Second molar	25–33 mo	12–13 y
Third molar		17–21 y
Lower Teeth		
Third molar		17–21 y
Second molar	23–31 mo	11–13 y
First molar	14–18 mo	6–7 y
Second premolar		11–12 y
First premolar		10–12 y
Canine (cuspid)	17–23 mo	9–10 y
Lateral incisor	10–16 mo	7–8 y
Central incisor	6–10 mo	6–7 y

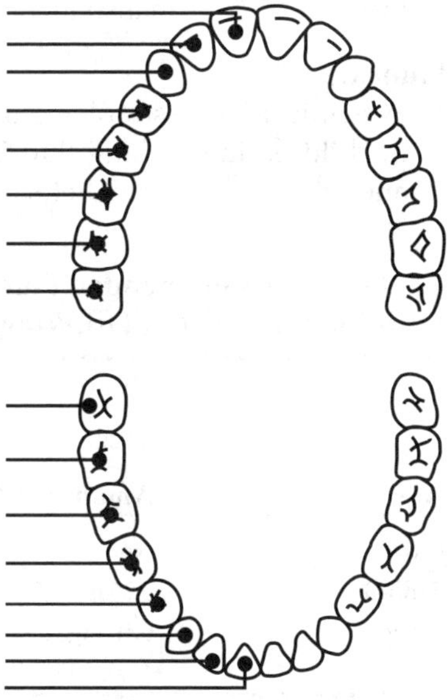

Figure 12-1. Diagram of tooth eruption sequence by age.

- There is wide variance in the eruption age of primary and permanent teeth; however, primary teeth usually erupt between 6 months and 2½ years, with the mandibular incisors erupting first. Permanent mandibular incisors erupt around 6 years of age, and permanent teeth continue until eruption of the third molars between 17 and 21 years of age
- In the past, tooth decay was primarily associated with industrialized countries and diets high in processed sugar. However, the availability of processed sugar in developing countries is on the rise, with a concomitant increase in the incidence of dental caries. This is a particular problem in developing countries because access to dental care is extremely limited and costly. Using bottles and "sippy" cups with juice or milk for long periods of time can put children at high risk for caries, especially in the maxillary anterior teeth. This is particularly true if children are given the bottles or cups when they are put in bed and allowed to fall asleep while holding them in their mouths. Frequent consumption of snacks and drinks containing fermentable carbohydrates (eg, juice, milk, formula, soda) can also increase a child's caries risk

Fluoride

- Systemic fluoride supplementation should **only** be considered in children in drinking fluoride-deficient water (< 0.6 ppm) and when a complete dietary history is available (Table 12-1)

Table 12-1. Recommended Fluoride Dosages According to Fluoride Ion Level in Drinking Water

	Fluoride Ion Level in Drinking Water (ppm*)		
	< 0.3	0.3–0.6	> 0.6
Age	**Amount of Fluoride to Prescribe**		
0–6 mo	None	None	None
6 mo–3 y	0.25 mg/day†	None	None
3–6 y	0.50 mg/day	0.25 mg/day	None
6–16 y	1 mg/day	0.50 mg/day	None

*1 ppm = 1 mg/L.
†2.2 mg sodium fluoride contains 1 mg fluoride ion.

- Many areas with well water have natural fluoride
- Well water must be tested prior to prescribing fluoride supplementation
- The lethal dose of fluoride is 30–36 mg/kg in a single dose. The probable toxic single dose of fluoride is 5–10 mg/kg of body weight. Toxicity begins with gastric signs and symptoms
- Over-the-counter toothpaste has approximately 1 mg of fluoride per 1 inch

- Improper fluoride supplementation often leads to fluorosis of permanent teeth, which makes them more prone to dental decay
- Professional applications of fluoride, especially in high-concentration varnishes, have proven safe and effective for reducing dental decay

Toothache

- Toothaches are most frequently caused by dental caries or trauma
  - If dental caries involves the inner pulp of the tooth, the infection may progress to an irreversible pulpitis or abscess and may require tooth extraction
  - If dental caries does not directly involve the tooth's inner pulp (reversible pulpitis), it may be treated by debridement of the decay and placement of intermediate restorative material (IRM)
  - Temporary toothache pain caused by hot or cold stimuli is an indication of reversible pulpitis amenable to treatment with IRM; spontaneous, severe toothache of longer duration or severe pain that wakes the patient up at night are signs of irreversible pulpitis requiring tooth extraction if follow-up root canal care is unavailable
- Emergency treatment of dental caries and reversible pulpitis is as follows:
  - Gently remove as much visible decay as possible
  - Mix and place IRM, which contains eugenol to reduce pain, into the cavity
  - For severe deep caries with associated pain that obviously extends to the inner pulp, extract the tooth

- Local anesthetic for palliative care of toothache pain (also for extraction; see "Extraction Basics") is as follows:
  - 2% lidocaine with or without 1:100,000 epinephrine; maximum dose 4.4 mg/kg
  - 0.5% bupivacaine for long-acting local anesthesia; maximum dose 1.3 mg/kg
  - Use either local infiltration (Figure 12-2) or inferior alveolar nerve block
  - Always aspirate before injecting
  - Posttreatment, self-inflicted lip and tongue trauma are common from a child sucking or chewing on an anesthetized lip or tongue; posttreatment observation of the anesthetized child is required

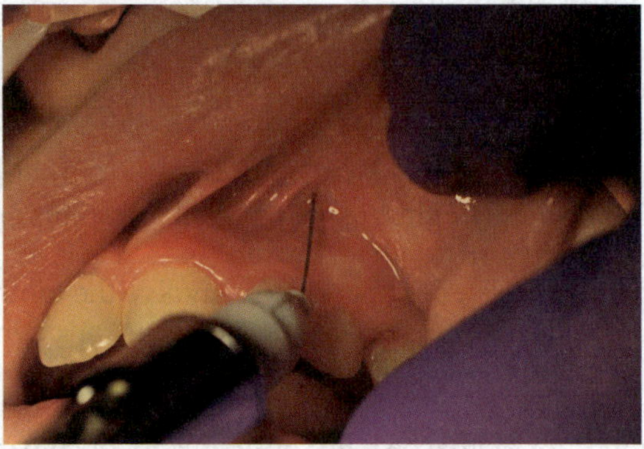

Figure 12-2. Local infiltration anesthesia.

Dental Abscess

- Abscesses may be localized or involve facial spaces
- Definitive treatment consists of extracting the offending tooth
- If the tooth cannot be extracted and intraoral swelling is present, use an 18-gauge needle and syringe to aspirate purulent material or incise and drain with a #15 scalpel
- Antibiotics are usually not indicated after extracting a primary tooth with localized swelling because the source of the infection is no longer present. For larger, diffuse swelling or cellulitis, antibiotics can be prescribed as follows:

  - Mild to moderate infection: clindamycin (10 mg/kg/day) orally every 6 hours for 7 days; amoxicillin (50 mg/kg/day) orally every 6 hours for 7 days
  - Severe infection: clindamycin (20 mg/kg/day) intravenous (IV) every 6 hours for 7 days
- Hospitalization is indicated for severe trismus, dehydration, descending neck infection, inability to protrude tongue, and swelling involving the eye orbit

Extraction Basics

- Indications for extraction include severe tooth pain, abscess, severe periodontal (gum) disease, and traumatic injuries
- Anterior teeth have single roots, premolars have one or two roots. Maxillary molars usually have three roots, mandibular usually have two
- Technique:
  - If possible, take a radiograph to look for multiple roots or root fracture
  - Anesthetize the area
  - Use a 301 Apexo elevator (Hu-Friedy, Chicago, Ill) to loosen the selected tooth (Figure 12-3)
  - Firmly grasp the tooth with the forceps beak under the gingival margin. For anterior teeth, use a screwdriver-type

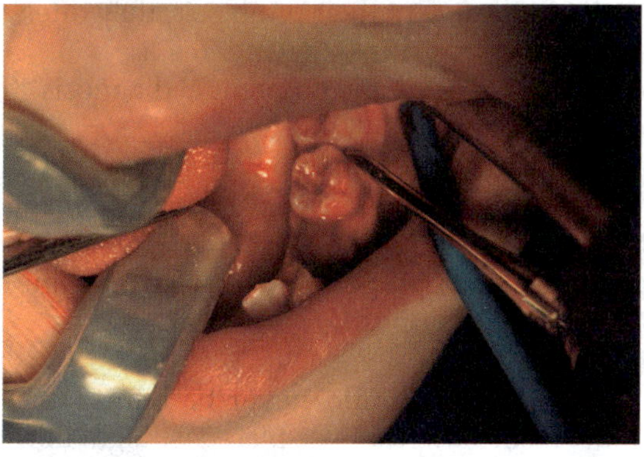

Figure 12-3. A 301 elevator may be used to loosen selected tooth.

(rotating) motion to extract the tooth; for posterior teeth (premolars and molars), with a firm grasp, roll the forceps in a facial direction to extract the tooth (Figure 12-4)

- If a root fractures during extraction, leave it in place if it cannot be easily removed

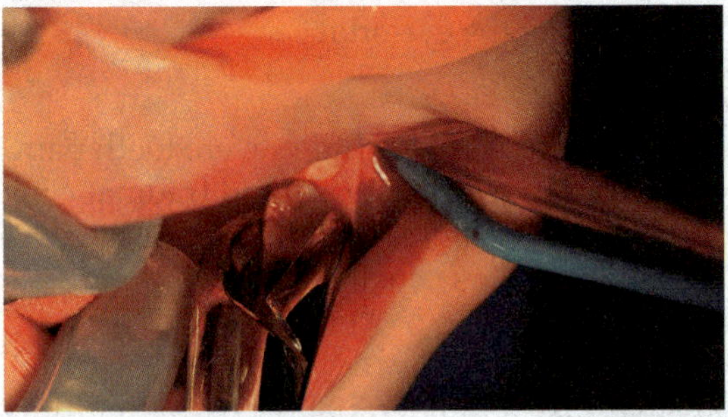

Figure 12-4. Roll the forceps in a facial direction to extract tooth.

Trauma

- Check tetanus status. Neurological examination is required if there is trauma to the head or face
- Primary teeth may darken when traumatized, but this is not necessarily indicative of their prognosis; they often return to their original color within 6 to 9 months
- Include abuse as part of the differential diagnosis
- **Fractured tooth**
  - Enamel fracture only: smooth with file
  - Enamel and dentin fracture: apply protective filling material (IRM or dental composite)
  - Fracture to tooth pulp: apply protective filling material (IRM or dental composite)
- **Avulsed tooth**
  - A primary tooth should never be reimplanted. When primary teeth are apically displaced (straight down into the tooth socket) from trauma, they often reerupt in the correct position; primary teeth displaced other than apically will not reerupt in the correct position

- Reimplant a permanent tooth within 2 hours of the incident. Avulsed permanent teeth reimplanted within the first hour have a greater chance of a successful outcome; after that the chance of complication increases. Because of the high likelihood that extensive treatment (eg, root canal) will be needed following reimplantation, permanent teeth should only be reimplanted if the patient has access to good follow-up care
- Reimplantation technique:
  - Do not scrub the tooth; lightly rinse it with saline to remove debris
  - Store the tooth in milk or balanced saline solution if reimplantation will be delayed
  - Radiograph the area if possible
  - Reimplant the tooth as soon as possible
  - Stabilize the reimplanted tooth with flexible wire (0.018 inch) for 1 week. The wire can be bonded with composite dental material to the adjacent teeth and the injured tooth
  - Check the occlusion of reimplanted teeth with opposing arch (ensure reimplanted teeth do not interfere when the patient bites teeth together)
  - Prescribe antibiotics for 7 to 10 days following a traumatic avulsion (Figures 12-5–12-8)

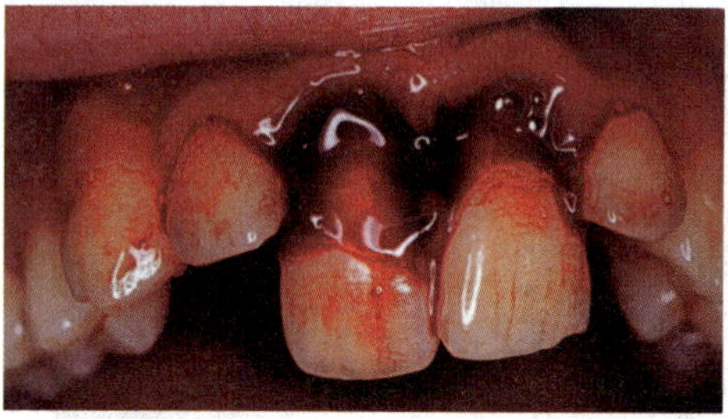

Figure 12-5. Severely displaced maxillary incisors.

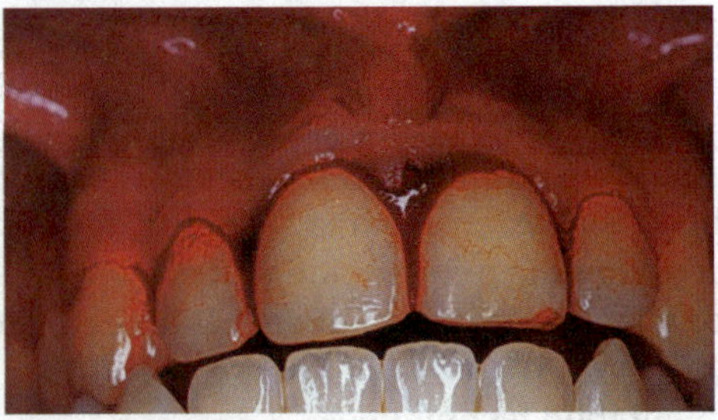

Figure 12-6. Repositioned maxillary incisors (always check occlusion with mandibular teeth).

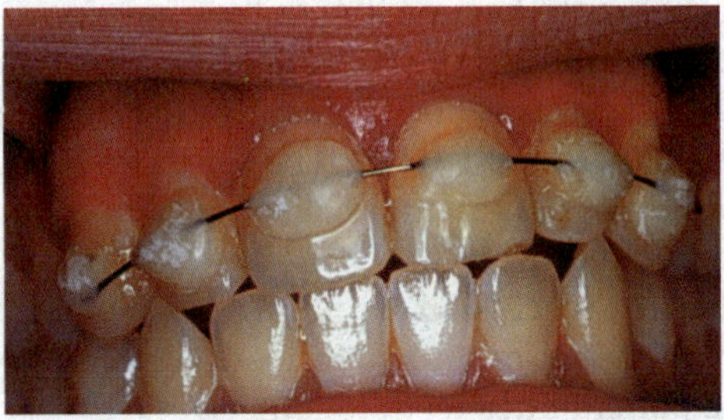

Figure 12-7. Splint made of flexible orthodontic wire (0.018 inch) bonded with composite.

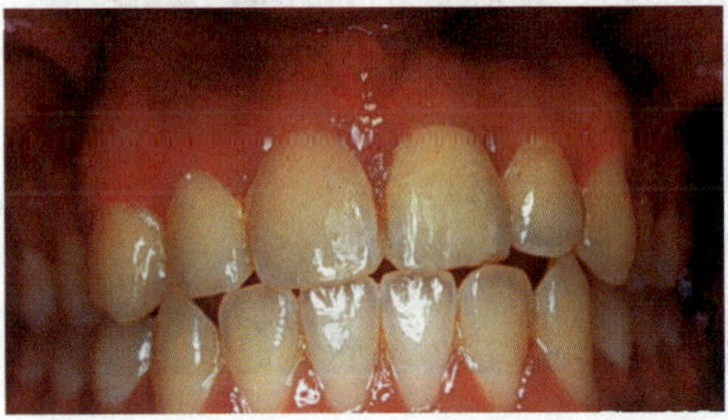

Figure 12-8. Maxillary incisors after splint removal.

Oral Pathology

- **Primary herpetic gingivostomatitis** (Figures 12-9 and 12-10)

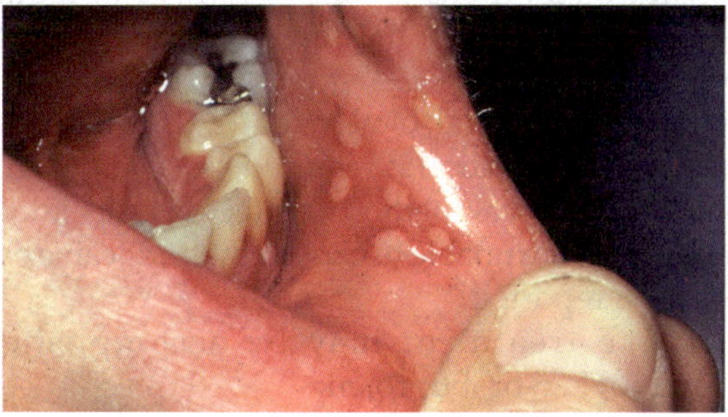

Figure 12-9. Primary herpetic gingivostomatitis on inner surface of cheek.
Photograph courtesy of Harvey P Kessler, DDS, MS, Baylor College of Dentistry.

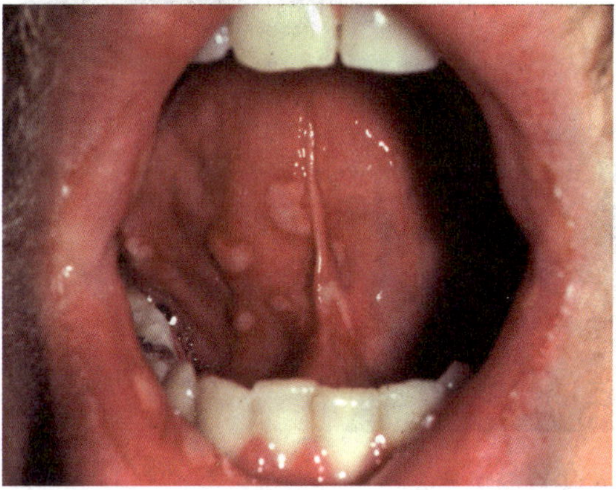

Figure 12-10. Primary herpetic gingivostomatitis on ventral surface of tongue.
Photograph courtesy of Harvey P Kessler, DDS, MS, Baylor College of Dentistry.

- Manifests with multiple vesicles or ulcers on lips, gingiva, and palate
- Patient is febrile, often dehydrated, irritable, and lethargic
- Antiviral medications are only effective in reducing the duration of infection if they are given within the first few days of the outbreak
- Hydration is essential. Oral hydration is usually sufficient; however, IV hydration is required for severe infections
- Do not give topical medications (eg, viscous lidocaine) to patients who are unable to expectorate; lidocaine overdoses have been reported
- Palliative treatment may be accomplished with acetaminophen or ibuprofen
- Continue implementing oral hygiene practices as much as possible

• **Aphthous ulcers** (Figure 12-11)

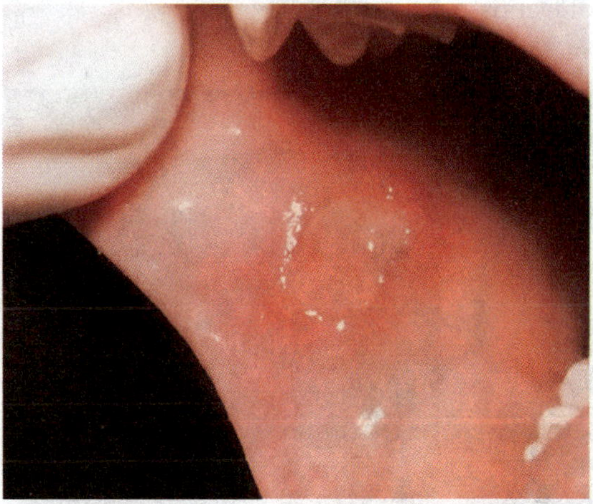

Figure 12-11. Aphthous ulcer.

- Painful oral lesions located on unattached oral mucosa; red halos with pale centers that occur in fewer numbers than with herpetic gingivostomatitis
- Causes include allergic or immunological response or

streptococci infection
  - Treatment is palliative. Lesions usually disappear in 10 to 14 days without treatment
  - For pain, administer benzocaine topical dressing twice daily or chlorhexidine gluconate 0.12% oral mouth rinse twice daily. Amoxicillin may be used for very large, painful lesions (50 mg/kg/day for 10 days)
- **Neonatal sublingual traumatic ulceration**
  - Ulceration on ventral portion of tongue caused by the lower incisors
  - Often seen with natal or neonatal teeth in the first several months of life
  - Can cause pain and limit an infant's breast-feeding and nutrition intake
  - Treatment: extract tooth or smooth edges of offending tooth
- **Pyogenic granuloma**
  - Localized mass, sometimes on gingiva, associated with traumatic irritation from calculus deposits
  - Treatment: remove calculus; lesion will disappear with the removal of the cause
- **Other pathology**
  - In addition, noma—an opportunistic, rapidly spreading oral infection related to poor hygiene and patients who are immunocompromised—and oral manifestations of human immunodeficiency virus and autoimmune deficiency disorder are more prevalent in developing than industrialized countries

Chapter 13

Face and Neck

Disorders of the Upper Airway

- Choanal atresia
  - Congenital obstruction of the posterior nasal choana
  - Can be bony or membranous
  - Involvement
    - Unilateral: mild respiratory symptoms
    - Bilateral: intermittent respiratory distress in infants (obligate nasal breathers)
  - Diagnosis
    - Inability to pass a nasal catheter into the pharynx
    - Use computed tomography (CT) scan
    - Perform direct nasopharyngoscopy
  - Initial management
    - Insert an oropharyngeal airway
    - Administer orogastric tube feeds
- Intraoral obstruction
  - Mandibular hypoplasia (micrognathia)
    - Associated with Pierre Robin syndrome and Treacher Collins syndrome
    - A normal-sized tongue falls posteriorly, obstructing the supraglottic airway
    - Treatment: placing patient in a prone position is usually all that is required; nasopharyngeal tube is rarely needed
    - The mandible grows faster in children, so by 3 months of age, the condition is usually resolved
  - Macroglossia
    - Associated with Beckwith-Wiedemann syndrome
    - Treatment
      - Place patient in the prone position to keep tongue forward
      - Tracheostomy and gastrostomy tube may be necessary

- Intraoral neoplasms
  - Types: lymphangiomas, teratomas, aberrant thyroids, rhabdomyosarcomas
  - Treatment approaches vary
- Laryngeal obstructions
  - Malformations
    - Laryngomalacia: anatomic malformation of the supraglottic larynx, resulting in collapse of supraglottic structures on inspiration (the vocal cords, subglottic larynx, and trachea are normal)
      - This is the most common obstructing lesion of the infant airway
      - Symptoms include inspiratory stridor, but not cyanosis
      - May not be present for days to weeks
      - Worsens with agitation and supine positioning
      - Milder when patient is in prone position with neck extended
      - Diagnose with lateral neck radiograph or direct laryngoscopy (will reveal Ω-shaped epiglottis)
      - Treatment is usually nonsurgical; place infant in prone position with neck extended
      - Temporary tracheotomy may be required for severe symptoms
      - Symptoms will resolve by 2 or 3 years of age
    - Clefts: incomplete separation of trachea and esophagus, associated with esophageal atresia
      - Symptoms: respiratory distress, cyanosis, and aspiration pneumonia
      - Diagnosis: endoscopy
      - Treatment: endotracheal (ET) intubation and gastrostomy tube, later surgical reconstruction
    - Webs: thin, membranous, obstructing diaphragms usually located at the glottic level
      - Symptoms: airway obstruction at birth
      - Diagnosis: laryngoscopy
      - Treatment: endoscopic excision
    - Atresia: requires immediate tracheostomy
    - Foreign bodies

        - Symptoms: sudden choking, loss of voice, dyspnea, inspiratory stridor, retractions
        - Initial treatment: modified Heimlich maneuver
        - Surgical treatment: removal by direct laryngoscopy
- Cysts and tumors
    - Laryngocele: fluid-filled cyst of the larynx
        - Symptoms: inspiratory stridor
        - Diagnosis: laryngoscopy
        - Treatment: ET intubation and needle aspiration of the cyst, surgical unroofing
    - Lymphangioma
        - Pathology: usually multiloculated and lined with endothelium
        - Symptoms: airway obstruction
        - Treatment: staged excision
    - Hemangioma
        - Usually seen in infants < 1 year old
        - Subglottic location
        - Often associated with cutaneous hemangiomas
        - Symptoms: inspiratory stridor
        - Diagnosis: laryngoscopy
        - Treatment: may regress spontaneously; administer steroids (if symptomatic)
    - Papillomas: benign neoplastic lesions associated with condyloma acuminatum in mother at the time of birth
        - Symptoms: hoarseness, stridor, dyspnea
        - Treatment: surgical excision
- Acquired obstructions
    - Acute epiglottitis (supraglottitis): acute inflammatory swelling of the epiglottis, caused by *Haemophilus influenzae* type b
        - Occurs in children ages 2–6 years old
        - Symptoms: inspiratory stridor, "sniffing" head position, systemic illness, drooling, dyspnea, muffled voice; patients appear toxic with fever, tachycardia, tachypnea, and increased white blood cell count
        - Diagnosis: radiograph of the lateral neck; **never attempt to visualize the throat in the emergency department**

  - Treatment: ET intubation (usually for 3 days) in an operating room under general anesthesia with a surgeon present; tracheostomy if necessary (rare); intravenous antibiotics (cefotaxime or ceftriaxone)
- Croup (acute laryngotracheobronchitis): viral inflammation producing subglottic edema, caused by parainfluenza viruses A and B
  - Pathology: subglottic edema
  - Occurs in children ages 3 months to 3 years old
  - Symptoms: barking cough, inspiratory and expiratory stridor, substernal retractions, no drooling
  - Laboratory findings show increased white blood cell count with right shift of differential (ie, lymphocytosis)
  - Diagnosis: neck radiographs show subglottic narrowing
  - Treatment: humidification (croup tent) and racemic epinephrine (occasionally dexamethasone for severe cases)
- Foreign bodies
  - The most common site affected is the right mainstem bronchus
  - Symptoms: stridor, aphonia, cyanosis, hypoxia, coughing, wheezing, fever, rhonchi
  - Diagnosis: anterior-posterior and decubitus chest radiographs with nonobstructed side down; radiograph will show hyperaeration on the side with obstruction due to air trapping
  - First aid: Heimlich maneuver, cricothyroidotomy, oxygen
  - Surgical treatment: extraction using rigid bronchoscopy under general anesthesia
- Postintubation subglottic tracheal stenosis: cricoid forms the only complete ring in the airway and the area of smallest tracheal diameter; stenosis usually occurs at the level of the ET tube balloon cuff
  - Diagnosis: laryngoscopy
  - Prevention: ensure there is a small air leak around the ET tube, stabilize ET tubes, and avoid reintubations

Surgical Procedures for Procuring an Emergency Airway

- Cricothyroidotomy (avoid in children < 12 y old)
- Tracheostomy
  - Avoid in an emergency setting
  - Never excise cartilage from the anterior tracheal wall
  - Make longitudinal tracheal incisions through the second and third rings
- Laryngoscopy
  - Most common indication is inspiratory stridor
  - Unique anatomical features of the infant larynx to note before performing laryngoscopy:
    - Infant larynx is situated more anteriorly at birth
    - It is the narrowest in the subglottic region
  - Indications
    - Laryngomalacia
    - Subglottic hemangiomas, papillomas, webs, foreign bodies, cysts
    - Most common complication is laryngeal edema; treat with humidification, racemic epinephrine, and steroids
- Bronchoscopy (flexible or rigid)
  - Diagnostic uses
    - Tracheomalacia and stenosis
    - Extrinsic compression
    - Tracheobronchial lavage (in cystic fibrosis patients)
    - Foreign body retrieval (rigid bronchoscopy)
- Establishing an airway
  - Rapid sequence intubation: etomidate plus succinylcholine (except in burns or crush injuries)
  - In patients < 12 years old, perform a tracheostomy through the second tracheal ring instead of cricothyroidotomy
  - ET tube size (estimate): (16 + age in years)/4, or approximately the size of the child's little finger
  - Distance (in centimeters) from lips to midtrachea: 12 + (age in years/2)

Trauma

- Airway issues
  - Fractures of the mandible (particularly subcondylar

fractures) or maxilla (Le Fort fractures) can result in free-floating bone or soft tissue, which can prolapse and obstruct the airway
  - Dislocated teeth or debris can obstruct the airway
  - Initial maneuvers to secure an airway may include jaw thrust, nasal trumpet (**do not use** if a fracture at the base of the skull is suspected), or oral airway
- Managing facial bone fractures
  - In the absence of fractures leading to airway obstruction or severe bleeding, facial bone fractures do not need to be managed acutely, but can be addressed up to 2 weeks after injury
  - Mandibular fractures can result in free-floating segments, causing tongue prolapse and airway obstruction
    - If this occurs, the mandible can be maneuvered anteriorly to allow airway management and fractures can be addressed later
    - Presenting symptoms include pain upon jaw opening, inability to open jaw (trismus due to masseter muscle spasm), and malocclusion (top and bottom teeth do not match up correctly)
    - Most mandibular fractures involve more than one site; isolated fractures are uncommon
    - Many mandibular fractures are of the greenstick (incomplete) type and can be managed conservatively by closed reduction
    - Subcondylar fractures are generally managed with a soft diet and close observation
    - Nongreenstick body, angle, ramus, and parasymphysis fractures are managed with open reduction and internal fixation, along with mandibular maxillary fixation via intraoral wiring
    - Care must be taken to avoid injuring permanent tooth roots when placing screws
    - When wiring the jaws together, consider possible airway obstruction, emesis, and suitable caloric intake; wire cutters should be available at the bedside at all times
  - Maxillofacial fractures
    - Le Fort classification (these fractures can wait up to 2

weeks for repair and are **not** urgent once bleeding is controlled and the airway is stable)
    - Le Fort I: maxillary and alveolar fracture
    - Le Fort II: pyramidal, nasal, and orbital fracture
    - Le Fort III: craniofacial disassociation
  - Presenting symptoms: distorted facial appearance, facial swelling or bruising, malocclusion, diplopia
  - Significant hemorrhage often accompanies fractures of the maxilla; it can be managed with nasal and oral packing **after** the airway has been secured
  - May be accompanied by cervical spine trauma and orbital or ocular trauma
  - Use caution when considering placing nasal tubes (eg, nasogastric tubes, nasal trumpets) in patients with nasal or maxillary fractures because of the possible presence of a basilar skull fracture; this can result in inadvertent placement into the brain
  - Assess the hard palate for fracture by palpation
  - Management is limited to the facial support buttresses (medial and lateral), which are repaired with open reduction and internal fixation, and possible mandibular maxillary fixation (temporary, short term)
- Nasal fractures
  - Most common facial fractures of the face, but the least important
  - The decision to repair is based upon cosmetic considerations and is not urgent (can be delayed 10–14 days)
  - Septal hematoma
    - May be associated with a fractured nasal septum
    - Treatment: incision and evacuation of the clot; suture the mucoperichondrial flap in place over bolsters; administer antibiotics

- Base of the skull and temporal bone fractures
  - Presenting symptoms
    - Postauricular bruising (Battle's sign)
    - Orbital bruising (raccoon eyes)
    - Auditory deficits
    - Facial nerve injury
    - Hemotympanum

    - Cerebrospinal fluid otorrhea or rhinorrhea
  - If facial nerve function is absent, determining and documenting the time frame (ie, delayed versus immediate) is important to optimize future facial nerve function; complete immediate-onset nerve damage requires direct nerve repair once life-threatening injuries have been addressed
    - Managing incomplete facial nerve injuries (ie, some movement is visible) is not of acute interest and management can be delayed for up to 2 weeks
    - Facial nerve repair, when indicated, is performed after decompression and under magnification with 9-0 suture
  - Hearing loss can be conductive (mechanical) or sensorineural (nerve) and is distinguished using a tuning fork
  - Treat tympanic membrane perforation by keeping the ear clean and dry
  - Cerebrospinal fluid leak often presents with a clear, salty-tasting drainage that is exacerbated by sitting upright and leaning forward
    - Drainage should be stopped with pressure or packing and broad-spectrum antibiotics to limit the possibility of meningitis
    - Repair can be deferred until appropriate otolaryngological or neurosurgical expertise is available
- Laryngeal trauma
  - Uncommon in pediatric patients because of the elevated position of the larynx underneath the mandible and the cartilaginous structure of the pediatric larynx (which is commonly ossified in adults)
  - Presenting symptoms
    - Hoarseness
    - Stridor
    - Crepitation and subcutaneous emphysema
  - Acute management consists only of appropriately securing the airway
  - Definitive management can then be performed by the appropriate specialists
- Penetrating neck trauma: hemorrhage and airway injury are

the primary concerns

- The neck is divided into three anatomic zones to aid in management:
  - Zone 1
    - Boundaries: clavicle to cricoid membrane
    - Critical structures: common carotid artery, subclavian artery, apices of the lung, and the brachial plexus
  - Zone 2
    - Boundaries: cricoid to angle of the mandible
    - Critical structures: common and internal carotid arteries, internal jugular vein, esophagus, and trachea
  - Zone 3
    - Boundaries: angle of mandible to base of the skull
    - Critical structures: internal carotid artery, jugular vein
- If the platysma muscle is not transgressed, no surgical management is initially indicated, and close observation is warranted
- Diagnostic measures
  - Esophagoscopy
  - Bronchoscopy
  - Contrast swallow
  - CT angiogram
- Zone 1 and 3 injuries
  - Management is selective based on clinical evidence of significant structural injury, such as significant bleeding, expanding hematoma, subcutaneous emphysema, hoarseness or stridor, hemoptysis, decreased pulses in the arm or neck, or mental status changes
  - If the above are present, exploration with the appropriate expert (ie, vascular surgeon, otolaryngologist, neurosurgeon) is indicated to manage injury of involved structures
- Zone 2 injuries
  - Presenting symptoms
    - Air bubbling from the wound
    - Subcutaneous emphysema
    - Stridor

      - Dyspnea
      - Hypoxia
    - Management includes initial neck exploration to evaluate vascular structures, trachea, and the esophagus; repair as indicated
    - Tracheal injury: after the airway is secured, repair can be performed with 5-0, 6-0 nylon sutures, being careful not to enter the lumen of the trachea (if the airway is secure, evacuation to a suitable expert is strongly encouraged)
  - Esophageal injury may be difficult to diagnose because of delayed presentation, but should be considered in patients with unexplained fever or tachycardia and penetrating neck trauma in Zone 1 or 2
    - Presenting symptoms include fever, tachycardia, and dysphagia
    - Diagnosis: chest radiograph, esophagoscopy, diatrizoate meglumine and diatrizoate sodium solution swallow
    - Initial management: nothing by mouth, exploration and drainage, antibiotics, and referral if necessary to the appropriate surgical specialty (general surgery, thoracic surgery, etc)
    - Definitive management: debridement with primary repair and feeding tube placement

Masses

- Cervical lymphadenitis
  - Most common cause of a neck mass in a child
  - Etiology: usually *Staphylococcus* or *Streptococcus*
  - Treatment
    - Initial: antibiotics (eg, third-generation cephalosporin) to treat the primary cause (otitis media, pharyngitis)
    - Incision and drainage of fluctuant nodes
    - Excision for chronic lymphadenitis
    - Differential diagnosis includes tuberculosis, atypical mycobacteria, and cat-scratch fever (*Bartonella henselae*)
- Lymphoma
  - Most common malignant neoplasms of the head and neck
  - Firm, fixed nodes with generalized involvement (especially

  if present in the neck, axilla, or groin)
  - Diagnosis: excisional lymph node biopsy
- Thyroglossal duct cyst
  - Etiology
    - Development of the thyroid gland originates at the base of the tongue in the foramen cecum and passes between the genioglossus muscles and through the hyoid bone to its normal anatomic position
    - Most common congenital lesion of the neck
  - Symptoms
    - Usually discovered at 2–4 years of age, when baby fat starts to diminish
    - Usually asymptomatic, but recurrent infection is a characteristic problem due to communication with the pharynx
  - Physical
    - Located in the midline at or below the level of the hyoid bone
    - Moves up and down with swallowing
    - Differential diagnosis: lymphadenopathy, dermoid cyst, thyroid gland (obtain thyroid scan if any question exists regarding the presence of a normal thyroid gland)
  - Treatment
    - Antibiotics for infection
    - Needle aspiration of abscesses
    - Elective surgical excision of the cyst and tract to the pharynx, in continuity with the central portion of the hyoid bone (Sistrunk operation), and ligation of the foramen cecum
- Branchial cleft cysts
  - Congenital fistula resulting from malformation or persistence of the second (most common) or third branchial cleft; abnormalities of the first brachial arch are associated with facial clefts (eg, cleft palate)
  - First branchial cleft sinuses communicate with the eustachian tube
  - Second branchial cleft cysts extend from the anterior border of the lower third of the sternocleidomastoid muscle

superiorly, then inward between the carotid bifurcation, entering the posterolateral pharynx just below the tonsillar fossa
  - The third branchial cleft tracts lateral to the carotid bifurcation
  - Symptoms
    - Painless nodule at anterior border of the sternocleidomastoid
    - Drainage from external auditory canal (third cleft sinus)
    - External fistula with drainage of clear fluid from the lateral neck (second cleft)
    - Abscess formation in the lateral neck
  - Pathology: lined with squamous and columnar epithelium, cartilaginous remnants, and cystic dilatations
  - Treatment of second branchial cleft anomalies
    - Initial: treat infection (if present) with antibiotics to cover *Staphylococcus* and *Streptococcus*
    - Perform complete surgical excision of the cyst and tract
      - A lacrimal duct probe inserted through the external opening, as well as injection of methylene blue, will help define and facilitate dissection of the tract
      - Use a series of small, transverse, "stair step" incisions, rather than a long, oblique incision
      - The marginal branch of the facial nerve may be injured by intraoperative retraction
- Cystic hygroma (lymphangioma)
  - Etiology
    - Congenital malformation resulting in sequestration or obstruction of developing lymphatic channels
    - Usually posterior to the sternocleidomastoid muscle of the neck (posterior triangle)
    - Other sites include:
      - Axilla
      - Groin
      - Mediastinum
      - Retroperitoneum
  - Cysts are usually multiple, may "infiltrate" deep structures of the neck (tongue, mouth floor), and are lined by endothelium
  - Infected cysts may cause airway compromise by compressing

the trachea
      - May contain nests of vascular tissue (benign lesions)
   - Physical characteristics
      - Soft and compressible
      - Transilluminate
      - Usually apparent at birth, sudden enlargement later may be due to hemorrhage into the lesion
   - Diagnosis: ultrasound, chest radiograph, CT scan
   - Complications
      - Airway compromise
      - Disfigurement
      - Hemorrhage into the cyst may cause a purplish discoloration
      - Infection (*Staphylococcus* or *Streptococcus*) may cause rapid enlargement and airway compression
   - Treatment
      - Conservative surgical resection
         - Rarely complete because the lesion is usually multilocular and there is no well-defined cleavage plane between the lesion and normal tissue
         - May require repeated partial excisions with preservation of all adjacent critical structures
         - Wound is drained postoperatively by closed suction
         - Needle aspiration of accumulated fluid may be required postoperatively
      - Injury to the facial nerve (cranial nerve VII) must be avoided
      - Injection of sclerosing agents (eg, OK-432, which is derived from group A *Streptococcus pyogenes*) may yield good results in cases with primarily macrocystic disease; sclerotherapy may also be used in conjunction with operative excision before and after the operation

Miscellaneous Conditions

- Congenital wryneck (torticollis)
   - Evident in early months of life due to fibrosis of the sternocleidomastoid muscle
   - Physical examination reveals tender, palpable swelling in

lower part of the sternocleidomastoid, head rotated toward the opposite side of the mass

- Treatment
    - Perform neck radiograph to exclude vertebral anomalies (Klippel-Feil syndrome)
    - Active and passive stretching exercises
    - Surgical transection of the belly of the sternocleidomastoid muscle if above is unsuccessful (rarely necessary)
- 20% will have associated hip dysplasia

- Epiglottitis
    - Age group: 3–6 years old
    - Etiology: *Haemophilus influenzae B*
    - Symptoms
        - High fever
        - Inspiratory stridor
        - Drooling
        - Head in sniffing position
        - Cherry red epiglottis
    - Diagnosis
        - Lateral neck radiograph shows edema (evident with "thumbprinting") of the epiglottis
        - If epiglottitis is suspected, **never** attempt direct examination of the throat, except in the operating room
    - Treatment
        - Intubation in the operating room, under general anesthesia, by the most experienced airway endoscopist available; a surgeon should be present, scrubbed, and prepared to perform an emergency tracheostomy if necessary
        - Give antibiotics
- Epistaxis
    - If anterior vessel is the source, it can usually be treated by pinching the nasal ala for several minutes
    - Apply hemostatic packing or tamponade using a balloon device if bleeding persists

Chapter 14

Orthopaedics

- **Triage**

The general categories of care (ie, immediate, delayed, expectant, minimal, and urgent) apply to civilian pediatric casualties in a mass casualty situation. In a combat setting, it is possible that a traditionally defined pediatric patient (< 18 years old) may be an enemy combatant and in a special category that places medical personnel at risk. Although these patients are treated the same as "friendly casualties," it is mandatory to carefully screen for ordnance and weapons before moving the casualty to patient care areas.

- Resource constraints
    - Utilization: it is imperative to constantly reassess resources to conserve necessary equipment and personnel
    - Standard of care: treating pediatric orthopaedic problems in theater may be different than in a noncombat environment
        - Resources in roles 1–3 military medical treatment facilities are focused on adult orthopaedics; equipment tailored to pediatric sizes and specific problems may not be available
        - Weather, sanitation, and ease of transport may alter treatment; for instance, external fixation of closed long-bone fractures may be elected over open fixation to obviate infection, or external fixation may be more practical than closed treatment in a heavy cast
        - Medical providers should familiarize themselves with local medical care resources for follow-on treatment; the treatment regimen chosen must be compatible with available local civilian resources

        - General knowledge of the indigenous cultural views on health, gender, and specific conditions (eg, amputations and congenital deformities) is helpful in directing care for pediatric civilian casualties; chaperones may be necessary when examining a patient's unclothed extremity
  - Disposition. Local pediatric civilian patients will typically stay in country and are not usually evacuated to a higher level of care (occasionally a local patient is transferred). The judgment of when to end care in the military system may be difficult and will usually be resource and safety dependent. Liaison with local resources and avenues to the International Committee of the Red Cross should be investigated
  - Outcomes. Medical personnel delivering humanitarian care should be aware of, but not disappointed by, the limitations in orthopaedic care. Short-term intervention may have limited impact and cultural norms may affect efforts to improve outcome
- **Epidemiology**
  - Types of orthopaedic care
    - Trauma. Children are subjected to the same mechanisms of injury as war fighters. In the past two decades, the leading etiologies of pediatric orthopaedic trauma seen in deployed military facilities are:
      - Blast injury (ie, direct contact with an explosive device)
      - Penetrating injury
      - Thermal injury
      - Blunt force injury
    - Congenital malformations / reconstruction. Deployed orthopaedic surgeons may be asked to evaluate and treat mild to severe congenital anomalies. Healthcare providers must use good judgment when initiating reconstructive treatment because there may be limited means for follow-up or follow-on treatment
    - Infection. Pediatric musculoskeletal infections may be caused by pathogens endemic to the geographic area of operations

- ▹ Wound infections may be caused by common environmental microorganisms
  - *Staphylococcus aureus* remains the most common cause of musculoskeletal infection throughout the world
  - *Salmonella typhi* has been reported to be the most common infecting organism in Africa
  - *Acinetobacter baumannii* is common in southwest Asia. It is found in soil and can live on open surfaces for a number of days, enabling it to spread. Patients with open wounds and on ventilators are susceptible to this multiple drug-resistant organism
  - *Klebsiella pneumoniae,* an organism that lives in water, is typically acquired in a hospital setting and is often associated with people with poor nutrition and those with slightly depressed immune systems
  - *Pseudomonas aeruginosa* thrives in moist environments and is a threat to patients with several kinds of injuries, including burns. *Pseudomonas* and *Staphylococcus epidermidis* are the most common causative agents of infection in extramedullary implants in local hospitals in Iraq
  - Clostridia are gram-positive, anaerobic, spore-forming bacilli found in high density in cultivated rich soil. *Clostridium perfringens* is the most common cause of gas gangrene and food poisoning. *Clostridium difficile* is responsible for pseudomembranous colitis after long-term antibiotic usage
- ▹ Osteomyelitis and septic joints can be hematogenous in origin or result from direct inoculation. The causative organisms are those found in the particular environment. The first principle of treatment is to evacuate purulent material when it is entrapped. Eradication of osteomyelitis or a septic joint will require long-term antibiotic therapy

○ Difference in levels of trauma. Although common pediatric orthopaedic trauma may present to the military medical facility, most cases will be more complex. In the civilian and military settings in the continental United States, the receiving facility often provides emergency care and transports the patient to a higher-level facility for definitive care. In theater, the major orthopaedic care for local civilians will occur at the military facility, followed by transportation to a lower-level facility

- **Amputations**
  - Children sustain amputations from the same mechanisms of injury as war fighters
    - Exsanguination is the immediate concern
    - Explosive munitions with penetration and concussive blast effects create a large zone of injury with extensive contamination that may affect the level of final amputation
  - Indications for amputation
    - Partial or complete traumatic amputation
    - Irreparable vascular injury or failed vascular repair with an ischemic limb
    - Life-threatening sepsis due to local infection, including clostridial myonecrosis
    - Severe soft tissue or bone injury beyond functional recovery
  - Principles of amputation
    - Amputations should be done at the **lowest level of viable tissue** (in contrast with traditional amputation levels; eg, below the knee, above the knee, etc) to preserve as much limb as possible; a longer residual limb is most desirable for prosthetic fitting and will serve the amputee best if prosthetic fitting is not possible
    - Open length-preserving amputation has two stages:
      - Initial: the bone is completed at the lowest possible level; the residual limb is left open
      - Reconstructive: this involves the process of healing to reach optimum function and prosthetic fitting; civilian pediatric amputees will undergo this phase in country, unlike military patients who will be evacuated out of the combat zone for reconstruction in a stable environment

  - All viable skin and soft tissue distal to the amputated bone should be preserved for future wound closure. These "flaps of opportunity" can be used to add length to the residual limb regardless of irregularity
- Amputation technique
  - Apply tourniquet. It is necessary to limit blood loss and preserve volume in trauma patients. There is very little literature on the use of tourniquets in the pediatric population (see Further Reading at the end of this chapter). General guidelines are as follows:
    - Place the tourniquet on the most proximal portion of the limb
    - Use the widest cuff possible suitable for the limb, location, and procedure
    - Use a specifically designed limb protection sleeve for the cuff, if available. If not, use two layers of tubular stockinette, slightly stretched but not tight
    - Apply the tourniquet snugly over the sleeve
    - Determine the occlusion pressure and set the tourniquet pressure to 50 mmHg above that (average is 175 mmHg)
    - Exsanguinate by elastic bandage or gravity, as appropriate for the case
    - If bleeding persists after cuff inflation, increase the cuff pressure in increments of 25 mmHg until it stops
    - Minimize tourniquet time (no more than 2 h without 15 min deflation time)
    - Remove the cuff and sleeve as soon as possible after the tourniquet is deflated
  - Prepare entire extremity
  - Excise nonviable bone and soft tissue that has been devascularized
  - Ligate major arteries and veins
  - Locate major nerves, provide gentle traction, and transect proximal to the level of amputated bone; ligate major nerves
  - Preserve muscle flaps, but do not suture
  - Full debridement of a blast injury may require extending

incisions longitudinally to remove contamination along fascial planes

- Differences in managing local amputees
  - Definitive care will be provided in theater. Following the principles of the Red Cross surgeons working in relatively stable environments, the local civilian pediatric patient will undergo delayed primary closure when the wound is clean. Skin retraction of open residual limbs should be prevented, using skin traction until closure is possible. Skin traction may be accomplished through a classic technique of benzoin-secured stockinette and 1–2 lb of weight (Figure 14-1). In select situations, skin retraction can be prevented by placing large, loose trauma sutures with bolsters or vessel loops and skin staples at the wound margins. Preserving viable skin flaps, even if they are irregular, aids in closure and is preferable to skin grafting

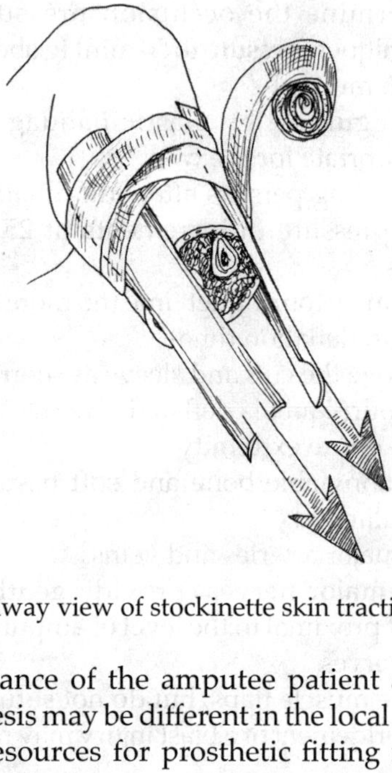

Figure 14-1. Cut away view of stockinette skin traction.

  - Acceptance of the amputee patient and the type of prosthesis may be different in the local culture. Existing local resources for prosthetic fitting may be limited.

When applicable, early prosthetic fitting, especially in upper-extremity amputations, promotes best functional use of the prosthesis. Frequent prosthetic changes are expected

- Because of growth and the quantity of young healing bone, various long-term problems may arise, especially in below-the-knee amputations, such as:
  - Anterior bowing associated with the distal element pointing medially; varus bowing with the distal element pointing medially
  - Heterotopic bone formation, requiring revision
  - The fibula may outgrow the tibia, resulting in the formation of bursa overlying the fibula and prominent bone spicules projecting beneath the skin
  - These problems can be prevented or controlled by synostosis of the distal fibula and tibia, which results in an end-bearing residual limb (this procedure should **not** be performed until the soft tissues have fully healed)

- **Fractures**
  - Evaluating fractures
    - Obtain history, perform a physical examination to fully assess injuries, and establish vascular and neurologic status of the extremities
    - Obtain radiographs of the adjacent joints (above and below the fracture in the case of a long-bone fracture), with images in two planes
    - Examine and cover open wounds, preferably with a sterile dressing
    - Splint the involved extremity, including the joints above and below, for a long-bone fracture
    - Fracture reduction should be done with adequate anesthesia or analgesia
    - After reduction and application of a cast or external fixator, reevaluate vascular status and nerve function of the limb
    - Children's fractures remodel 1°/mo for the first 24 months
  - Open fractures

- Open fractures sustained in a combat area are produced by small arms (bullets) and explosive munitions (improvised explosive devices, mortars, artillery, land mines, grenades, or bombs)
- The most common battlefield injury is multiple fragment wounds that involve only the soft tissue
- Open fractures caused by weapons of war are more severe than those seen in a noncombat setting
- Initial treatment for open fractures
  - Evaluate the wound while the patient is under anesthesia
  - Surgically incise the skin and fascia to inspect the soft tissues and fracture site
  - Excise devitalized tissue or debris
  - Copiously lavage with a physiological solution to decontaminate and remove debris, dead tissue, or hematoma
  - All wounds should initially be left open and closed at a later date
  - Negative-pressure (wound vac) wound dressings may be a useful adjunct, especially for more extensive wounds
  - Administer systemic antibiotics appropriate for the wound
  - If a skin defect is present, perform coverage as a second, staged, operative procedure only after the wound is clean and free of necrotic tissue
  - Coverage procedures should be planned and performed in a stable environment

- Long-bone fractures
  - General
    - Internal fixation of pediatric fractures in theater is rarely, if ever, indicated because of operative conditions and potential for infection
    - Based on the patient's size and available equipment, external fixation may be desirable for stabilizing long-bone fractures in theater. Appropriately sized fixators may not be available; the "pins in plaster" technique may be used to maintain length

- Casting remains an acceptable treatment option, provided alignment can be maintained; skeletal traction is also a useful means to care for some fractures
- See Figure 14-2 for fracture classification

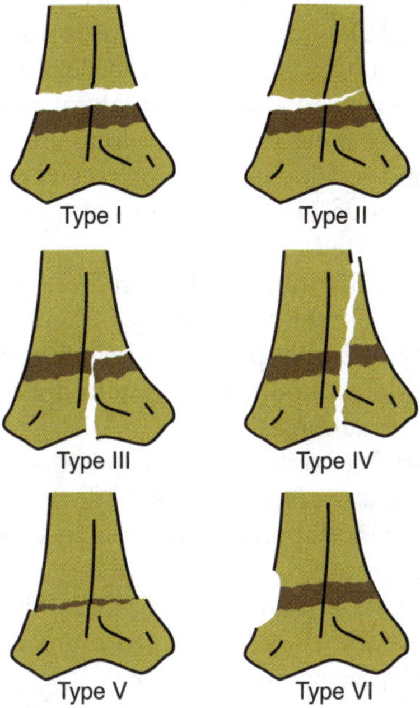

Figure 14-2. Salter-Harris classification of fractures involving the growth plate. Type I: transverse fracture through the physis. Type II: fracture through the physis and metaphysis. Type III: fracture through the physis and epiphysis. Type IV: fracture through all three (physis, metaphysis, and epiphysis). Type V: physeal compression fracture. Type VI: peripheral physeal injury.

- Upper extremity fractures
  - Proximal humerus fractures. The majority of proximal humerus fractures in the pediatric age group are treated conservatively with a sling and swathe for roughly 2 weeks. Gradual return to normal function is allowed once pain subsides
  - Midshaft humerus fractures. Use a coaptation splint

with a sling and swathe for comfort; this may be changed to a Sarmiento-type brace at 2 weeks (if available) instead of definitive treatment in long-arm cast

- Supracondylar humerus fractures
  - Significantly displaced fractures (Gartland types 2 and 3) require closed reduction and percutaneous pinning; crossed medial and lateral pins (rather than two or more divergent lateral pins) are adequate
  - Place the extremity in a long-arm cast for 3 weeks and consider a bivalving cast if swelling is present; remove pins at 3 weeks and begin activities as tolerated
  - Avoid immobilization in more than 90° of elbow flexion; this may lead to ischemic contracture
  - Type 2 fractures can sometimes be reduced and held without pinning with a long-arm cast (see precautions above)
- Lateral condyle fractures
  - These are often difficult to diagnose in the younger population; when in doubt, use an arthrogram to diagnose
  - Open reduction is indicated if the fracture enters the joint and there are more than 2–3 mm of displacement
  - Use a lateral approach; do not strip posterior soft tissue attachments off the fragment because blood supply enters posteriorly
  - A headlight is often useful
  - Reduce the fragment and pin with 2 or more Kirschner wires
  - Use a long-arm cast for 4–6 weeks, then remove pins
- Medial epicondyle fractures rarely require treatment, regardless of displacement, unless they are entrapped in the joint (in which case, open reduction and pin fixation is indicated)
- Forearm and wrist fractures
  - These may involve the radius, ulna, or both, and may occur at the distal, middle, or proximal forearm

- Remodeling potential is greatest in younger patients and in distal areas near the physis
- Expect an angular correction of approximately 1°/mo or 10°/y for 2 years
- Rotational deformities do not correct with growth; bayonet apposition of up to 1 cm is acceptable if the patient is < 8–10 years old
- If initial displacement is outside this range, fracture reduction and casting are recommended
- In general, immobilization consists of 4 weeks in a long-arm cast, followed by 2 weeks in a short-arm cast; immobilization duration varies depending on fracture healing and age
- Wrist fractures (at the distal ⅓ of the forearm) can be treated with 3–6 weeks of short-arm casting, depending on the age of the child and the fracture type

- ► Lower extremity fractures
  - ▹ Femur fractures
    - Certain current acceptable and standard treatments, such as internal fixation with plates, may not be not be reasonable in an austere environment because of risk of infection and limited equipment availability
    - Treatment is typically based on the age and size of the patient and the availability of equipment in theater (Table 14-1)

Table 14-1. Guidelines for Acceptable Reduction in Femur Fractures

Age (y)	Varus/Valgus	Procurvatum/Recurvatum	Shortening
0–2	30°	30°	15 mm
2–5	15°	20°	20 mm
6–10	10°	15°	15 mm
11 and older	5°	10°	10 mm

- Birth–6 months old: casting. Use a spica cast for diaphyseal fractures and a long-leg cast for supracondylar fractures. The Pavlik harness that is recommended in the noncombat environment may not be available

- 6–12 years old: external fixator or pins in plaster. Submuscular bridge plating is a good option in a developed healthcare system, but may not be appropriate in theater. Skeletal traction may be used where external fixation is not available or not advised (eg, while a child is confined to bed); it requires limited operating room technology
- 12 years and older: external fixator. Intramedullary nailing or bridge plating are good options in a developed healthcare system, but may not be appropriate in theater

▹ Tibia fractures
- The majority of tibia fractures are treated with reduction and long-leg casting
- Acceptable alignment: 50% apposition, < 1 cm shortening, and 5°–10° of angulation in the sagittal and coronal planes
- A long-leg cast is applied with slight (10°–20°) ankle–plantar flexion and 45° of knee flexion
- Time to healing is based on age; neonates heal in 2–3 weeks, children in 4–6 weeks, and adolescents in 8–12 weeks
- External fixation and open reduction internal fixation may be used if clinically indicated (ie, in the case of severe comminution, open fractures, etc)

▹ Ankle fractures
- The majority of ankle fractures are Salter-Harris–type injuries and can be treated with closed reduction and a short-leg cast
- Displaced fractures (> 2 mm) that traverse the physis and involve the joint may require reduction and internal fixation
- Physis may be crossed if the patient is near skeletal maturity
- Tillaux fractures and triplane fractures are more complex ankle fractures and may need evaluation by computed tomography (CT) scan to discern

fracture pattern and displacement. Displaced Tillaux or triplane fractures are treated with open reduction and internal fixation. In an austere setting, open reduction with Kirschner wires and casting is an option

- Pelvic fractures (see Further Reading for additional guidance)
  - Overall, pelvic fractures in pediatric patients are rare
  - Usually caused by a high-energy mechanism that results in other life-threatening injuries. Comprehensive workup is indicated using advanced life support principles
  - Children have greater plasticity, thick cartilage, and more mobile joints than adults, and their vessels tend to spasm and not bleed (life-threatening hemorrhage is rare)
  - Low mortality rate (compared to adults)
  - The majority can be treated nonoperatively and have a much better prognosis than when in adults
  - Imaging
    - Radiographs (anterioposterior pelvis, inlet and outlet, Judet views)
    - CT scan is best, especially with image reconstructions
  - Treatment is based on age; fracture location, type, and stability; and concomitant injuries
    - Most are treated nonsurgically and heal uneventfully
    - Surgical indications include intraarticular acetabular or triradiate cartilage displacement of > 2 mm, and pelvic ring displacement with > 2 cm of limb length discrepancy
    - External fixation may be used for unstable fractures
  - Complications
    - Acetabular fracture or triradiate injury may lead to a dysplastic acetabulum and early degenerative changes
    - Sacroiliac joint pain

Further Reading

1. Lieberman JR, Staheli LT, Dales MC. Tourniquet pressures on pediatric patients: a clinical study. *Orthopedics.* 1997;20:1143–1147.
2. Tredwell SJ, Wilmink M, Inkpen K, McEwen JA. Pediatric tourniquets: analysis of cuff and limb interface, current practice, and guidelines for use. *J Pediatr Orthop.* 2001;21(5):671–676.
3. Holden CP, Holman J, Herman MJ. Pediatric pelvic fractures. *J Am Acad Orthop Surg.* 2007;15:172–177

Chapter 15

Thoracic Cavity

Chest Trauma

- General chest trauma
    - Incidence
        - Penetrating: rare
        - Blunt: common
    - Compliant chest wall transmits impact forces to intrathoracic structures, often without external evidence of injury to the chest wall (ie, no rib fractures)
    - Types
        - Pulmonary contusion
            - Most common thoracic injury in children
            - Pathology: parenchymal hemorrhage and edema produce intrapulmonary shunting (alveolar ventilation and pulmonary perfusion [V/Q] mismatch) that results in hypoxia, atelectasis, and pneumonia
        - Intrapulmonary hemorrhage
        - Cardiac contusion
    - Diagnosis
        - Physical examination
        - Chest radiograph
        - Computed tomography (CT) scan
    - Treatment
        - Oxygen
        - Fluid restriction
        - Antibiotics
        - Analgesics
        - Assisted ventilation when clinically indicated
- Tension pneumothorax and hemothorax
    - Not well tolerated due to a child's mobile mediastinum
    - Symptoms
        - Breath sounds are decreased
        - Percussion
            - Hyperresonance (pneumothorax)

            - Dullness (hemothorax)
        - Tracheal shift to the contralateral side
        - Tachypnea, tachycardia, pallor, and cyanosis
    - Treatment
        - Immediate needle aspiration
            - Place the needle just over the top of the third rib into the second intercostal space, in the midclavicular line
            - Use a size 16 or smaller gauge over-the-needle catheter in infants and small children to prevent lung laceration
        - Thoracostomy tube
            - Place in the fifth intercostal space, just anterior to the midaxillary line
            - Tunnel subcutaneously over the fifth rib
            - Refer to the table on the inside front cover for age-appropriate thoracostomy tube sizes
        - Indications for thoracotomy
            - Rapid blood drainage of > 20 cc/kg
            - Bleeding continues at > 3 cc/kg/h for 2–4 hours
- Posterior flail
    - Not well tolerated in children
    - May be associated with an underlying pulmonary contusion, hemothorax, or pneumothorax
        - Hypoxia
        - Intrapulmonary shunting (V/Q mismatch)
        - Atelectasis and pneumonia
    - Treatment may require supplemental oxygen; endotracheal intubation; ventilatory support with continuous positive airway pressure (CPAP) or positive end-expiratory pressure (PEEP) on assisted ventilation; or intercostal blocks
- Bronchial injuries and traumatic diaphragmatic hernias
    - More common than great vessel injury
    - Symptoms
        - Respiratory distress
        - Hypoxia
        - Massive air leak from the chest tube
        - Failure of the lung to reexpand after chest tube placement
    - Diagnosis
        - Chest radiograph

    - Bronchoscopy (flexible)
  - Treatment
    - If injury covers > ⅓ of the circumference of the airway, perform an emergent thoracotomy and operative repair with fine, absorbable suture
    - Buttress with a muscle flap
- Aortic injury
  - Rare in children
  - Etiology: rapid deceleration
  - Pathology: the tear is usually at the ligamentum arteriosum or the takeoff of the left subclavian artery
  - On chest radiograph, findings consistent with aortic injuries include:
    - Fractures in the first to third ribs or the scapula
    - Mediastinum widening
    - Pleural or apical cap
    - Deviation of the trachea to the right
    - Deviation of the esophagus (or nasogastric tube) to the right
    - Obliteration of the aortopulmonary window
    - Obliteration of the aortic knob
    - Widened paratracheal stripe
    - Elevation of the right mainstem bronchus
    - Depression of the left mainstem bronchus
    - Left hemothorax
  - Diagnosis: arch aortogram, spiral CT scan
  - Treatment: surgical repair
- Pericardial tamponade
  - Symptoms (Beck triad)
    - Systemic arterial **hypo**tension
    - Central venous **hyper**tension
    - Muffled heart sounds
  - Diagnosis
    - Clinical
    - Ultrasound
  - Treatment
    - Needle pericardiocentesis is a temporizing measure **only**
      - For pneumopericardium: create subxiphoid pericardial window and place a pericardial tube

- For hemopericardium:
  - Traumatic: perform thoracotomy
  - Nontraumatic: place drainage catheter

- Myocardial contusion
  - Diagnosis
    - Electrocardiogram (ECG) will show nonspecific ST-T wave changes (most helpful)
    - Creatine phosphokinase, muscle band (CPK-MB); troponin (most accurate)
    - Echocardiogram will show traumatic ventricular septal defect and ruptured chordae
  - Treatment
    - Continuous cardiac rate and rhythm monitoring
    - Serial ECGs
    - Assess serial cardiac enzymes (especially troponin)
- Diaphragmatic rupture
  - 80% are on the left
  - Associated with injury to the spleen or kidney
  - Symptoms: respiratory distress (may be delayed)
  - Diagnosis: chest radiograph (nasogastric tube in the chest)
  - Treatment
    - Immediate diagnosis: midline abdominal incision
    - Delayed diagnosis: thoracotomy instead of laparotomy
- Penetrating chest wound with tracheal and esophageal injury
  - Treatment: primary repair with interposition of cervical strap muscle between the repair suture lines

Infections of the Lung and Pleura

- Bacterial pneumonias (see Chapter 29, Infectious Diseases)
- Complications of pneumonia
  - Pneumatocele
    - Usually seen in young children with *Staphylococcus aureus* pneumonia
    - Etiology: necrosis and liquefaction of the lung parenchyma
    - Diagnosis: chest radiograph or CT scan will show intrapulmonary air pockets without air–fluid levels
    - Differential diagnosis: congenital lung cysts
    - Treatment: pneumatocele usually regresses in response

to antibiotics

- Lung abscess
  - Etiology
    - The most common cause is pulmonary aspiration
    - Operations on upper respiratory tract (eg, tonsillectomy, tooth extractions)
    - Most common sites are the superior segment right lower lobe (supine position), posterior segment of the right upper lobe (lying on right side), basilar segments of lower lobes (upright position)
    - Typical organism causes are anaerobes (most common), *S aureus*, *Pseudomonas*
  - Symptoms include fever, malaise, and cough
  - Diagnosis: chest radiograph and CT scan show an intrapulmonary cavity with an air–fluid level
  - Treatment
    - Antibiotics for 6–8 weeks
    - Bronchoscopy with direct aspiration of fluid
    - Chest physical therapy
    - Indications for surgical resection (usually a segmental resection)
      - Chronic (> 3 mo), thick-walled (> 4–6 cm) abscess
      - Progression to empyema
      - Massive hemoptysis
- Empyema
  - Pathogenesis
    - Stages
      - Exudative or acute: thin pleural fluid, pH < 7.2, low cell count
      - Fibropurulent: many polymorphonuclear leukocytes, pH < 7.2, decreased glucose, deposition of fibrin, fluid loculations
      - Organizing: thick exudates, fibrous peel
    - Organisms: *Streptococcus pneumoniae* (most common), *S aureus*, *Haemophilus influenzae*
    - Early treatment with intravenous antibiotics may prevent the effusion from becoming infected and forming an empyema

        - Anaerobic empyemas are associated with the highest mortality rate
    - History
        - Tachypnea
        - Fever
        - Cough
    - Diagnosis
        - Physical examination
        - Chest radiograph
        - Thoracentesis (differential diagnosis of transudate)
            - pH < 7
            - Appearance: fibropurulent
            - Glucose < 40
            - Lactate dehydrogenase > 1,000 units / mL
            - Cell count: large numbers of polymorphonuclear leukocytes
            - Gram stain showing organisms
    - Treatment: intravenous antibiotics and either of the following:
        - Nonloculated fluid: thoracostomy tube drainage
        - Loculated fluid: video-assisted thoracoscopic surgery (VATS)
- Mediastinal masses
    - Anterior mediastinum
        - Ectopic thyroid
        - Lymphoma
        - Sarcoma
        - Teratoma
        - Thymus (cyst, thymoma, normal thymus)
    - Middle mediastinum
        - Bronchogenic cyst
        - Cardiac tumor
        - Cystic hygroma
        - Lymphadenopathy
        - Lymphoma
        - Pericardial cyst
        - Vascular abnormalities
    - Posterior mediastinum
        - Esophageal duplication
        - Meningomyelocele

    - Neurenteric abnormalities
    - Neurogenic tumors (eg, neuroblastoma)
- Miscellaneous conditions
  - Spontaneous pneumothorax
    - Etiology: ruptured subpleural apical bleb
    - Typical patient is a thin, lean, adolescent male, often a smoker
    - Physical
      - Diminished breath sounds on the ipsilateral chest
      - Tympany to percussion
      - Shift of the mediastinum to the contralateral side (if under tension)
      - Shift of mediastinal structures may decrease the venous return, resulting in hypotension and tachycardia
    - Diagnosis
      - Obtain posteroanterior and lateral chest radiographs
      - Perform chest CT scan to assess for the presence of apical blebs
    - Treatment
      - If under tension: emergent needle decompression through the second intercostal space, midclavicular line
      - If < 15%: observation and oxygen by mask
      - If > 15%: small intrathoracic catheter and Heimlich valve
    - Treatment for recurrence or persistent air leak: VATS for apical pleurectomy (endostapler) and pleurodesis (mechanical and/or chemical)
  - Pneumomediastinum
    - Etiology: esophageal or tracheal perforation
    - Symptoms: chest pain (possible)
    - Diagnosis: chest radiograph, chest CT scan, esophagram
    - Treatment: treat the inciting condition
  - Pneumopericardium
    - Etiology: usually associated with dissection of air from a tension pneumothorax in infants on assisted ventilation with high mean airway pressures
    - Treatment: if cardiac output is impaired, perform needle aspiration, place a pericardial tube, and decrease the mean airway pressures, if possible

- Hemothorax
  - Etiology
    - Trauma (blunt or penetrating)
    - Injury to subclavian vessels or the heart during insertion of a central venous catheter
  - Sources of bleeding
    - Intercostal artery
    - Internal mammary artery
    - Lung parenchyma
    - Mediastinal vessel
    - Great vessels
    - Heart
  - Physical: dullness to percussion, tachycardia, pleuritic pain, tachypnea
  - Diagnosis: chest radiograph, CT scan, thoracentesis
  - Treatment (initial): thoracostomy tube in the fifth intercostal space, just anterior to the axillary line
- Chylothorax
  - Etiology
    - Congenital anomalies of the thoracic duct
    - Blunt, penetrating, or birth trauma
    - Neoplasms (lymphomas, lymphangioma, neuroblastoma)
    - Operative injury during a thoracotomy, especially on the left (eg, patent ductus arteriosus, coarctation of the aorta, Blalock shunt)
    - Thoracic duct enters the left internal jugular vein posteriorly at the junction with the left subclavian vein
  - Symptoms
    - Acute respiratory distress (dyspnea, tachypnea, cyanosis)
    - Decreased breath sounds, dullness to percussion
    - Effects of a prolonged loss of chyle
      - Malnutrition (loss of fat)
      - Immunodeficiency (lymphopenia), which predisposes patient to opportunistic fungal infections
      - Hypoproteinemia
      - Fluid and electrolyte abnormalities
  - Diagnosis
    - Chest radiograph shows pleural effusion

        - Thoracentesis of chyle (high fat, high protein, 80%–90% T lymphocytes)
            - Clear, straw-colored in a fasting patient
            - White, milky after feedings containing fat
    - Treatment
        - Nonoperative
            - Thoracostomy tube drainage
            - Nothing by mouth; peripheral or central total parenteral nutrition, medium chain triglycerides
            - Octreotide (decreases gastric, pancreatic, and intestinal secretions)
        - Operative indications
            - Persistence > 2–3 weeks
            - Daily chyle loss > 100 cc/year of age for 5 days
            - Nutritional complications
        - Operative treatment
            - Technetium-99m lymphangiography to identify the site of leakage preoperatively
            - Preoperative administration of cream into the gastrointestinal tract
            - Ipsilateral thoractomy
            - Identification and ligation of leaking ducts, proximally and distally
            - When the site of leakage cannot be identified, ligate all tissues surrounding the aorta at the hiatus
            - Fibrin glue
            - Pleurodesis
            - A Denver pleuroperitoneal shunt (Denver Biomaterials, Surgimed Inc, Golden, Colo) is sometimes (but rarely) used
- Hemoptysis
    - Etiology
        - Pulmonary hypertension
        - Bronchiectasis
        - Foreign body
        - Congenital pulmonary malformations
        - Pneumonia
    - Treatment of massive hemoptysis
        - Usually stops spontaneously

- Bronchoscopic localization and selective bronchial artery embolization
- Perform lobectomy if the above measures are unsuccessful

Chapter 16

Vascular Surgery

Hemangiomas

- Benign tumors of vascular tissue, vascular birthmarks, and vascular malformations are the most common tumors of infancy. They are considered a type of hamartoma and develop from abnormal angiogenesis
- Hemangiomas are usually solitary, located on the head or neck, and occur most often in females
  - Typically appear within a week after birth
  - Superficial lesions are raised, bright red, and bosselated
  - Deep lesions are raised and appear blue-purple
  - The proliferating phase is characterized by 8–12 months of rapid growth
  - Involution occurs over 1–5 years
  - Complete resolution is usually achieved by age 5–7 years
- Classification
  - Neonatal staining ("stork's bite"): light pink lesion on the back of the neck in the midline; usually fades spontaneously
  - Salmon patch: a light pink variety of intradermal hemangioma that sits level with the skin surface, blanches with pressure, and does not change over years. Can be treated with cover-up creams or laser treatment
  - Capillary hemangioma (port-wine stain, nevus flammeus): hyperkeratotic patches (abnormal nerve endings) on the facial skin (deep in the dermis) that are supplied by cranial nerve V (trigeminal). These lesions are permanent (they do not enlarge or regress) and may be associated with Sturge-Weber syndrome (indicating central nervous system involvement). Can be treated with laser ablation
  - Spider angioma: small, central arteriole with a network of radiating intradermal capillaries; these usually appear at age 3–4 years and regress spontaneously

  - Juvenile hemangioma: congenital vascular malformations that usually regress spontaneously after a period of rapid growth. This is a soft, spongy, nontender, reticular pattern of blood vessels in skin over a mass. Treatment consists of observation
  - Strawberry (capillary) hemangioma: these intensely red lesions undergo a period of very rapid growth; complications may develop before regression
  - Congenital arteriovenous (AV) fistulas: multiple and diffuse lesions, 50% of which occur in the head and neck. Treatment consists of intermittent pneumatic compression and complete surgical resection
  - Arterial hemangioma: pulsatile masses that exhibit bruits or thrills and may be associated with sign bleeding or marked regional gigantism. Treatment consists of surgical resection of all AV shunts
  - Venous malformations (cavernous hemangioma): spongy, subcutaneous swellings with a bluish discoloration; these do not regress and may grow to gigantic size, causing disfigurement. Treat with injections of sclerosing agents (eg, tetradecyl sulfate)
  - Kasabach-Merritt syndrome: rapidly enlarging, solitary lesion that presents with hemolytic anemia, thrombocytopenia, and coagulopathy. Treat with interferon
  - Visceral hemangioma: most commonly occurs in the liver and manifests with hepatomegaly, anemia, coagulopathy, and high-output heart failure. Treatment is indicated for large and symptomatic lesions; use steroids, interferon, or embolization
- Diagnose with complete blood count, platelet count, computed tomography scan with intravenous (IV) contrast, magnetic resonance imaging (MRI), or angiogram (rarely indicated)
- Complications
  - Ulceration (most common complication)
  - Bleeding from ulceration
  - Cosmetic concerns
  - Infection
  - Platelet trapping (in Kasabach-Merritt syndrome)
  - Compromise of vital structures (eg, airway, eye)

- Disseminated intravascular coagulation after surgical resection
- Internal organ involvement
    - Liver: hepatomegaly, congestive heart failure
    - Lung: hemoptysis, recurrent pneumonia
    - Treatment for internal organ involvement includes administering prednisone or cyclophosphamide and performing hepatic artery embolization or ligation

- General treatment principles
    - True hemangiomas, if persistent, may require surgical excision
    - Observe uncomplicated hemangiomas
    - Provide compression
    - Sclerosis can provoke an inflammatory reaction, leading to fibrosis and obliteration of vascular channels; inject tetradecyl sulfate
    - Chemotherapy
        - Give steroids (oral or intralesional for periorbital hemangiomas; administer intravenously for life-threatening lesions or when patient's airway or vision are at risk)
        - Isolated cases have shown regression after receiving cyclophosphamide and interferon
    - Embolization can be useful in treating liver lesions and as a preoperative adjunct to surgical resection
    - Surgical treatment is only indicated for complications, including visual impairment, thrombocytopenia, luminal obstruction, uncontrollable ulceration, hemorrhage or infection, atypical growth, congestive heart failure (due to AV fistula), small lesions that can be easily excised, and vascular malformations (do not involute)
    - Laser (argon) treatment is especially useful for port-wine stains, but is not indicated for strawberry capillary or cavernous hemangiomas

Lymphangiomas

- The lymphatic vessels drain protein-rich fluid leaked from capillaries and return it to the blood. Lymph travels through the cisterna chyli, to the thoracic duct, and on to the left internal jugular vein at its junction with the subclavian vein.

Lymphangiomas develop as a result of abnormal embryologic development of the lymphatic system. Unlike hemangiomas, lymphangiomas do not regress spontaneously. Types include cystic hygroma and lymphedema

- Types of benign lymphatic tumors
  - Cystic hygroma (see Chapter 13, Face and Neck)
  - Lymphedema: an abnormal accumulation of lymphatic fluid in interstitial fluid due to abnormal development (aplasia or hypoplasia of lymphatic channels) or obstruction. There are three types: congenital (Milroy's disease; present at birth), praecox (appears in adolescence), and tarda (occurs in middle age)
    - Complications include infection (eg, lymphangitis, cellulitis) and lymphangiosarcoma
    - Diagnose using MRI and nuclear scans (lymphangiograms are rarely performed because of the risk of lymphangitis)
    - Nonsurgical treatment includes diuretics and compression stockings
    - Although staged excision of subcutaneous lesions and skin is sometimes undertaken, surgical treatment is rarely satisfactory

Venous Disorders

- Embryology: right umbilical vein regresses before birth (this may account for a gastroschisis defect occurring to the right of the umbilicus)
- AV malformations
  - Truncal malformations arise from major arterial branches. They are hemodynamically active with large communications, and often form on the upper extremities, head, or neck
  - Diffuse malformations have multiple small communications, are seldom hemodynamically active, and a bruit is common
  - Malformations are bright red, exhibit increased skin temperature, and manifest an audible bruit
  - Complications include bleeding, distal ischemia, and congestive heart failure
  - Diagnose by arteriography
  - Treatment can include surgical excision (high recurrence

rate), compression garments, selective embolization, and proximal ligation (contraindicated, but ligating multiple small feeding vessels may help)

- Congenital anomalies of central veins
  - Duplication of superior vena cava
  - Anomalous pulmonary venous return (total or partial)
    - Infant is cyanotic at birth and has a right-to-left shunt
    - Associated with atrioseptal defect
  - Absence of inferior vena cava, resulting in venous drainage through azygos system; associated with situs inversus
  - Preduodenal portal vein: often associated with duodenal anomalies and malrotation, but also associated with situs inversus
  - Diagnose above disorders with Doppler ultrasound
  - Treat thrombotic complications of congenital anomalies of central veins with heparin anticoagulation or, in the case of acute thrombosis of major veins that is life- or organ-threatening, use thromboplastin

Arterial Disorders

- AV malformations (AVMs)
  - Usually occur in lower limbs and are associated with unilateral limb hypertrophy (hemihypertrophy)
  - A hepatic AVM in a newborn may produce congestive heart failure
  - Intestinal AVM may produce bleeding
  - Physical findings include increased warmth, swelling, and pulsating varicosities
  - Diagnose by Doppler ultrasound, angiography, or MRI
  - Treat by surgical resection (if possible), compression, excision, or angiographic embolization
- Visceral aneurysms (rare)
  - Most common in the renal and splenic arteries
  - Treat by resection and reanastamosis if the aneurysm is >2 cm

Connective Tissue Disorders

- Marfan syndrome
  - Physical findings include tall, thin, body habitus, arachnodactyly and lens dislocation
  - Symptoms include inguinal hernias, spontaneous pneu-

mothorax, pectus carinatum, and aneurysms of the ascending aorta, which results from cystic medial necrosis that ruptures the intima and initiates aortic dissection (sudden aortic insufficiency is a common early manifestation of aneurysm)

- Acquired disorders
    - Kawasaki disease: manifested by skin rash, erythema, edema of the hands and feet, arthritis, cervical adenopathy, and conjunctivitis and aneurysms of the coronary and peripheral arteries
    - Thrombi and emboli: occur in infants of diabetic mothers and manifest with dehydration and polycythemia, which may produce a state of hyperviscosity and result in thrombosis
        - Umbilical artery catheters may be associated with aortic and renal artery thrombosis that leads to hypertension and heart failure
        - Treat with heparin, hydration, and, in some cases, total parenteral nutrition
- Occlusive syndromes
    - Intracranial and extracranial arteries (eg, sickle-cell disease, which is the most common cause of stroke in children)
    - Renal artery stenosis (resulting from fibromuscular dysplasia)
        - Symptoms include hypertension producing headache, visual disturbance, and congestive heart failure
        - Second most common cause of surgically correctable hypertension (coarctation is first)
        - Usually bilateral
        - Diagnose using aortogram with renal angiography
        - Treat with reconstruction using a hypogastric artery graft from aorta to distal renal artery
            - Saphenous vein grafts are contraindicated because of the potential for aneurysmal dilatation when used in children
            - Transaortic balloon dilatation may be effective if stenosis is in branches, but not if stenosis is at a renal orifice (eg, ostium)

Traumatic Vascular Injury

- Due to the laxity of soft tissue, vascular injuries in children may be associated with greater blood loss from third spacing as compared to adults; collateral blood flow is also more extensive in children because of the lack of atherosclerotic narrowing in their vessel lumens

- Vasospasm is common. Carefully perform a thrombectomy with a small Fogarty balloon and continuously flush repair with heparinized (1 unit/mL) saline and papaverine (30–60 mg in 100 cc)
- Computed tomography angiography with 3-dimensional reconstruction may be useful to detect occult vascular injury and avoid conventional angiography
- Catheter-directed angiography is useful for localizing injuries with abnormal physical examinations (ankle-brachial index < 0.9) or soft signs of injury; hard signs of injury (eg, expanding hematoma, pulselessness, bruit or thrill) should be explored
- The greater saphenous vein makes an ideal conduit, although small vessel size may contribute to technical challenges or necessitate a panel or spiral graft
    - Blood vessels will grow with the patient, so an autogenous graft with an interrupted suture line is favored over prosthetic conduits of fixed diameter
    - The most common injured vessels are the brachial, superficial femoral, and popliteal arteries (Tables 16-1 and 16-2)
- A primary end-to-end anastomosis has the best patency and

Table 16-1. Arteries to Ligate Versus Arteries to Reconstruct

Arteries That May Routinely Be Ligated	Arteries That Should Be Reconstructed
Digital, radial or ulnar (not both, preserve ulnar when possible)	Common/internal carotid
External carotid	Subclavian
Brachial (if distal to profunda and adequate signal is present at wrist)	Axillary
Subclavian branches	Brachial (if there is no Doppler signal at the wrist)
Internal iliac and profunda femoral arteries*	Common iliac
	External iliac
	Superficial femoral
	Popliteal
	Tibioperoneal trunk
	Celiac
	Superior mesenteric

*Preserve at least one tibial vessel. The posterior tibial artery is the most critical to repair, followed by the dorsalis pedis and the peroneal arteries, respectively.

Table 16-2. Veins to Ligate Versus Veins to Reconstruct

Veins That May Routinely Be Ligated	Veins That Should Be Reconstructed
Internal and external jugular	Popliteal for prevention of extremity venous hypertension and potential for compartment syndrome
Brachiocephalic	Common and external iliac, if time and patient condition permits
Left renal	Portal vein
Infrarenal inferior vena cava (to control damage)	Right renal vein
Internal iliac	
Tibialis	
Mesenteric	
Subclavian	

can be performed when segmental loss is limited to < 2 cm; a patch repair is an option when > 50% of the native wall is preserved to avoid a residual stenosis

- Classic extremity fractures that contribute to vascular injury are those in the humerus (brachial artery), tibial plateau, and proximal tibia (tibioperoneal trunk)
- A continuous Doppler assessment should always confirm the pulse examination; an ankle-brachial index < 0.9 is abnormal and should be investigated; C-arm and fluoroscopy units should be available for focal vascular visualization, but complete angiography is rarely necessary
- Micropuncture needles with intrinsic guide wires are helpful for emergent arterial and venous access
- Assess grafts for flow every 3 months for 2 years, then biannually for 3 years, and then annually for life
- Intraluminal shunts may be used as a temporizing measure to prevent tissue ischemia, with revision if patient demonstrates symptoms of ischemia
- Revascularization of an extremity after > 6 hours of ischemia necessitates a fasciotomy
- Common technical pitfalls
  - Excessive graft length, resulting in kinking and graft thrombosis
  - Inadequate graft length, resulting in anastomosis disruption
  - Failure to adequately cover the graft with viable soft tissue,

  leading to desiccation and disruption
  - A break in sterile technique, resulting in graft infection
  - Inadequate debridement may create an intimal flap, leading to occlusion
  - Poor distal runoff, resulting in occlusion or vasospasm
  - Inadequate immobilization of the associated bony injury, resulting in graft disruption
  - Failure to prevent, recognize, or treat a compartment syndrome after revascularization, resulting in graft occlusion and tissue loss from ischemia
- Postoperative management (all records should include time of observation and name of observer)
  - Frequently monitor distal pulses by palpitation and Doppler ultrasound
  - Assess capillary filling, warmth, and sensation
  - Monitor for hematoma formation
  - Observe for compartment syndrome

Chapter 17

Abdominal Wall, Peritoneum, and Diaphragm

Abdominal Wall Defects

- Gastroschisis (Greek for "belly cleft")
  - Bowel is histologically normal, but thickened and shortened due to prolonged contact with amnionic fluid; these changes are reversible with time and after reduction into the abdominal cavity
  - Defect is almost always to the right of the umbilical cord (which is normally positioned) and separated from it by a skin bridge
  - Midgut, stomach, and gonads are the most commonly herniated organs (liver rarely herniates in gastroschisis)
  - There is no sac covering the herniated viscera
  - Malrotation is always present (in both gastroschisis and omphalocele)
  - Associated anomalies are rare (except intestinal atresia)
- Omphalocele
  - In most cases, the bowel is covered by an intact membrane, from which the umbilical cord arises (ie, herniation into the base of the umbilical cord) so gastrointestinal tract function is usually normal; in a "ruptured" omphalocele, the membrane is not intact
  - Malrotation is present
  - Often contains liver
- Incidence
  - Gastroschisis-to-omphalocele ratio: 2–3:1
  - Both are associated with prematurity
- Anomalies
  - Gastroschisis
    - Associated conditions
      - Undescended testicles (common)
      - Atresias due to vascular compression in utero

        - Hypoperistalsis
        - Necrotizing enterocolitis
  - Omphalocele
    - 60% have associated abnormalities (cardiac and chromosomal; eg, trisomy 13, 18, or 21)
    - Associated with Beckwith-Wiedemann syndrome, which can result in:
      - Macroglossia, which may cause airway problems
      - Visceral hypertrophy (cardiomegaly, pancreatic β-cell hyperplasia that results in hypoglycemia)
    - Associated with Meckel's diverticulum, gastrointestinal tract duplications, and ambiguous genitalia
    - Increased association of malignant tumors (Wilms, neuroblastoma, adrenal)
- Diagnosis: prenatal ultrasound (> 13 wk) is usually accurate
- Delivery: vaginal delivery is not associated with more complications than cesarean delivery, with the exception of large omphaloceles
- Treatment
  - General
    - Set orogastric tube to low suction
    - Use a "bowel bag" or plastic cling film to conserve body heat, minimize evaporative heat loss, and prevent traction or twisting of the mesenteric blood supply—the most important aspects of pretransport and preoperative preparation
    - Antibiotics
      - Ampicillin (100 mg/kg/day)
      - Gentamicin (5–7 mg/kg/day)
    - Intravenous (IV) fluids
      - 20 cc/kg Ringer's lactate or 5% albumin
      - 150–175 cc/kg Ringer's lactate during the first 24 hours
      - If not adequately hydrated, the child may become hypotensive on induction of anesthesia due to hypovolemia
    - Vitamin K
      - Premature infant: 0.5 mg intramuscular (IM)
      - Full-term infant: 1 mg IM

- Omphalocele and gastroschisis
  - Steps for primary closure
    - Excise the sac (except if attached to liver)
    - Inspect the umbilical cord and number of umbilical arteries (presence of a single artery may be associated with an absent kidney)
    - Inspect the bowel for atresias or perforations
    - Manually stretch the abdominal wall
    - In gastroschisis, if a larger opening is required to reduce the herniated viscera, open the fascia cephalad in the midline
    - Manually extrude meconium from the colon after anal dilatation and saline irrigations (**do not** perform an enterotomy to evacuate meconium)
    - A silicon-plastic silo or bioprosthetic may be used to retain the herniated viscera
    - Do not excise a Meckel's diverticulum
    - The liver must be reduced carefully to avoid torsion of the hepatic veins or occlusion of portal vein inflow that results in hemodynamic instability and injury to capsule
    - Complications of an excessively tight closure include:
      - Respiratory insufficiency (secondary to excessive pressure on the diaphragm; peak inspiratory pressure should be < 35 cm H_2O after fascial closure, abdominal compartment pressure should be < 15 cm)
      - Vena cava compression, resulting in decreased venous return
      - Decreased renal vein flow, resulting in decreased glomerular filtration rate
      - Decreased mesenteric artery flow, resulting in bowel ischemia (an immediate primary repair in an infant with respiratory distress syndrome is **contraindicated** due to resultant high mortality)
      - If there is any question about bowel viability, place a silo and perform a second look in 12–24 hours
      - **Do not** attempt definitive repair until chromosomal abnormalities and possible cardiac defects have been evaluated

        - Delayed primary closure
            - Sew silicon-plastic or Gore-Tex (WL Gore & Associates, Inc, Newark, Del) sheets to the edges of the fascia; a silicon-plastic bag (with an integrated spring to hold the base open) can also be used, and does not require suturing
            - Gradually reduce the silo over several days
            - Remove the silo and perform primary fascial closure after about 7 days
            - Allow the sac (which must be intact) to thicken and epithelialization to occur before applying escharotic or desiccating agents
                - Use Acticoat (Smith & Nephew, London, England) dressing and change every 4–5 days
                - Povidone-iodine may be associated with iodine absorption and suppression of thyroid-stimulating hormone
                - 0.5% silver nitrate may be associated with hyponatremia
                - Apply silver sulfadiazine twice a day for 2 weeks, and perform primary skin closure in about 2 months
                - Indications for applying escharotic agents include suspected chromosomal syndromes (eg, trisomy 13 or 18); severe, unstable cardiac defects (eg, hypoplastic left heart, hypoplastic aortic arch); and, in premature infants, hyaline membrane disease, primary pulmonary hypertension, and sepsis
    - Intestinal atresia
        - Conserve bowel when feasible
        - Perform ileostomy
- Postoperative considerations
    - Respiratory: ventilator support for 48–72 hours, pharmacological paralysis (using pancuronium bromide)
    - Provide total parenteral nutrition (TPN) until full enteral feeds can be resumed
        - Normal intestinal absorption may be delayed for weeks
        - Dysmotility problems may persist for weeks to months

        - If gastrointestinal contrast studies show no evidence of obstruction, do not operate; operating will only create new adhesions
        - Place a gastronomy tube, continue TPN, administer physical therapy for sucking, give erythromycin to increase motility, and be patient
  - Administer 5% albumin infusions as needed
  - Give antibiotics until the silicon-plastic silo has been removed
  - Patient may experience increased gastroesophageal reflux due to increased intraabdominal pressure; this rarely requires fundoplication
  - After successful skin closure of a giant omphalocele, a ventral hernia repair may be associated with hemodynamic instability due to hepatic venous anatomy
- Long-term complications
  - Stricture may result in a small-bowel obstruction
  - Ventral hernia
  - Undescended testicles
- Survival depends on prematurity, size of the defect, and severity of associated anomalies

Disorders of the Umbilicus

- Umbilical drainage
  - Omphalitis
    - Etiology
      - Poor hygiene
      - Most commonly caused by *Staphylococcus aureus*
      - *Clostridium perfringens* (purple wound) is rare, but is associated with high mortality
    - May result in portal vein thrombosis, leading to portal hypertension and, eventually, to upper gastrointestinal bleeding (treated nonoperatively)
  - Granuloma
    - Small: treat with silver nitrate
    - Large: treat by surgical excision (electrocautery)
  - Polyp
    - Physical appearance: glistening, cherry-red nodule

- Pathology: vitelline duct remnant consisting of a small piece of intestinal mucosa
- Treatment: surgical excision with central core of umbilicus (**silver nitrate does not work!**)

- Persistence of vitelline duct structures: omphalomesenteric sinus, fistula, Meckel's diverticulum, cysts, bands

- Urachal sinus
  - Definition: cord-like, mucosal-lined structure extending from the dome of the bladder to the lower border of the umbilical ring
  - Symptoms: urinary fistula
  - Associated conditions
    - Bladder outlet obstruction (eg, posterior urethral valves)
    - Recurrent cystitis
  - Diagnosis: voiding cystourethrogram
  - Treatment: excision of entire tract down to the bladder via an infraumbilical incision
- Urachal cyst
  - May occur anywhere along urachal tract, from the umbilicus to the bladder
  - Symptoms: enlarging suprapubic or infraumbilical mass, which may become infected, resulting in an urachal abscess
  - Diagnosis: ultrasound, voiding cystourethrogram
  - Treatment: drain abscess, excise cyst (infraumbilical incision) after infection is resolved
- Patent omphalomesenteric sinus
  - Etiology: persistent vitelline duct, usually at the site of a Meckel's diverticulum (located in the ileum)
  - Symptoms
    - Contents of small bowel draining through the umbilicus
    - Obliterated cord may become fixed to the umbilicus and may be associated with a closed-loop intestinal obstruction
  - Diagnosis: ultrasound, sinogram
  - Treatment: surgical excision via an infraumbilical excision
- Umbilical hernias
  - Most occur through the umbilical vein (cephalad) portion of the ring, where the cicatricial scar is less dense
  - Most important factors in assessing likelihood of closure

include:

    - Age of the patient
    - Size of the fascial defect (fascial defects > 1.5 cm are unlikely to close after 4–5 years of age)
  - Indications for operation
    - Absolute: incarceration (rare in infants), strangulation, evisceration
    - Relative: fascial defect persisting after age 5, a herniation that is proboscis-like (repair at 2 years)
  - Repair technique
    - Infraumbilical incision
    - Excision of the sac
    - Transverse fascial closure
    - Attachment of fascial skin to underlying fascia
    - Pressure dressing for 72 hours to prevent a hematoma
- Epigastric hernia
  - Location: linea alba above the umbilicus
  - Etiology: congenital fascial defect
  - Pathology: protrusion of preperitoneal fat
  - Symptoms: pain, tenderness
  - Physical appearance: small, palpable, irreducible mass in the midline (usually supraumbilical, often multiple)
  - Treatment: operative repair via transverse incision
- Spigelian hernia
  - Location: between semilunar line and lateral border of the rectus sheath
  - Physical appearance: prominent when patient is crying and straining
  - Sac may contain omentum or bowel
  - Diagnosis: computed tomography (CT) scan, ultrasound
  - Treatment: surgical repair

Inguinal Disorders

- Anatomy
  - Processus vaginalis
    - Defined as peritoneal diverticulum that extends through the internal inguinal ring
    - In an indirect hernia, hernia sac is anterior and medial to the cord structures, lateral to the epigastric vessels

- Communicating hydrocele
  - Defined as intraperitoneal fluid that has tracked down the patent processus vaginalis into the tunica vaginalis
  - In females, a hydrocele may occur along the round ligament (canal of Nuck), presenting as a bulge or mass in the labia majora
- Incidence of inguinal hernias
  - ~ 3% overall
  - Male:Female ratio = 10:1
  - Right = 50%; left = 25%; bilateral = 15%, due to later descent of the right testis and delayed obliteration of the processus vaginalis
  - Increased in premature infants (~ 20% incidence)
  - Increased-risk patients include those with cystic fibrosis, chronic lung disease, connective tissue disease, and those on peritoneal dialysis or with a ventriculoperitoneal shunt
  - Treatment: routine bilateral explorations are recommended
  - Direct and femoral hernias are rare in children
- Hydrocele
  - Noncommunicating hydroceles usually resolve by 12 months of age; if not, they should be considered hernias and repaired
  - Diagnosis
    - Usually absent upon waking, and most prominent once the child is ambulatory due to movement of intraperitoneal fluid through the processus (resulting from gravity)
    - Transillumination or ultrasound
  - Treatment (if hydrocele is present after 12 months of age)
    - Ligate patent processus vaginalis, excise hydrocele
    - Aspiration is not recommended
      - If the processus is patent, the hydrocele will recur
      - If the hydrocele is encysted, it will resolve spontaneously
- Symptoms of inguinal disorders
  - Indirect hernia (most common)
    - Groin bulge extending toward the top of the scrotum
    - A palpable mass in a female in the labia majora usually represents an ovary (if the mass is bilateral, suspect tes-

ticular feminization syndrome; strangulation is rare)
    - Visibility is better during periods of increased intraabdominal pressure (eg, crying, stooling)
    - Cord thickens as it crosses pubic tubercle ("silk glove" sign)
    - Hernia sac is anteromedial to cord structures and lateral to the epigastric artery and vein
  - Direct hernia
    - Rare in children
    - May result from an injury to the floor of the inguinal canal during a previous hernia operation
    - Occurs medial to epigastric vessels
  - Hydrocele
    - Communicating: intermittent scrotal swelling
    - Noncommunicating: remains the same size
- General principles of treatment
  - Patients needing treatment include:
    - Those with a hernia on physical examination, or with a convincing history consistent with a hernia
    - Patients who present with incarcerated hernias that can be reduced; these should be admitted and have semielective repair before discharge (waiting 24 hours from time of reduction to operation permits edema to subside)
    - Hernias in premature infants (usually indirect) should be repaired prior to the child's discharge
    - If a patient has an undescended testicle at the time of hernia repair, perform an orchiopexy at the same time
    - Infants < 50 weeks old (corrected gestational age) who were premature should be admitted for overnight observation postoperatively to monitor for residual effects of anesthesia (apnea and bradycardia)
    - Excise an appendix testis to prevent torsion
- Complications
  - Incarceration: sac contents (usually bowel) cannot be reduced nonoperatively
    - Most common in infants < 1 year old
    - Symptoms
      - Severe irritability
      - Cramping abdominal pain

        - Vomiting
    - Physical manifestation: firm, nontender mass in groin
    - Pathology
        - Decreased venous/lymph drainage increases edema and pressure
        - This leads to decreased arterial perfusion and eventual gangrene and necrosis, which presents as scrotal redness, edema, or a mass (strangulation)
    - Treatment
        - Attempt reduction
            - Sedate (using midazolam 0.05–0.1 mg/kg, or chloral hydrate)
            - Elevate the lower body
            - Apply ice to the hernia sac
        - If nonoperative reduction is successful, admit the patient for repair in 24 hours
        - If nonoperative reduction is unsuccessful, perform immediate operative reduction
        - If patient's bowel is infarcted, perform a resection through the groin incision if possible; if not, perform a laparotomy
    - Complications of incarceration
        - Gonadal infarction
        - Intestinal obstruction
        - Gangrenous bowel
            - Physical appearance: erythematous scrotum
            - Attempts at reduction are usually unsuccessful
    - Recurrence
        - A direct hernia may occur at the site of repair of a previous indirect hernia if there has been an intraoperative injury to the floor of the inguinal canal
        - Excessively tight closure of the internal inguinal ring can result in recurrence
            - Symptoms: tender, swollen testis
            - Treatment: reexploration and inspection of the testis

Disorders of the Peritoneum and Peritoneal Cavity

- Abdominal compartment syndrome
    - Etiology: increased intraabdominal pressure due to an

inflammatory process (eg, perforated appendix) or any space-occupying condition (eg, bleeding, edema) that increases the volume of the abdomen

- Symptoms
  - Sepsis
  - Respiratory distress due to pressure on the diaphragm
  - Oliguria due to renal vein compression
  - Hypotension due to compression of vena cava and decreased venous return
  - Vasomotor changes
  - Acidosis due to hypoperfusion
- Physical appearance: abdominal distension
- Diagnosis: intraabdominal pressure > 20 cm H_2O, as determined by measuring bladder pressures
- Treatment
  - Assisted ventilation
  - IV fluids
  - Treatment of underlying cause
  - Abdominal decompression using a silo or wound vacuum device

- Meconium peritonitis
  - Frequently associated with cystic fibrosis as the etiology of obstruction
  - Types
    - Pseudocyst: meconium is contained by necrotic bowel and omentum; cyst wall is lined with calcium
    - Plastic: free perforation causes marked generalized inflammatory reaction and adhesions
    - Generalized: prenatal perforation with continuing leak produces meconium ascites
  - Etiology
    - Intrauterine volvulus of meconium-filled loop of bowel, leading to intestinal vascular compromise
    - This results in bowel ischemia then atresia, which leads to obstruction and, finally, perforation
  - Symptoms: polyhydramnios, abdominal distension, and bilious vomiting
  - Diagnosis
    - Prenatal ultrasound shows polyhydramnios, dilated

bowel loops, or calcifications
    - Abdominal radiograph shows dilated loops of intestine and intraabdominal calcifications (linear calcifications may line the processus vaginalis and scrotum)
  - Treatment
    - For obstruction or pneumoperitoneum, perform laparotomy with conservative resection
    - In asymptomatic cases, observe patient closely
- Omental and mesenteric cysts
  - Pathology: usually lymphangiomas
  - Symptoms: pain, vomiting, and abdominal mass
  - Diagnosis: CT scan or ultrasound
  - Treatment: excision
- Ascites
  - Etiology
    - Urinary tract malformation (eg, ureteropelvic junction obstruction, posterior urethral valves) resulting in obstruction (most common etiology in the neonate)
    - Immune hydrops (Rh incompatibility, cardiac anomalies)
    - Pancreatitis
    - Ovarian cyst or tumor
    - Chyle due to lymphatic abnormality
  - Treat underlying abnormality
- Peritoneal adhesions
  - Immediate postoperative bowel obstruction is usually due to small bowel intussusception
  - Diagnosis: upper gastrointestinal study with small bowel follow through
  - Treatment (initial): nasogastric tube, IV fluids, antibiotics, laparotomy with adhesion lysis for complete obstruction

Congenital Diaphragmatic Hernia

- General
  - Normal openings in the diaphragm occur at the aorta, vena cava, and esophagus
  - Late-onset diaphragmatic hernias
    - Diagnosis: chest radiograph in an asymptomatic patient
    - Symptoms

      - Gastrointestinal obstruction
      - Respiratory distress (severe hypercarbia, hypoxia)
    - Treatment: repair
    - Differential diagnosis: congenital cystic adenomatoid malformation, sequestration
  - Defects
    - Esophageal hiatus (Morgagni): stomach prolapses into the mediastinum
    - Congenital posterolateral defect (Bochdalek)
    - Anomalous attachment of diaphragm to sternum and ribs
    - Epigastric omphalocele and retrosternal defect in the diaphragm and pericardium (Pentalogy of Cantrell), producing herniation within the pericardium
    - Attenuation of the tendinous or muscular portion of the diaphragm produces eventration (phrenic nerve injury)
  - Incidence
    - Associated with malrotation
    - Occurs more frequently in females than males
    - Occurs most often on the left (90%)
- Diagnosis
  - Prenatal diagnosis
    - Polyhydramnios (75%)
    - Associated with major central nervous system, cardiac, and chromosomal abnormalities (eg, trisomy 13 and 18); many are stillborn
  - Postnatal diagnosis
    - View prenatal ultrasound
    - Chest radiograph will show tip of the nasogastric tube to be above diaphragm, indicating herniation of the viscera into the chest and a mediastinum shift
    - Rule out associated abnormalities (occur in 15%–25% of cases) in the following:
      - Central nervous system: head, spine (meningomyelocele)
      - Heart (most common): patent ductus arteriosus, ventricular septal defect
      - Kidneys
      - Lung: sequestration (occurring most commonly in left lower lobe)

  - Rule out chromosomal (trisomy 13) and metabolic abnormalities
- Pathophysiology
  - Herniated viscus becomes distended with air, displacing the mediastinum
  - Increased pulmonary artery pressure and pulmonary vascular resistance resulting from decreased pulmonary artery branches and thickened muscularis of bronchioles
  - A right-to-left shunt through a patent ductus arteriosus and the foramen ovale results in hypoxia, hypercarbia, and acidosis; these lead to increased pulmonary vasoconstriction
  - Acidosis and hypercarbia lead to pulmonary vasodilation
  - Alkalosis and hypocarbia lead to pulmonary vasoconstriction
- Physical appearance
  - Respiratory distress is evident by grunting, flaring, retracting, and cyanosis
  - Scaphoid abdomen
  - Shifted heart sounds, decreased bowel sounds
  - Tracheal deviation
  - Bilateral pulmonary hypoplasia (more severe on the side of herniation)
- Treatment
  - Support spontaneous respiration; provide sedation with paralysis only if necessary
  - Endotracheal intubation (avoid bag-mask ventilation to prevent insufflation of air into the stomach and small bowel)
  - Insert repogle nasogastric tube
  - Ventilatory settings
    - Peak inspiratory pressure < 25 cm H_2O
    - Positive end expiratory pressure < 6 cm H_2O (to minimize barotrauma)
    - 100% oxygen
    - Adjust rate and inspiratory–expiratory ratio to maximize partial pressure of oxygen (PaO_2), decrease partial pressure of carbon dioxide ($PaCO_2$)
    - Maintain pH > 7.20 (permissive hypercapnea)
  - Place umbilical venous catheter, umbilical arterial catheter (postductal), or right radial A line (preductal)

- When placing an umbilical arterial catheter, ideal arterial blood gas levels should be as follows: $PaO_2 > 40$ mmHg, $PaCO_2 < 30$, pH > 7.5

◦ Administer sodium bicarbonate or trimethamine drip
◦ Provide volume replacement (Ringer's lactate or 5% albumin)
◦ Maintain oxygen content between aorta and right atrium < 5%

Oxygen content (CaO_2) = (SaO_2 × HgB × 1.34) + .003(PaO_2)

SaO_2: arterial oxygen saturation

PaO_2: mixed venous oxygen saturation

◦ Maintain mixed venous (from right atrium) saturation > 65%
◦ Administer dopamine / dobutamine as needed
◦ Tolazoline enhances histamine release, but can result in hypotension and peptic ulcers
◦ Nitric oxide (an endothelium-derived relaxing factor), which decreases pulmonary vasoconstriction, may be helpful
◦ Perform surgical repair after pulmonary hypertension has resolved
◦ Appropriate pulmonary vasodilators to administer include prostaglandin E1 and E2; appropriate pulmonary vasoconstrictors include prostaglandin F, thromboxane A1 and B2, and leukotrienes

- Surgical repair
  - Perform when patient is physiologically stable, not as an emergency measure
  - A diaphragmatic hernia is not an indication for fetal surgery
  - Administer general anesthesia (eg, pancuronium)
  - Make a subcostal abdominal incision for right-sided or left-sided defects or thoracoscopy
  - Reduce herniated viscera by excising sac; a hernia sac is present in 10%–20% of patients and may be easily missed
  - Primary repair
    - Small defect: use pledgets
    - Large defect: use bioprosthetic or synthetic prosthesis
  - Place a thoracostomy tube to underwater seal
  - A purple-brown mass near or in the left lower lobe may represent a sequestration
    - Blood is usually supplied from a branch of the abdomi-

nal aorta below the diaphragm
    - Treatment consists of excision with repair of the diaphragm
- Postoperative care
  - Administer IV fluids (dopamine or dobutamine may be added)
  - Anticipate pneumothorax
- Results
  - Overall mortality ~ 50% (unchanged for past 20 y)
  - Prognosis is determined by the degree of hypoplasia
  - Lung volumes approach equality on a ventilation/perfusion scan
  - Residual volume and functional residual capacity are increased
  - Vital capacity, forced expiratory volume, and minute ventilation volume are normal or slightly decreased

Eventration of the Diaphragm
- Most common cause is injury to the phrenic nerve from stretching of the neck at the time of birth or from direct operative trauma
- Symptoms
  - Inspiration leads to negative intrathoracic pressure, which causes herniation of viscera into the ipsilateral chest
  - This leads to mediastinum shift to the contralateral side, which results in respiratory distress and/or pneumonia
  - Occurs more frequently in the left diaphragm than the right
- Diagnosis
  - Chest radiograph will show elevated hemidiaphragm
  - Fluoroscopy of the diaphragm or ultrasound shows elevated diaphragm with paradoxical motion
  - Differential diagnosis: congenital diaphragmatic hernia with hernia sac
- Treatment
  - Intubation with assisted ventilation initially
  - Perform transthoracic (seventh intercostal space) plication **only** if patient is symptomatic (ie, ventilator support required for > 2 wk)

Chapter 18

Gastrointestinal Tract

Esophageal Conditions

- Tracheoesophageal fistula (TEF) and esophageal atresia (EA)
  - Symptoms
    - Copious salivation (drooling) and aspiration at first feeding
    - Choking, coughing, respiratory distress, and atelectasis
    - Aspiration of acidic gastric secretions results in chemical pneumonia (the most common cause of death)
    - Abdominal distention as the stomach fills with air passing through the TEF
  - Diagnosis
    - In a newborn, a nasogastric (NG) tube (radiopaque) cannot be passed into the stomach and polyhydramnios is evident (more common with a pure atresia)
    - A bowel gas pattern can be seen on a chest radiograph and plain abdominal radiographs
      - Pure atresia will present with a gasless abdomen
      - A fistula between the trachea and esophagus appears as a gas-filled stomach and bowel
    - A contrast swallow is not indicated unless the diagnosis cannot be established by other means
    - A chest radiograph shows the NG tube curled in the blind upper esophageal pouch
  - Initial treatment
    - Give nothing by mouth
    - Pass an NG tube (Repogle sump type, low suction)
    - Provide intravenous (IV) fluids
    - Elevate the patient's head to minimize aspiration
    - Administer antibiotics
    - Evaluate for associated vertebral, anorectal, cardiac, tracheoesophageal fistula, renal, and radial limb (VACTERRL) anomalies
    - Take plain radiographs to rule out vertebral and limb

anomalies
      - Perform an echocardiogram to define anatomy
      - Perform a renal ultrasound to detect anomalies
      - Operative repair is best performed at a tertiary medical facility
- Corrosive injury of the esophagus
   - Strong liquid alkalis (hydroscopic) are the most common cause of corrosive injury to the esophagus, coagulating protein and causing liquefaction necrosis (solids are more difficult to swallow and are usually expectorated). Agents become firmly attached to a moist mucosal surface and may involve the entire thickness of the esophageal wall, but perforation is rare
   - Common injury-causing agents
      - Potassium hydroxide, sodium hydroxide, and sulfuric acid are associated with severe injury
      - Sodium hypochlorite (bleach) and detergents seldom cause clinically significant injuries
   - Injury to the esophagus is much more common than injury to the stomach in alkali burns, but acidic corrosives will injure the stomach by coagulation necrosis
   - Symptoms
      - Vomiting
      - Dysphagia
      - Drooling, inability to swallow saliva
      - Abdominal or upper abdominal pain
      - Burns of the mouth or pharynx
   - Diagnosis
      - Perform esophagogastroduodenoscopy using a flexible endoscope, with the patient under general anesthesia, within 24 hours of injury
         - This is the most accurate means of identifying the extent and severity of the burn
         - Injured areas appear as a whitish coagulum surrounded by an area of hyperemia
         - The endoscope should be passed only up to (but not through) the level of injury
         - Avoid instrumentation after 24–36 hours following injury

        - Remember that deep, circumferential burns have a high incidence of stricture
    - Cineesophagram is the most accurate means of assessing the extent of esophageal injury and motility and can help predict later stricture formation
    - Perform chest and abdominal radiographs
- Treatment
    - If patient does not have a burn, discharge with follow-up in 3–4 weeks
    - If patient has a minimum to moderate burn, give antibiotics (ampicillin and gentamicin) and perform esophagram within 48 hours
    - If motility is undisturbed:
        - Give clear liquids for 72 hours
        - Advance to regular diet
        - Stop antibiotics on the 14th day
        - Discharge with regular follow-ups on the 21st day
    - In severe cases:
        - Pass a string at the time of esophagogastroduodenoscopy
        - Place a gastrostomy tube
        - Steroids have no therapeutic value; give antibiotics (ampicillin, 150 mg/kg/day)
        - If the cineesophagram is normal:
            - Give nothing by mouth until the patient can swallow saliva, then clear liquids; advance to a regular diet
            - Stop antibiotics and repeat the contrast swallow; discharge if normal on the 21st day
        - If the cineesophagram is abnormal:
            - Give nothing by mouth until a gastrostomy tube can be used
            - On the 21st day, stop antibiotics and repeat contrast swallow; if swallow is normal, discharge with monthly follow-up for 1 year; if a stricture is present, start dilatations
    - Long-term complications
        - Stricture (treat with monthly dilatations for 1 y)
        - Achalasia

        - Squamous cell carcinoma (latency may be > 20 y)
- Esophageal perforation
    - Etiology is most commonly iatrogenic
    - Symptoms
        - Respiratory distress (newborns and infants)
        - Drooling
        - Subcutaneous emphysema
        - Substernal chest pain
        - Septic shock
        - Pleural effusion
    - Diagnosis
        - Chest radiograph will show pneumothorax, pneumoperitoneum, pneumomediastinum, and pleural effusion
        - Perform contrast study with water-soluble contrast
    - Treatment
        - For traumatic perforation of the cervical esophagus in a newborn, place an NG tube and give broad-spectrum antibiotics
        - For submucosal perforation of the intrathoracic esophagus with symptoms of mediastinitis (increased temperature, increased white blood count):
            - Perform left posterolateral thoracotomy at the sixth intercostal space (for a low esophageal perforations)
            - Administer broad-spectrum antibiotics
            - Perform primary repair of the esophagus if the perforation is < 24 hours old (interpose pericardial, pleural, or strap muscle patch)
            - Place a chest tube for mediastinal drainage
        - For submucosal perforation of the intrathoracic esophagus without symptoms of mediastinitis, antibiotics alone are often sufficient
        - If the perforation is > 24 hours old with marked contamination, treat as above and perform end cervical esophagostomy and gastrostomy; provide mediastinal drainage
- Gastroesophageal reflux
    - Antireflux barriers
        - Several anatomic factors serve as antireflux barriers, including the sling formed by right crus of the diaphragm, the phrenoesophageal membrane, the Angle of Hiss

(formed by the sharp angle between the lower esophagus and the gastric fundus), and the rosette-like configuration of gastric mucosa
    - Physiologic factors that serve as antireflux barriers include the high-pressure zone, which includes the intraabdominal esophagus and a segment of the supradiaphragmatic thoracic esophagus
    - The intraabdominal length of the esophagus (3–4 cm is optimal), intraabdominal pressure, and hormonal and pharmacological factors can also serve as antireflux barriers
- Etiology: reflux is normal in infants until 10–15 months of age, when children assume a more upright posture, ingest a more solid diet, and develop increased lower esophageal sphincter tone
- Symptoms
    - Recurrent vomiting with failure to thrive, coughing, stridor, and laryngospasm
    - Recurrent aspiration pneumonia
    - Asthma-like symptoms
    - Esophagitis (occult blood loss causing iron-deficient anemia; may result in eventual stricture)
    - Apnea, sudden infant death syndrome, retrosternal burning (older children)
    - Sandifer syndrome (voluntary contortions of the head, neck, and trunk associated with reflux esophagitis, producing iron-deficiency anemia)
- Diagnosis
    - Use cineesophagram, contrast swallow, upper gastrointestinal (UGI) series, or gastric emptying scan
    - Perform esophagoscopy with biopsies (to diagnose esophagitis and Barrett esophagus)
    - 24-hour pH-probe testing is the preferred diagnostic study; esophageal pH should be < 4.0, $< 4\%$ of the probe test time
    - Use a radioisotope "milk scan" to assess gastric emptying time; the normal quantity emptied over 1 hour should be greater than 30%; over 2 hours, quantity emptied should be $> 80\%$

- Perform esophageal manometry
- Nonsurgical treatment (80% success rate)
  - Thicken feedings
  - Position patient upright
  - Give bethanechol or metoclopramide (0.1 mg/kg/dose, bid–qid before meals) to increase lower esophageal sphincter tone, oral erythromycin (2–3 mg/kg/dose before meals), an antacid or H2-blockers (eg, ranitidine) to decrease acidity, and proton pump inhibitors (eg, omeprazole)
  - Give frequent, small-volume feeds
- Treatment (surgical)
  - Nissen fundoplication (360° wrap)
    - Indications
      - Esophageal stricture (especially if it occurs following a TEF repair and does not respond to dilatations)
      - Severe esophagitis (especially with secondary anemia)
      - Barrett's metaplasia (a metaplasia of esophageal mucosa resulting from chronic irritation secondary to gastroesophageal [GE] reflux)
      - Recurrent aspiration pneumonia
      - Failure of medical management
      - Repeated vomiting with failure to thrive
      - Severe apneic spells
    - Intellectually disabled children with GE reflux who need a gastrostomy tube for feeding have a high incidence of delayed gastric emptying and may require pyloromyotomy or pyloroplasty at the time of fundoplication; erythromycin (10 mg/kg tid) may increase gastric emptying
- Postoperative complications
  - Wrap breakdown resulting in recurrent reflux
  - Excessively tight wrap resulting in dysphagia (usually responds to dilation)
  - Slippage of the wrap onto the stomach
  - Herniation of the wrap into the mediastinum

- Strictures

- Etiology
  - Reflux esophagitis
  - Corrosive ingestion
  - Anastomotic scarring (may be aggravated by GE reflux)
- Treatment
  - Serial dilatations
  - Antireflux procedure
  - Local resection (if stricture is short and circular)
  - Esophageal substitution (as a last resort)
- Types of dilators
  - Tucker (passed over a string)
  - Hurst, Maloney (mercury-weighted)
  - Jackson
  - Pneumatic balloon

Stomach and Duodenum

- Infantile hypertrophic pyloric stenosis (HPS)
  - Etiology: multifactorial with proven X-linked factor
  - Male-to-female ratio is 4:1 (most common in firstborn male); occurs more frequently in Caucasians than African Americans
  - Symptoms
    - Usually occurs at 2–6 weeks of age
    - Nonbilious, projectile vomiting
    - Ravenous appetite shortly after an episode of emesis
  - Physical examination
    - Visible peristaltic waves (left to right) during a test feed of glucose water
    - A palpable olive (hypertrophied pyloric musculature) above and to the right of the umbilicus is felt in 80% of cases
  - Diagnosis
    - Physical examination findings as above
    - If physical examination is doubtful, perform an ultrasound
    - HPS ultrasound criteria for pyloric stenosis are as follows:
      - Diameter of pyloris > 14 mm
      - Muscular thickness > 4 mm
      - Length > 16 mm

    - Contrast UGI series should be performed only if the physical examination and ultrasound are not diagnostic; "string sign" shows a thickened, narrow pyloric canal
- Laboratory tests
    - Typically, the patient's electrolytes show a hypochloremic, hypokalemic metabolic alkalosis
        - Hydrogen and chlorine are lost by vomiting, producing a metabolic alkalosis
        - Because chlorine is depleted, bicarbonate is reabsorbed with sodium to increase the metabolic alkalosis
    - Paradoxical aciduria: sodium is conserved because of extracellular fluid loss, and potassium is lost in the urine to compensate for sodium reabsorption
        - The resulting hypokalemia enhances excretion of hydrogen in the urine
        - Decreased potassium induces a worsening alkalosis, resulting in a further decrease in potassium and increased hydrogen excretion
        - This results in paradoxical aciduria, which is a late sign indicating depletion of total-body potassium
    - Increased bilirubin (indirect) is due to decreased glucuronyl transferase activity
- Treatment
    - Correct fluid, electrolyte, and acid-base abnormalities using D_5½ normal saline plus potassium chloride (2–4 mEq/kg after patient urinates) at 150–175 cc/kg/day
    - Resuscitation is adequate when patient achieves a urine output about 2 cc/kg/h, electrolytes are normal, and serum bicarbonate is < 27 mEq/L (patients with uncorrected metabolic alkalosis are at risk for dysrhythmias and apnea from general anesthesia)
    - An anesthesiologist should aspirate the stomach before giving anesthesia to decrease the risk of aspiration on intubation
    - Ramstedt pyloromyotomy
        - Surgical approaches include transverse right upper-quadrant incision, periumbilical incision, and laparoscopic pyloromyotomy (a longitudinal incision is made through the hypertrophied muscle to relieve

the constriction while avoiding mucosal perforation)

- Postoperative feeding
  - Initiate small-volume oral feedings of glucose and water at 4–8 hours following operation. For example:
    - 15 cc oral electrolyte solution every 2 hours × 3, then
    - 30 cc oral electrolyte solution every 2 hours × 3, then
    - 30 cc full-strength formula or breast milk every 2 hours × 3, then
    - 60 cc full-strength formula or breast milk every 3 hours × 3, then
    - 90 cc full-strength formula or breast milk every 4 hours
  - If vomiting occurs, wait 2 hours and retry the last volume tolerated
- Treating complications
  - Mucosal perforation
    - Close in two layers using a polyglactin 919 (absorbable, synthetic, braided) suture over an omental patch
    - Consider a second myotomy at a different site 45° from the first site
    - Give nothing by mouth and maintain an NG tube on suction for 24 hours before starting feeds
  - Vomiting is usually secondary to gastritis or reflux and resolves in 1–2 days in almost all cases
  - In the case of wound infection, prescribe antibiotics
  - Bleeding may indicate the need for reexploration
  - Consider incomplete myotomy only if vomiting continues for > 7–10 days postoperatively, is forceful, or follows every feeding. Redo the myotomy at a site 45° from the original site
  - Arrhythmias and apnea are associated with general anesthesia in patients with uncorrected metabolic alkalosis (ie, serum bicarbonate < 27 mEq/L); monitor pulse oximetry and apnea postoperatively

- Gastric antral web
  - Produces incomplete obstruction with an insidious delay in symptoms
  - Pathology: submucosal web in the distal antrum is covered by gastric mucosa (no muscular layer present)

- Symptoms include postprandial, nonbilious vomiting; failure to thrive; and epigastric pain
- Diagnosis: UGI series
- Treatment
  - Intraoperatively place a balloon-tipped catheter through the web, inflate the balloon, and gently retract the catheter to identify the site on the gastric wall where the web originates
  - Make a longitudinal gastrotomy incision over the site, excise a portion of the web, and close the gastrotomy transversely

- Gastric volvulus
  - Pathology: abnormal rotation of one part of the stomach around another
    - Organoaxial: rotation occurs around a plane joining the hiatus and pyloris
    - Mesentericoaxial: rotation occurs around a line joining the greater and lesser curvatures (most common)
  - Usually seen in infants
  - Symptoms: Borchardt triad (acute gastric distention, difficulty passing an NG tube, and nonproductive vomiting)
  - Diagnosis must be made early to prevent hemorrhage and necrosis of the stomach. Mesentericoaxial UGI series shows obstructed, upside down stomach, with antrum often in the chest
  - Treatment
    - Fluid resuscitation
    - Emergency operation to prevent necrosis; perform Stamm gastrostomy with fixation of the stomach to the anterior abdominal wall
- Gastric perforation
  - Spontaneous neonatal
    - Neonate is usually healthy in first week of life
    - Symptoms include poor feeding, abdominal distention, lethargy, and peritonitis
    - Abdominal radiograph shows massive pneumoperitoneum
    - Usually occurs on the greater curvature
    - Treatment

      - Give nothing by mouth
      - Place NG tube
      - Give IV fluids
      - Give antibiotics
      - Perform 2-layer closure
      - Perform gastrostomy for prolonged obstruction or perforation
  - Posttraumatic (eg, secondary to an NG tube or postoperative endoscopy)
    - Diagnose using water-soluble contrast
    - Usually occurs on the lesser curvature
    - Treatment
      - Provide IV fluid resuscitation (20 cc/kg bolus Ringer's lactate)
      - Place an NG tube under fluoroscopy
      - Give antibiotics (ampicillin plus gentamicin)
      - Perform operative closure (2 layers)
      - Perform gastroduodenostomy (Billroth I operation) if distal stomach is necrotic
- Bezoars
  - Types
    - Trichobezoar (hair; usually seen in intellectually disabled children)
    - Phytobezoar (vegetable fibers)
    - Lactobezoar (milk; caused by improper milk preparation, such as with powdered formulas or concentrated milk requiring reconstitution or dilution)
  - Symptoms: nonbilious vomiting, dehydration, and failure to thrive
  - Palpable epigastric mass is evident on physical examination
  - Diagnosis: UGI, endoscopy
  - Treatment: gastrotomy and surgical removal if patient is symptomatic and endoscopic removal is not possible
- Duodenal obstruction
  - Etiology
    - Duodenal atresia or web
    - Annular pancreas
    - Preduodenal portal vein
  - Anomalies associated with duodenal atresia

  - Down syndrome (30%)
  - Cardiac, renal, central nervous system, annular pancreas, malrotation, and anterior portal vein
- Symptoms
  - Bilious vomiting after starting feeds
  - Infants have usually passed meconium by 24 hours of age
- Diagnosis
  - Plain abdominal radiographs will show "double bubble" sign, representing air in the stomach and duodenum
- Treatment
  - Emergency operative correction
  - Malrotation discovered while fixing an intestinal atresia must be repaired (see Intestinal atresias, page 204)
- Preoperative preparation
  - Place an NG tube; suction to decompress the stomach and duodenum
  - Administer IV fluid resuscitation (10–20 mL/kg of crystalloid or 5% albumin); urine output should be about 2 mL/kg/h
  - Administer antibiotics (eg, ampicillin and gentamicin)
  - Rule out cardiac anomalies
- Operation
  - Perform transverse, right supraumbilical incision, extending to the midline
  - If a "windsock web" is present,
    - Pass a Foley catheter (about size 8 Fr) through the length of the duodenum into the proximal jejunum and slowly withdraw
    - Perform duodenotomy along the lateral aspect to avoid injury to the ampulla of Vater, which is located medially
    - Excise the web
  - In the case of duodenal atresia and annular pancreas
    - "Kocherize" the duodenum
    - Perform a duodenoduodenostomy (one layer, diamond-type anastomosis) if possible, or duodenojejunostomy (often required for annular pancreas); never perform a duodenogastostomy, which carries a risk of marginal ulceration

        - ▹ If the proximal duodenum is significantly dilated, consider suture plication (interrupted Lembert sutures) or stapled tapering duodenoplasty (using an endostapler) on the antimesenteric side
    - Return of normal bowel function is frequently delayed; consider using a central venous catheter for total parenteral nutrition (TPN)

Small Intestine

- Malrotation with volvulus (rotational anomaly)
  - Anatomy: ligament of Treitz extends from the second lumbar vertebrae to the sacroiliac joint in the right lower quadrant
  - Etiology: mesenteric fixation failure permits the midgut to rotate the last 90° counterclockwise around the narrow mesenteric pedicle, which contains its entire blood supply (superior mesenteric artery and superior mesenteric vein)
  - The risk of volvulus in patients with malrotation does not decrease with age and should be surgically corrected, even in asymptomatic patients
  - Symptoms of midgut volvulus
    - Bilious vomiting (always rule out malrotation with volvulus and duodenal atresia in a newborn with bilious vomiting)
    - Abdominal distention is possible
    - Painful, tender abdomen
    - Hematemesis, hematochezia
    - Child appears acutely ill
    - Sepsis
    - Shock (hypoperfusion state)
  - Diagnosis of midgut volvulus
    - Plain abdominal radiographs show dilated stomach (double bubble), gasless abdomen
    - Ultrasound may be used to determine the relative positions of the superior mesenteric artery and superior mesenteric vein
    - UGI is only indicated if acute abdominal findings are absent on physical examination, but will show duodenum and jejunum lying to the right of the spine,

entire opacified bowel on the right side, and duodenal obstruction with the proximal duodenum appearing as a corkscrew at the obstruction point

- Treatment of midgut volvulus
    - Perform a transverse upper-abdominal incision
    - Eviscerate and inspect the entire small bowel for areas of atresia or perforation
    - Reduce a volvulus by counterclockwise rotation of the midgut
    - Divide Ladd bands, which extend from the cecum across the first and second portions of the duodenum to the retroperitoneum at the right gutter
    - Widen the mesentery (the most important step to prevent recurrence)
    - Separate the duodenum from the cecum and place the cecum in the left lower quadrant; position the duodenum, the proximal jejunum in the right lower quadrant, and the ascending colon in the left upper quadrant
    - Perform an appendectomy (because of the potential delay in the future diagnosis of acute appendicitis that results from the new, nonanatomical location of the cecum and appendix)
- Treatment of ischemic or necrotic small bowel
    - If a short segment is necrotic but the remainder is normal, perform conservative resection and primary anastamosis
    - If a short segment is necrotic but the remainder is of questionable viability, perform conservative resection with stoma formation
    - Reexamine in 12–24 hours if large portions of the gut or stomas appear ischemic

- Intestinal atresias
    - General
        - Most common cause of congenital intestinal obstruction in the newborn
        - Etiology: fetal gut infarction (mesenteric vascular accidents)
        - Esophageal atresia
        - Duodenal atresia

- Small-intestinal atresia: distal ileum is the most common site; diagnose using UGI series with small-bowel follow through
- Colonic atresia: represents only 5% of intestinal atresias, most commonly occurring at the transverse colon; diagnose using contrast enema

- Diagnosis
  - Prenatal: ultrasound will show polyhydramnios (> 2,000 mL total amniotic fluid volume)
  - Postnatal
    - Early, bilious (85%) vomiting is associated with duodenal and proximal jejunal obstruction
    - Delayed (hours to days) vomiting is associated with distal intestinal obstruction
  - Failure to pass meconium in the first 24–48 hours of life
  - Presence or absence of abdominal distention depends on the level of the obstruction
  - Jaundice: increased indirect bilirubin; β-glucuronidase in the intestinal mucosa deconjugates direct bilirubin and enhances enterohepatic recirculation of bilirubin in the presence of bowel obstruction
  - Radiographs
    - Double-bubble sign is associated with duodenal obstruction (atresia, annular pancreas)
    - Triple-bubble sign shows air in the stomach, duodenum, and bowel proximal to the area of atresia
      - Perform limited UGI series to rule out malrotation or volvulus
      - There will be a paucity of gas in the distal bowel
      - Contrast enema will show microcolon; dilated, air-filled proximal bowel
- Treatment
  - Preoperative
    - Place an NG tube
    - Administer IV fluids
    - Type and cross-match blood
    - Administer antibiotics
    - Rule out associated anomalies
  - Perform operative treatment for duodenal atresia (see

Duodenal obstruction, see page 201), small bowel atresia, or colonic atresia

- In the case of small bowel atresia, take the following steps:
  - Inspect the entire small bowel for areas of atresia or stenosis
  - Flush saline into the distal bowel to rule out additional areas of atresia or stenosis
  - Resect dilated proximal bulbous tip to avoid postoperative functional obstruction
  - Perform primary end-to-end oblique anastomosis (a stapled, antimesenteric tapering duodenoplasty [duodenal atresia] or enteroplasty [small bowel] of the dilated proximal bowel is preferred over resection of a significant length of bowel)
  - Preserve distal ileum and ileocecal valve, if possible, to prevent vitamin B_{12} and fat malabsorption
  - If primary anastomosis is not possible (eg, in premature infants or in the case of peritonitis), perform an ileostomy with exteriorization of both limbs
- In the case of colonic atresia, use primary anastomosis if possible; use temporary proximal end colostomy if there is a large size discrepancy

- Postoperative
  - Place an NG tube
  - Parenteral nutrition may be required because of the high incidence of prolonged postoperative ileus (lasting weeks to months)
  - Give elemental formulas (Nutramigen or Pregestimil [Mead Johnson Nutrition, Glenview, Ill])
  - Mortality is usually associated with complex congenital heart disease (especially Down syndrome with endocardial cushion defect)
  - Duodenojejunostomy may be associated with blind loop syndrome; treat by converting to a duodenoduodenostomy

- Complications
  - Sepsis resulting from pneumonia or an anastomotic leak
  - Functional obstruction

- Meckel's diverticulum
  - Anatomy
    - Located on the antimesenteric border of the ileum
    - Associated with omphalocele, malrotation, atresias, and many other congenital anomalies
    - Called a "disease of twos"
      - 2 inches long
      - Occurs 2 inches from the ileocecal valve
      - 2% of cases are symptomatic
      - Condition affects 2% of the population
      - There are 2 potential types of ectopic mucosa (gastric more common than pancreatic)
      - Occurs as a 2:1 ratio in males to females
  - Symptoms
    - The most common presentation in pediatric patients < 5 years old is sudden, painless, lower gastrointestinal (GI) bleeding
    - Occurs secondary to peptic ulceration in the adjacent ileal mucosa
    - Rarely results in a life-threatening hemorrhage
    - Causes grossly bloody or occasionally black, tarry stools resulting in anemia
    - Most common cause of massive rectal bleeding in pediatric patients (esophageal varices secondary to a history of omphalitis is the most common cause of massive hematemesis in this age group, and can be managed conservatively in almost all cases)
    - In Meckel's diverticulitis, pain is indistinguishable from that caused by acute appendicitis
  - May cause intestinal obstruction by acting as a lead point for intussusception
  - Littré hernia is a Meckel's diverticulum trapped in an incarcerated umbilical or inguinal hernia
  - In a hostile environment, diagnose using ultrasound, computed tomography scan, and clinical observation
  - Complications
    - Hemorrhage (most common in children)
    - Obstruction (most common in adults)
      - A common lead point for ileocolic intussusception

      - Attachment of diverticulum to abdominal wall by fibrous bands
    - Perforation
    - Volvulus
  - Treat symptomatic cases with surgical excision (treatment of asymptomatic cases is controversial, but most pediatric surgeons feel that incidental diverticulectomy is not indicated)
    - In the presence of a narrow base, perform a wedge resection with transverse closure
    - In the case of a wide base or significant degree of inflammation in the adjacent intestine, perform a sleeve resection with end-to-end ileoileostomy
    - In the case of intussusception, manual reduction is rarely possible; perform segmental resection
- Necrotizing enterocolitis
  - Most common surgical emergency in the neonate (infants < 30 days old)
  - Usually occurs after the tenth day of life when coliform bacteria colonize the GI tract, but can occur at any time in the neonatal period
  - Pathophysiology
    - Ischemic intestinal mucosa is susceptible to reperfusion injury and bacterial translocation of gut flora, especially involving *Escherichia coli, Klebsiella, Clostridium difficile, Enterobacter,* and *Proteus,* which produce hydrogen gas within the gut wall (pneumatosis intestinalis)
    - The most commonly affected sites are the terminal ileum and right colon
  - Histology
    - Most common pathology is bland ischemic necrosis of the superficial mucosa
    - Microthrombi occur secondary to platelet aggregation throughout the mesentery
    - Characterized by "skip areas" of involvement
    - Pneumatosis intestinalis
  - Reperfusion triggers agents that produce cellular injury (eg, anion radicals, superoxide, hydrogen peroxide)
  - Radiographic findings
    - Plain abdominal films demonstrate intramural gas

    - In the presence of pneumatosis intestinalis (pathognomonic), hydrogen gas (from *E coli*) will be evident
    - Air in the portal venous system (pylephlebitis) is a poor prognostic sign (however, these findings alone are not indications for operative intervention and are reversible with medical management)
    - Pneumoperitoneum may be present (secondary to GI perforation)
    - Static intestinal loops (persistent loops of adynamic or edematous bowel) can be seen on serial abdominal radiographs
    - The earliest, most common finding is distention of multiple bowel loops
    - Bowel gas is diminished
    - Ascites is a grave sign
    - Abdominal wall ecchymosis is usually indicative of underlying dead bowel
- Physical examination
    - Patient's first symptom will be feeding intolerance (high feeding residuals)
    - Abdominal distention is the most common sign
    - Lethargy
    - Bilious vomiting
    - Rectal bleeding (plus guaiac-positive stool)
    - Coagulopathy
    - Bradycardia
    - Apnea
    - Edema and erythema of the abdominal wall
    - Thermal instability
    - Carbohydrate intolerance, causing the presence of reducing substances in the stool
- Laboratory studies
    - Thrombocytopenia (secondary to microvascular plugging and binding to gram-negative endotoxin) is the most relevant
    - Leukopenia (especially in severe cases)
    - Metabolic acidosis (pH < 7.2, with an anion gap), especially with decreased serum sodium
    - Increased breath hydrogen excretion

- Medical treatment
  - Nothing by mouth for at least 10 days
  - NG tube decompression of the UGI tract
  - IV (not enteral) antibiotics (ampicillin, gentamicin, clindamycin) to cover *E coli*, *Klebsiella*, and *C difficile*
  - Parenteral nutrition
  - Serial abdominal radiographs
- Surgical treatment
  - Pneumoperitoneum is an absolute indication for surgical management
  - Relative indications for peritoneal drainage or laparotomy include:
    - Positive peritoneal lavage (brown color, positive Gram stain), which suggests a gangrenous or perforated bowel
    - Palpable abdominal mass
    - Progressive peritonitis (edema or erythema of the abdominal wall)
    - Deterioration on medical management (increasing acidosis, decreasing platelets)
    - Intestinal obstruction
    - Fixed, dilated loop of intestine (unchanged after 24 h) on serial abdominal radiographs
    - Portal vein gas
    - Ascites
  - Perform a right, transverse, supraumbilical incision
  - Conservative resection of frankly gangrenous bowel to prevent short-bowel syndrome
  - Preserve the ileocecal valve if possible
  - Take a second look at marginally viable bowel at 24–48 hours
  - Administer antibiotics and TPN postoperatively
  - In very small, ill, premature infants, set up peritoneal drainage using a ¼-inch Penrose drain placed while patient is under local anesthesia (this may be an effective temporary or permanent measure in an unstable, high-risk, premature infant with peritonitis, respiratory failure, or shock)
  - If resection of multiple necrotic segments is necessary,

perform a proximal stoma and multiple anastamoses of the distal, defunctionalized bowel

- Postoperative complications
  - Most common complication is stricture due to cicatricial healing of the injured mucosa (usually involving the left colon)
    - This often presents weeks to months later with a bowel obstruction
    - Diagnose by contrast enema
    - Treat with segmental resection and primary anastomosis
  - Short-bowel syndrome resulting from extensive bowel resection
    - This may be prevented by conservative resection and "second look" operations
    - Treatment includes TPN and dietary manipulation
  - Malabsorption (usually reversible) resulting from extensive mucosal injury
  - Interloop fistulae: treat with octreotide (3–5 μg/kg/h IV) or 1 mg/kg bid (up to 4 mg/kg/8 h)
  - Survivors of severe necrotizing enterocolitis remain at high risk for growth and neurologic morbidity

- Intussusception
  - Seen in healthy children 6–24 months old, usually due to hypertrophy of Peyer's patches in the terminal ileum from an antecedent viral infection (eg, rotavirus, reovirus, or echovirus); seasonal incidence (midwinter and early summer) corresponds with upper respiratory infections and GI viral disease
  - Lead points (only 5% of children)
    - Polyps (juvenile, hamartoma)
    - Malignant tumors (eg, lymphoma, lymphosarcoma)
    - Meckel's diverticulum (most common), appendix
    - Peutz-Jeghers syndrome
    - Intestinal duplications
    - Hemangioma
    - Cystic fibrosis (due to inspissated feces in the terminal ileum)
    - Henoch-Schönlein purpura (hamartomas in the intesti-

nal wall act as lead points for ileal-ileal intussusception)

- Site
  - Most common site in the pediatric age group is ileocecal and ileocolic
  - When resulting from postoperative abdominal and thoracic operations, ileal-ileal site is the most common
- Pathophysiology
  - Proximal portion of bowel (intussusceptum) is drawn into the distal loop (intussuscipiens) by peristaltic activity
  - Mesentery of the proximal bowel is strangulated and compressed, leading to venous obstruction that results in edema of the bowel wall; this causes arterial obstruction, leading first to gangrene and then perforation and peritonitis
- Symptoms
  - Characteristically seen in an otherwise healthy, robust child
  - Child experiences paroxysms (lasting around 10–15 minutes) of abdominal cramps and intermittent vomiting (may or may not be bilious); screams and pulls legs up to abdomen
  - Dark red (bloody) mucoid ("red currant jelly") stools
- Physical findings
  - Elongated (sausage-shaped) mass in the right upper quadrant, absence of bowel in the right lower quadrant (Dance sign)
  - Hyperperistaltic rushes during episodes of pain
  - Symptoms include tachycardia, fever, and hypotension
  - If peritoneal symptoms are present, perform a laparotomy (do not attempt radiographic reduction)
  - Radiographic diagnosis: take flat and upright abdominal films; cecal gas shadow will be absent in right iliac region and small bowel obstruction will be evident (air–fluid levels may be present on upright abdominal radiograph)
  - Ultrasound will show target sign
  - Perform air enema or contrast enema (will show coiled spring appearance of the lead point)
- Treatment

- Initial stabilization
  - Administer IV fluids (10 mL/kg of 5% albumin solution or Ringer's lactate)
  - Give nothing by mouth
  - Administer antibiotics (ampicillin, gentamicin, and metronidazole)
  - Place NG tube to suction
- Laboratory tests: complete blood count, electrolytes, blood urea nitrogen, glucose, and creatinine; type and cross-match blood
- Attempt hydrostatic reduction using diatrizoate sodium or air enema (do not attempt in the presence of peritonitis or pneumoperitoneum)
  - Suspend enema bag < 1 meter (~ 3 ft) above the level of the anus
  - Water-soluble contrast is preferred
  - Other methods of reduction include insufflated air (preferred; maximum pressure of 80–120 mmHg) or saline enema under ultrasonography
- After successful reduction, contrast must be seen to pass into the terminal ileum; at the same time, feces and contrast should be expelled
- If reduction is unsuccessful, perform operative exploration
- Nonoperative treatment is effective > 80% of the time

◦ Incidence of recurrence is low (< 10%)
- Diagnose using air or contrast enema
- After the third episode, operative intervention is indicated because of the high likelihood of a pathologic lead point
- If contrast or air reduction is unsuccessful, or if physical examination reveals a tender or rigid abdomen
  - Perform laparotomy using a transverse, right, lower incision
  - Attempt manual reduction by gently milking the intussusceptum out of the intussuscipiens (never pull it out)
  - Perform appendectomy (usually) and resection of frankly gangrenous bowel or lead point (eg, Meckel's)
  - Perform primary ileocolic anastomosis

    - Postoperative intussusception is evident by a small bowel obstruction in the early postoperative period (around postoperative day 5)
        - Most commonly occurs as an ileo-ileal intussusception
        - Treat with manual, operative reduction
- Meconium disease
    - Meconium ileus
        - Generalized mucoviscidosis of exocrine secretions, resulting in inspissated meconium that may cause intraluminal intestinal obstruction in a newborn
        - Affects all exocrine glands and is usually associated with cystic fibrosis
            - Lung: air passages are obstructed by thick mucoid secretions
            - Pancreas: pancreatic ducts are obstructed
            - Intestine: obstruction by thick, viscous mucus as water migrates out of the intestinal lumen
            - Other organs affected include sweat and salivary glands, nasal mucus membranes, and reproductive organs
        - Differential diagnosis includes Hirschsprung disease (especially total aganglionosis), hypothyroidism, small left colon syndrome, colonic or ileal atresia, and meconium plug syndrome
        - Radiographic findings (on abdominal radiograph) include the following:
            - Multiple distended loops of intestine mimicking small bowel obstruction, but air–fluid levels are rarely present because of the viscosity of the intraluminal meconium and because the bowel is completely filled with fluid or meconium
            - Course, granular, soap-bubble ("ground glass") appearance (mixture of air within thick meconium; Neuhauser's sign)
            - Prenatal perforation with meconium peritonitis (due to liberated lipases and bile salts) results in calcium deposition (saponification)
            - Prominent air–fluid levels suggest intestinal atresia or volvulus

    - Ascites and pneumoperitoneum are indicative of postnatal colonic perforation
    - There is no clinical or radiographic evidence of perforation or peritonitis with uncomplicated meconium ileus
  - Nonoperative treatment
    - Ensure patient is well hydrated
    - Insert an NG tube
    - Administer anibiotics
    - Perform fluoroscopically visualized enema with a hyperosmolar agent (meglumine diatrizoate or *N*-acetylcysteine)
  - Operative treatment
    - Indicated for "complicated" patients (ie, those with perforation or peritoneal signs, volvulus, gangrene, or atresia) or after a failed attempt at nonoperative treatment
    - Technique
      - Perform enterotomy at ileum or appendectomy (with irrigation and drainage) through the appendiceal stump (to avoid an anastomosis or ileostomy)
      - Run entire length of bowel to rule out areas of necrosis or atresia; if any are discovered, they should be resected
      - Pass a red rubber catheter proximally and distally
      - Irrigate with saline or *N*-acetylcysteine (mucolytic)
      - Perform primary anastomosis, ileostomy and mucus fistula, or Bishop-Koop end-to-side (proximal dilated bowel to side) or Santuli anastomosis (avoided by irrigating through the appendiceal stump)
      - Administer antibiotics for 3 days
      - Continue NG suction
      - Initiate oral feedings and pancreatic enzymes 5–10 days following operation
- Meconium plug syndrome

    - Newborn infants with this condition sustain intestinal obstruction because the colon cannot rid itself of fetal meconium residue
    - Physical findings include an obstructing meconium mass and colonic hypomotility
    - Differential diagnosis includes Hirschsprung disease, decreased potassium, decreased calcium, and increased glycogen
    - Associated with decreased glucose in infants of diabetic mothers, but not usually associated with cystic fibrosis
    - Symptoms include abdominal distention and colonic obstruction (resulting from plug of inspissated meconium, which is usually whitish gray distally, green proximally)
    - Abdominal radiograph will reveal multiple loops of dilated small bowel
    - Diagnose and treat using diatrizoate sodium enema; operation is rarely necessary (rule out Hirschsprung disease by rectal biopsy)
  - Meconium ileus equivalent
    - Mechanical obstruction resulting from thick, putty-like, inspissated stool in the intestine
    - Seen at any age beyond the newborn period in patients with cystic fibrosis

Large Intestine

- The appendix arises from the posteromedial border of the cecum and has its own mesoappendix; blood supply flows from the superior mesenteric artery to the right colic artery, then from the ileocolic artery to the appendicular branch
- Acute appendicitis is the most common acute surgical condition of the abdomen; it parallels the amount of lymphoid tissue in the appendix (peak incidence is during the mid-teenage years)
  - Fecaliths, which obstruct the lumen, are the most common cause of luminal obstruction and the most common factor in the etiology of acute appendicitis; other causes include lymphoid hyperplasia, seeds, and worms (eg, pinworms, Ascaris)
  - Sequence of events in acute appendicitis

    - Begins with an obstruction of the lumen; normal mucosal secretion continues
    - Distention increases
    - Nerve endings of visceral afferent sympathetic pain fibers are stimulated through the celiac ganglion to the tenth thoracic segment, causing vague, dull, diffuse pain in the midabdomen or lower epigastrium; this pain is referred to the umbilical area (tenth dermatome)
    - The parietal peritoneum becomes irritated by the inflamed tip of the appendix, causing pain to be localized to the right lower quadrant
    - The stimulation of peristalsis leads to cramping
    - Appendiceal distention increases secondary to bacterial proliferation, which produces reflex nausea and vomiting
    - Venous pressure is exceeded while arterial inflow continues, resulting in engorgement and vascular congestion
    - Bacteria from the lumen translocate into the bloodstream
    - Reflex nausea and vomiting result, as does severe visceral pain from the increased distention
    - The appendiceal wall becomes infarcted, resulting in perforation and peritonitis
- Symptoms
    - Localized pain in the right, lower quadrant is the most important diagnostic finding on physical examination
    - Pain is initially centered in the lower epigastrium or periumbilical area (serosa of the appendix becomes inflamed and pain localizes to the right lower quadrant after 4–6 hours as a result of parietal peritoneum inflammation)
- Anatomical locations
    - A long appendix with an inflamed tip results in pelvic pain
    - Occurrence at the retrocecal (two thirds of all cases of appendicitis occur here) location results in flank or back pain (most commonly), nausea, vomiting, and increased white blood cell count; microscopic hematuria may occur if the inflamed appendix lies near the ureter
    - Occurrence at the pelvic location results in suprapubic pain from an inflamed tip lying against the bladder,

which causes urinary frequency and dysuria
    - If there is tenderness on a rectal examination, the inflamed tip is lying adjacent to the rectum
    - An abscess presents with severe urinary symptoms and diarrhea
  - Occurrence at the retroileal location results in testicular pain from irritation of the spermatic artery and ureter; anorexia almost always accompanies appendicitis (if a child is truly hungry, appendicitis is unlikely)
    - Vomiting (1–2 episodes) is frequent
    - Symptoms usually move from anorexia to abdominal pain to nausea with vomiting; if vomiting precedes the onset of abdominal pain, the diagnosis should be questioned (in favor of gastroenteritis)
    - Low-grade fever (> 100°F, 38°C) is rare
    - The individual will experience point tenderness over McBurney's point (at the junction of the lateral one third and medial two thirds of a line from the anterior superior iliac spine to the umbilicus), usually accompanied by guarding and muscle spasm; this is the most important physical finding
    - Individual may also show psoas sign (pain on extension of the right thigh, which, when patient is in side-lying position, stretches the irritated ileopsoas muscle)
    - Obturator sign may also be present (passive internal rotation of the flexed right thigh stretches the obturator internus muscle, producing pain)
    - Rovsing's sign (pain in the right lower quadrant upon palpation of the left lower quadrant) may be experienced by some individuals
    - Cutaneous hyperesthesia may be present in distribution of T10, T11, and T12 segments
    - Preoperative diagnosis should be correct in 85%–90% of cases
    - Symptoms secondary to bacterial toxins and absorption of dead tissue toxins include fever, tachycardia, and leukocytosis
- Laboratory findings
  - White blood cell count will be about 10,000–18,000, with

left shift (> 18,000 is consistent with a perforation)
    - Infants and elderly patients may be unable to increase white blood cell count, resulting in a delay in diagnosis and increased incidence of rupture
    - Perform urinalysis to rule out a urinary tract infection and pregnancy
    - Ultrasound will show the appendix diameter to be > 8 mm and appendix will be edematous with adjacent fluid (rule out gynecological problems such as ovarian cysts and tubal pregnancy)
      - A gas-filled appendix usually indicates appendicitis with proximal obstruction
      - Radiopaque fecalith is almost always associated with gangrenous appendicitis
      - A distended loop of small bowel will be evident in the right lower quadrant
    - Barium enema findings are pathognomonic of appendicitis; findings include nonfilling of appendix, mass effect on medial and inferior borders of the cecum, and mucosal irregularities of the terminal ileum
    - Obtain a chest radiograph to rule out right lower lobe pneumonia
    - Computed tomography scan will often reveal inflammation, fat stranding, and fluid
  - Appendiceal rupture is a common complication
- Appendicitis during pregnancy
  - This is the most common extrauterine surgical emergency (though incidence of appendicitis is not increased by pregnancy)
  - White blood cell count normally increases in pregnancy, but a left shift is abnormal
  - The appendix moves superiorly and laterally as pregnancy progresses
  - Laparoscopy may be helpful if diagnosis is uncertain
  - The infant mortality rate from maternal appendicitis is 8.5%; the rate of mortality from maternal perforation and peritonitis is 35%
  - Treat by inserting an NG tube and providing IV fluids and preoperative antibiotics appropriate to cover *Bacteroides*

fragilis (gram-negative rod; eg, cefotetan or clindamycin)
    - Nonoperative management may be appropriate to treat a periappendiceal abscess
    - Drain the abscess percutaneously or operatively
    - If symptoms regress, manage conservatively
    - If needed, perform an interval appendectomy at 5–6 weeks
  - If appendicitis is not found:
    - Rule out adnexal disease (if tuboovarian abscess is found, incise and drain only, do not resect tube or ovary)
    - Examine the mesentery for adenopathy (mesenteric lymphadenitis)
    - Examine the small bowel for a distance of about 3 feet to rule out Crohn disease, ulcerative colitis, terminal ileitis, and Meckel's diverticulitis
  - Complications (incidence approximately 5%)
    - Superficial wound or port-site infection. Treat by re-opening the skin and subcutaneous tissue, and begin saline wet-to-dry dressing (change tid); administer antibiotics
    - Pelvic abscess is the most common complication of a ruptured appendicitis; treat with antibiotics and drainage, depending on size and location
    - Ileus (place an NG tube and administer IV fluids)
    - Small bowel obstruction (place NG tube initially; may require lysis of adhesions)
    - Appendiceal stump blowout (drain or perform tube cecostomy)
    - Decreased fertility (due to scarring and fallopian tube obstruction)
  - Prognosis
    - The principal factor determining mortality is rupture
      - Unruptured: 0.1% mortality
      - Ruptured: 3% mortality
    - Cause of death is usually uncontrolled gram-negative sepsis
- Appendiceal rupture
  - Deaths from appendicitis are almost always secondary to complications of perforation, resulting in gram-negative sepsis (*E coli* and *Bacteroides* are the most common organ-

isms); incidence of appendiceal rupture is significantly higher in pediatric and geriatric age groups (due to a delay in diagnosis)

- Rectal or pelvic examinations are essential for all age groups
- Young children may not be able to form a phlegmon to wall off a perforation or abscess because of a paucity of omentum
- Symptoms
  - Temporary pain relief after perforation is rare; localized pain progresses to encompass the entire right lower quadrant
  - A tender, boggy mass in the peritoneal area indicates the presence of a phlegmon or abscess
  - Symptoms usually last > 36 hours and include temperature elevation to 102°F–104°F (39°C–40°C), increased white blood cell count (20,000–35,000 with extreme left shift), and hemoconcentration
- Pylethrombophlebitis (septic thrombophlebitis of the portal vein) is a complication of gangrenous appendicitis heralded by chills, spiking fever, right lower quadrant pain, and jaundice; septic clots may embolize to the liver, producing multiple pyogenic abscesses
- The most common sites of seeding from an appendiceal perforation are the pouch of Douglas (pelvic cul-de-sac) and the right subhepatic space (via the right gutter)
- The accuracy of the preoperative diagnosis should be approximately 85%–90% and depends on 3 major factors:
  - Anatomical location of the inflamed appendix
  - Stage of the process (simple or ruptured)
  - Age and sex of patient (harder to diagnose in young females)
- The most common erroneous diagnosis is acute mesenteric lymphadenitis (especially in children), which is usually associated with an antecedent upper respiratory infection. In acute mesenteric lymphadenitis, pain is less severe and not as sharply localized, there may be generalized lymphadenopathy, and complete blood count may show lymphocytosis
- To treat, observe the patient for a short time, perform serial abdominal examinations, then explore if the diagnosis is still in doubt

- Acute gastroenteritis
  - The viral form is evident by profuse watery diarrhea, nausea, and vomiting. Hyperperistaltic abdominal cramps precede watery stools, and vomiting precedes the onset of abdominal pain. Complete blood count is usually normal or shows a right shift (increased lymphocytes)
  - Bacterial (caused by *Salmonella*) often results from the ingestion of contaminated food. Symptoms include bloody diarrhea, skin rash, bradycardia, leukopenia, chills, and fever
    - Typhoid fever is usually due to *Salmonella typhosa*, which is cultured from stool or blood. Symptoms include maculopapular rash, inappropriate bradycardia, leukopenia, and ileal perforation (in 1% of cases)
    - Treat with chloramphenicol
  - Bacterial (caused by *Yersinia enterocolitica, Campylobacter*) results from ingesting food contaminated by feces or urine
    - Symptoms include cervical and mesenteric lymphadenitis, ileus, and colitis
    - Treat with ampicillin or gentamicin
- Gynecological disorders are important in the differential diagnosis of appendicitis
  - Gynecological disorders compose the highest rate of missed diagnosis in young adult females
  - Differential diagnosis includes pelvic inflammatory disease (the most common erroneous diagnosis), ruptured Graafian follicle (mittelschmerz), and ruptured ectopic pregnancy
- Diseases in the male include torsion of the testis and acute epididymitis (see Chapter 21, Genitourinary Tract)
- Urinary tract infection
  - Urinalysis shows pyuria
  - Symptoms include urinary frequency and dysuria
  - Suprapubic or costovertebral angle tenderness is evident on physical examination
  - Patient's temperature will be > 101°F (about 38°C)
- Ureteral stone
  - Pain is referred to pelvis
  - Laboratory findings show hematuria but neither fever nor increased white blood cell count

- Primary peritonitis
  - Diagnosis with peritoneal aspiration. If only a single species of cocci is seen, patient has primary peritonitis and needs medical treatment; if mixed flora are seen, patient has secondary peritonitis
- Henoch-Schönlein purpura
  - Usually occurs 2–3 weeks after a *Streptococcal* infection
  - Symptoms include joint pain, purpuric rash, and nephritis with albuminuria
  - Laboratory findings include increased platelets
- Hemolytic uremic syndrome
  - Main symptom is bloody diarrhea
  - Laboratory findings include anemia (due to hemolysis), increased white blood cells, decreased platelets, hematuria, and increased blood urea nitrogen
- Diverticulitis or perforating carcinoma of the cecum
- Constipation
  - Diagnose with abdominal radiograph
  - Treat with enemas
- Pneumonia
  - Physical findings show no point tenderness
  - Diagnose using chest radiograph
- Typhlitis (bacterial invasion of the intestinal wall)
  - Usually seen in oncology patients
  - Symptoms typically include right lower quadrant abdominal pain and neutropenia
- Hirschsprung disease (congenital megacolon)
  - Neural crest cells form neuroblasts, which migrate to the distal rectum in the twelfth week of gestation, becoming enteric ganglion cells (Auerbach myenteric plexus)
  - Pathology
    - Absence of ganglion cells in submucosa (Meissner plexus) and intramuscular plexus (Auerbach plexus)
    - Enlarged, hypertrophic, nonmyelinated nerve fibers in submucosa, muscularis mucosa, and Auerbach intramuscular plexus
    - Increased acetylcholinesterase in muscularis nerve fibers
  - Most common site of aganglionosis is the rectosigmoid due

to arrested migration of neuroblasts (80%)
- Symptoms
  - Decreased stool frequency, failure to pass meconium within 48 hours after birth
  - GI obstruction (distention, bilious vomiting)
  - Enterocolitis (the major cause of morbidity and mortality)
  - Fecal soiling is rare
- Differential diagnosis
  - In the neonate: sepsis, necrotizing enterocolitis-associated stricture, meconium plug or ileus, or intestinal atresias
  - Habit constipation associated with a full rectal ampulla and fecal soiling (whereas in Hirschsprung disease, the rectal ampulla is usually empty)
  - Functional constipation (infrequent, large, firm stools accompanied by pain and bleeding from anal fissures), a history of normal stool frequency during infancy is associated with functional constipation, not with Hirschsprung disease
  - Hypothyroidism

- Enterocolitis
  - Symptoms include abdominal distention, diarrhea, vomiting, sepsis, and perforation
  - Usually occurs in children < 3 years old and is the most common cause of death in affected children
  - May occur before or after colostomy or pull-through
  - Laboratory test results show high levels of C *difficile* toxin
  - Diagnosis
    - Perform rectal biopsy (suction or full-thickness)
    - Perform a contrast enema
      - Conical transition zone from the distal, nondilated, aganglionic colon or rectum to the proximal (ganglionic) dilated colon as demonstrated on contrast enema
      - A transition zone may be absent in neonates
      - Excludes other causes of colonic obstruction, including small left colon syndrome, meconium plug syndrome, and atresia
  - Nonsurgical treatment

- ▸ Perform NG tube decompression in the upper GI tract
- ▸ Administer IV fluids
- ▸ Administer antibiotics (ampicillin, gentamicin, or metronidazole)
- ▸ Perform rectal irrigations with 20 cc/kg warm Ringer's lactate tid using a soft, rubber catheter
- ▸ If the above measures are unhelpful and patient cannot be urgently transferred to the care of a pediatric surgeon, consider performing a colostomy

- ◦ Surgical treatment
  - ▸ Perform a leveling colostomy of normally innervated (biopsy-proven) bowel
  - ▸ If no clear-cut transition zone can be determined, the patient may have total colonic aganglionosis, and if a biopsy diagnosis is unobtainable, an ileostomy should be performed
  - ▸ Refer patient to a facility with pediatric surgery capability, if possible

Rectum and Anus

- Rectal prolapse (procidentia)
  - True prolapse: circular folds of full-thickness bowel
  - False prolapse: radial folds of mucosa only
  - Treatment
    - ▸ Rule out cystic fibrosis and parasites
    - ▸ Discourage patient from prolonged sitting or straining during a bowel movement
    - ▸ Prescribe stool softeners
    - ▸ Administer submucosal injection of 5% phenol in almond oil, hypertonic glucose (50%), or hypertonic saline (20%)
      - ▹ Administer 5 cc per treatment
      - ▹ Use a #18 spinal needle for four-quadrant sclerosis; inject 2 cc posteriorly and 1 cc in the other three quadrants (almost all cases will resolve spontaneously without an operative procedure)
- Anal fissure
  - Most common cause of rectal bleeding in the newborn
  - Symptoms include blood streaks on outside of stool and constipation

 - Physical examination will show a superficial tear of the anal mucosa, usually in the posterior midline. A sentinel skin tag indicates a chronic fissure. Fifty percent of anal fissures are associated with fistula-in-ano (see below)
 - Caused by stretching and tearing during evacuation of large, hard stools
 - Treatment consists of administering stool softeners, dilatation (may require manual stretch under sedation), and sitz baths
- Perianal and perirectal abscess
 - In infants, these can develop from an infected diaper rash. In children, rule out Crohn disease, leukemia, and immunodeficiency syndromes
 - Symptoms include fever and pain
 - Treat with incision, drainage, and sitz baths
- Fistula-in-ano
 - Results from a perianal abscess extending from a crypt to the perianal skin (suspect when an abscess recurs)
 - Tract is intersphincteric and lateral to the anus
 - Treat with fistulotomy (over a probe), tract curettage, or, if fistula is complex or high, place a seton tie
- Imperforate anus
 - Evaluate for associated VACTERRL defects
 - Initial approach consists of descending colostomy and mucus fistula
- Preoperative mechanical bowel preparation
 - Give polyethylene glycol electrolyte solution (25–35 cc/kg/h for 4–6 h via an NG tube; safe in infants and children)
 - Add oral erythromycin base and neomycin

Chapter 19

Hepatobiliary Tract

Liver Trauma

- Diagnosis
    - Computed tomography (CT) scan with oral and IV contrast
    - Focused assessment with sonography for trauma (FAST) examination
    - Diagnostic peritoneal lavage
- Treatment
    - As in adult patients, the primary goal of emergent operative therapy for liver injury should be to stop the bleeding and "get out" before the patient becomes coagulopathic, and return to the operating room in 24–48 hours when a definitive repair can be performed on a patient who is more physiologically stable
    - If the patient is hemodynamically stable, perform a serial physical examination and check hematocrit levels in the setting of an intensive care unit, using typed and cross-matched blood, if needed
    - Perform laparotomy if the patient is actively bleeding, or if blood loss is > 50% of blood volume (40 cc/kg packed red blood cells), or if > 12 cc/kg of Ringer's lactate (warmed if possible) is required to maintain hemodynamic stability
        - Pack initially with gauze sponges
        - Use compression to control venous bleeding
        - Perform resectional debridement of devitalized tissue using "finger fracture" technique, with direct suture ligation of bleeding vessels
        - Clamp the hepatoduodenal ligament, which contains the hepatic artery, portal vein, and common bile duct, (Pringle Maneuver) to help control bleeding
        - Parenchymal bleeding may be controlled with chromic sutures swedged on blunt liver needles and placed over omental pledgets
        - If the patient is unstable or has extensive hepatic bleed-

ing, pack with gauze sponges and hemostatic agents, apply a vacuum device to the abdomen, and reexplore in 24 hours; this will help prevent the factors exacerbating a coagulopathic state (hypothermia, acidosis, and hypotension)

- Hemobilia
  - Etiology: usually a sequella of hepatobiliary tract trauma
  - Symptoms include a triad of right upper quadrant pain, bleeding from the upper gastrointestinal tract, and jaundice
  - Diagnosis is made with CT scan or angiography
  - Treat with embolization instead of surgical exploration, if possible

Biliary Tract

- Trauma
  - Traumatic injuries to the gallbladder should be treated by cholecystectomy
  - Injury to the common bile duct should be repaired over a T-tube
  - Following extensive injury to the extrahepatic biliary tract, perform one of the following:
    - Damage control: tube choledochostomy
    - Definitive repair: choledochostomy or hepatojejunostomy
- Biliary atresia
  - A dynamic process of progressive obliteration and sclerosis due to a postnatal inflammatory process
  - Correctable: proximal extrahepatic bile ducts are patent; distal ducts are obliterated
  - Uncorrectable: gallbladder, cystic duct, and common bile duct are patent; proximal hepatic ducts are obliterated
  - Laboratory tests: direct (conjugated) hyperbilirubinemia (> 3 mg/dL; for patients ≥ 2 wk old); biliary atresia is the most common cause of conjugated hyperbilirubinemia in a 1-month-old
  - Physical examination
    - Icteric (jaundice or bilirubin > 10 at 7 days of life is pathologic)
    - Light (acholic), gray-colored stools
    - Dark urine

- Hepatomegaly
- Diagnosis
  - Liver biopsy
  - Technetium-99m
  - Iminodiacetate (diisopropyl iminodiacetic acid) scan
- Patient should be referred to a pediatric center for further work-up and operative treatment as soon as feasible

- Biliary hypoplasia
  - Not a specific disease entity, but a manifestation of a variety of hepatobiliary disorders including:
    - Neonatal hepatitis
    - α_1-Antitrypsin deficiency
    - Early intrahepatic biliary atresia
    - Alagille's syndrome (arteriohepatic dysplasia)
  - Treatment
    - Cannot be improved by operation
    - Perform a liver biopsy and close the abdomen without further treatment
    - Medications: choleretics (eg, ursodeoxycholic acid)
- Inspissated bile syndrome
  - Etiology
    - Massive hemolysis due to Rhesus factor and ABO incompatibility (resulting in obstruction from sludge in the biliary system)
    - Total parenteral nutrition cholestasis
    - Cystic fibrosis
  - Medications: choleretic agents (eg, phenobarbital, ursodeoxycholic acid, glucagon)
  - Treating an obstruction: remove stones and irrigate biliary tree via a catheter in the gallbladder
- Biliary ascites
  - Etiology: perforation of extrahepatic bile duct
  - Diagnosis: hepatobiliary iminodiacetic acid scan
  - Treatment: cholecystostomy, drainage
- Gallbladder disease
  - Hydrops
    - Pathology: severe edema around the gallbladder and common bile duct
    - Etiology: sepsis, scarlet fever, Kawasaki disease

- Diagnosis: ultrasound
- Treatment: usually resolves spontaneously

- Acalculous cholecystitis
  - Associated with sepsis, multisystem trauma, burns, total parenteral nutrition, and Kawasaki disease
  - Acute symptoms: fever, right upper quadrant tenderness, guarding, increased temperature, increased white blood cell count
  - Diagnosis: ultrasound showing gallbladder distention and echogenic debris
  - Treatment: may require cholecystectomy if severe

- Hemolytic cholelithiasis
  - Etiology
    - Hereditary spherocytosis (most common)
    - Sickle cell anemia
    - Thalassemia major
    - Hemolytic anemia
  - Treatment
    - Preoperative partial exchange or 2–3 transfusions preoperatively to decrease hemoglobin S to < 30%, and increase hemoglobin to 12 g/dL; intraoperatively, avoid hypothermia, acidosis, hypovolemia
    - Cholecystectomy is indicated in all patients with thalassemia major and spherocytosis who have symptomatic gallstones and in asymptomatic patients with gallstones who are undergoing splenectomy
- Choledocholithiasis
  - Commonly associated with sickle cell disease
  - Increased direct (conjugated) bilirubin, abdominal pain, fever, nausea
  - If amylase is also increased, consider choledocholithiasis with pancreatitis
  - Treatment
    - Endoscopic retrograde cholangiopancreatography (ERCP) and sphincterotomy preoperatively
    - Open or laparoscopic exploration

Chapter 20

Pancreas and Spleen

Pancreas

- Congenital variations
    - Ectopic pancreatic tissue
        - Pancreatic tissue may be functional, but patient is asymptomatic
        - Patient may have Meckel's diverticulum or intestinal duplications
        - Patient maintains exocrine function
        - Symptoms: bleeding and inflammation
        - Treatment: local resection if symptomatic
    - Annular pancreas
        - Etiology: pancreatic tissue circumferentially surrounds the second portion of the duodenum at the region of the sphincter of Oddi
        - Parenchymal and ductal structures are usually normal
        - Symptoms
            - Associated with atresia or stenosis of the underlying duodenum
            - Vomiting (may or may not be bilious) in newborns
        - Diagnosis
            - Antenatal polyhydramnios
            - Prenatal ultrasound and postnatal abdominal radiograph show "double bubble"
        - Treatment
            - Asymptomatic cases do not require treatment
            - Obstructive symptoms
                - Utilize right upper-quadrant transverse incision
                - Perform side-to-side duodenoduodenostomy (transverse incision in proximal duodenum, longitudinal incision in distal duodenum) as in correction of duodenal atresia
                - Duodenojejunostomy (alternate method)
                - Avoid gastrojejunostomy

- Pancreatic trauma
  - Etiology: blunt trauma (especially associated with bicycle or motorcycle handlebars; body may be transected when crushed over the spine)
  - Diagnosis
    - Check for persistent elevation of amylase; use magnetic resonance cholangiopancreatography (MRCP), or endoscopic retrograde cholangiopancreatography (ERCP) to rule out ductal injury (computed tomography [CT] scan may be normal)
    - Perform focused assessment with sonography for trauma (FAST) examination
    - Perform a CT scan (definitive study) with oral and intravenous (IV) contrast
  - Nonoperative management
    - Indications
      - Patient is hemodynamically stable
      - Transfusion requirement is < 50% of estimated blood volume (ie, < 40 mL / kg)
      - No transection of the pancreatic duct
    - Management
      - Admit to floor bed
      - Place patient under the care of a qualified pediatric surgeon
      - Ensure operating room and personnel are immediately available
      - Check serial hematocrit levels every 4 hours
      - Ensure there is cross-matched blood in the blood bank
      - Put patient on bed rest for 48 hours
      - Restrict patient's physical activity for 1 month
      - Perform ultrasound based upon clinical course and for follow up
  - Operative management
    - Injury to the body of the pancreas or pancreatic duct requires drainage; even if a ductal injury is not identified, it should be presumed and drained
    - Resect clearly nonviable pancreatic body or tail tissue
    - Treat transection or near-transection of the pancreatic duct

        - Oversew or staple the distal end of the proximal pancreas
        - Oversew or staple the proximal end of the distal segment and leave the entire distal segment in situ; resect the distal segment
        - Perform distal pancreatectomy (usually with splenectomy) if injury is in tail
        - Drain distal segment of pancreas by Roux-en-Y anastomosis to the jejunum
- Pancreatitis
    - Alcohol and biliary tract disease, common causes of pancreatitis in adults, are uncommon in children
    - Pathophysiology
        - Autodigestion (autolysis)
        - Exocrine secretions are stored in inactive forms in protective zymogens
        - Alkaline pH of exocrine glands and protease inhibitors assures protection
        - Pancreatic injury (trauma, obstruction, inflammation) can rupture protective membranes within the gland and activate digestive enzymes, causing autodigestion
    - Symptoms
        - Abdominal pain
        - Increased amylase
    - Diagnosis
        - Ratio of amylase to creatinine clearance > 6% indicates pancreatitis

$$\frac{\text{urine amylase} \times \text{serum creatinine} \times 100}{\text{serum amylase} \times \text{urine creatinine}}$$

        - Laboratory tests: serum amylase, lipase
        - Imaging methods: ultrasound, MRCP, ERCP (contraindicated in acute pancreatitis)
    - Etiology
        - The most common cause in children is blunt abdominal trauma
        - The most common cause of nontraumatic pancreatitis is idiopathic

    - Pancreatitis can also be caused by medications (eg, steroids, chemotherapy), infections, especially viral infections (eg, mumps), cystic fibrosis, underlying biliary tract disease, hemolytic disease resulting in stones (eg, spherocytosis, sickle cell disease), or cholelithiasis
  - Treatment
    - Medical
      - Stop offending medications
      - Control infection
      - Provide gut rest; insert nasogastric tube if patient is vomiting, administer total parenteral nutrition (TPN), and give analgesics (eg, meperidine, **not** morphine), volume replacement, antibiotics, H2-blockers, or somatostatin
      - Monitor arterial blood gasses for impending respiratory failure
      - Monitor lactate dehydrogenase and serum glutamic oxaloacetic transaminase, which indicate tissue necrosis
      - Monitor serum calcium for hypocalcemia (due to saponification); prescribe calcium gluconate as indicated
      - Monitor serum glucose for hyperglycemia; prescribe insulin as indicated
      - Monitor hematocrit for hemoconcentration or bleeding
    - Surgical
      - Debride obviously necrotic tissue
      - Drain (especially fluid in lesser sac)
      - Perform cholecystectomy for stones after resolution of the acute episode
- Pseudocysts
  - Trauma is the most common etiology in children
  - Cyst walls are composed of inflammatory tissue (**not** epithelium) and are usually located in the lesser sac
  - Symptoms: pain, compression or erosion of surrounding organs, secondary infection, hemorrhage, and perforation
  - Diagnosis
    - Upper gastrointestinal series will show anterior and superior displacement of stomach and downward displacement of colon

        - CT or ultrasound may also be useful in diagnosis
    - Treatment
        - Medical
            - 50% may resolve spontaneously in 3–4 weeks
            - Perform percutaneous drainage
            - Rest intestinal tract
            - Provide TPN
        - Surgical
            - Surgery is indicated in the case of persistence (>6 wk) or recurrence, and when pseudocyst communicates with a major duct
            - Provide external drainage (if infected)
            - Provide internal drainage by Roux-en-Y cystenterostomy (unless infected)
            - Perform distal pancreatectomy if pseudocyst is in tail
            - Perform cystogastrostomy (open or endoscopic) if pseudocyst is in the pancreatic body or adherent to the stomach (bleeding after operation is a common complication resulting from stomach acid)
            - Perform Roux-en-Y cystjejunostomy if pseudocyst is located at the head of the pancreas or not adherent to stomach

Spleen

- Physiology
    - The thymus is the primary lymphatic organ during intrauterine life
    - The spleen is the major site of hematopoiesis from birth to 6 months of age, when hematopoiesis is taken over by the bone marrow
    - The spleen produces immunoglobulin M (IgM) antibodies against encapsulated bacteria (eg, pneumococcus, hemophilus, meningococcus), and tuftsin and properdin, which enhance phagocytosis and stimulate production
    - Humeral immunity in neonates is transferred through the placenta (except IgM)
- Congenital anomalies
    - Asplenia (Ivemark syndrome): complete absence of the spleen
        - Also called asplenia syndrome or heterotaxia

        - Can be associated with situs inversus (with or without malrotation or volvulus), cardiac anomalies (which are associated with a high mortality rate), and three-lobed lungs
        - Symptoms
            - Congenital cyanotic heart disease, which results in cyanosis
            - Shortness of breath
            - Congestive heart failure
        - Diagnosis
            - Howell-Jolly bodies will be evident in a peripheral smear
            - Perform a spleen scan or ultrasound
    - Polysplenia
        - Multilobed spleen with 2–9 equal portions
        - Associated with situs inversus, cardiac anomalies, and biliary atresia
        - Patient exhibits normal splenic function
    - Accessory spleen
        - Small nodules of splenic tissue apart from a normal-sized spleen
        - These are most commonly located in the splenic hilum (gastrosplenic ligament)
        - Nodules must be removed when a splenectomy is performed for hypersplenia to prevent persistent hematologic disease
    - Cysts
        - Congenital cysts are rare
        - Epidermoid cysts are the most common type in pediatric patients
            - Symptoms: hemorrhage, left upper quadrant pain, infection
        - Echinococcal cysts are the most common type worldwide
        - Differential diagnosis: history, serology, scan
        - Diagnosis: ultrasound, spleen scan, CT scan
        - Treatment: perform partial cyst wall resection/marsupialization, rather than hemisplenectomy
- Trauma

- Diagnosis (see Pancreatic trauma)
- Nonoperative management (see Pancreatic trauma); patients who cannot be observed continuously in an intensive care unit (ICU) or who will be evacuated through multiple levels of care are **not** candidates for conservative management
- Operative management
  - Indications for operation
    - Patient requires transfusions of > 50% blood volume (~ 40 cc/kg)
    - Patient exhibits continued hypotension or evidence of continued hemorrhage
    - There is evidence of associated significant injuries
    - A patient with abdominal distension is in shock (immediate laparotomy is necessary)
  - Treatment
    - Splenorrhaphy is often possible
    - Perform splenectomy in an unstable patient with multiple injuries, or one who will not be continuously observed in an ICU setting or who will be transferred through multiple levels of medical care
    - Provide immunizations to protect against pneumococcus and vaccines to protect again *Haemophilus influenzae* and *Neisseria meningitidis*; give penicillin prophylaxis until the patient reaches 18 years of age

- Inflammation
  - Acute inflammatory splenomegaly
    - Etiology: infection is the most common cause
    - Treatment: treat the source of infection (do not perform splenectomy)
  - Abscess
    - Gram-negative anaerobic *Staphylococcus* is the most common cause
      - Hemoglobinopathy is associated with *Salmonella*
      - Leukemia is associated with *Candida*
    - Trauma
    - Infarction
    - Bacteremia
    - Immunosuppression

- Symptoms: fever, left upper-quadrant tenderness, and left shoulder pain
- Diagnosis: CT scan (best modality)
- Treatment
  - IV antibiotics
  - Percutaneous aspiration and drainage for large abscesses
  - Splenectomy (in the case of peristent infection)

- Hematologic disorders
  - Red blood cells (RBCs)
    - Hereditary spherocytosis
      - Autosomal dominant
      - Etiology: membrane is abnormal, which prevents RBCs from assuming discoid shape; deformity results in small, round, fragile RBCs
      - Symptoms: anemia, jaundice, splenomegaly, gallstones (gallstones occur in 75% of these patients)
      - Laboratory indicators: anemia, increased bilirubin, increased reticulocyte count, spherocytes, increased osmotic fragility
      - Treatment: splenectomy (deferred until age 3–4 years; most common indication) or cholecystectomy if stones present on preoperative ultrasound
      - If hemolysis recurs or if no Howell-Jolly bodies are seen in peripheral smear, suspect a residual accessory spleen
    - Elliptocytosis: rarely associated with RBC destruction sufficient to require splenectomy
    - Sickle cell anemia
      - Homozygous sickle cell gene produces severe, chronic, hemolytic anemia
      - Hemoglobin levels in individuals with sickle cell anemia are as follows:
        - HgB S: 90%
        - HgB F: 5%
        - HgB A2: normal
        - HgB A: absent
      - Sickling results in occlusion of small vessels ("sickle cell crisis")

- Etiology: infection, dehydration, hypoxia, acidosis
- Vasoocclusive crisis is a potential complication characterized by pain and swelling in the hands and feet ("hand / foot syndrome"), acute abdominal pain, pulmonary infarction
- Sequestration results in acute trapping of RBCs in the spleen, which leads to anemia, hypotension, and splenomegaly (if recurrent severe episodes [resulting in shock] occur, splenectomy is indicated after pneumococcal vaccine polyvalent and *H influenzae* type B [Hib] vaccine)
- Eventually the spleen becomes small, fibrotic, and infarcted (functional asplenia); most common infections are pneumococcal and *Salmonella osteomyelitis*
- Laboratory indicators:
  - HgB: 6–8 g / dL
  - Smear will show sickle, target, and nucleated RBCs; Howell-Jolly bodies; 5%–15% reticulocytes, increased white blood count, and increased platelets
  - Liver function tests: abnormal
  - Diagnosis: hemoglobin electrophoresis
- Treatment
  - Hydration
  - Packed red blood cell (PRBC) transfusion to decrease HgB S to < 40% (20 cc / kg type-specific Rh[–] PRBCs) from usual 90%
  - Analgesics

- White blood cells
  - Leukemia
    - Splenomegaly secondary to leukemic infiltrate is the most common cause of splenic rupture
    - Splenectomy is not indicated
- Platelets
  - Idiopathic thrombocytopenic purpura (ITP)
    - Etiology: antiplatelet antibodies attach to platelets, making the platelets more susceptible to destruction in the spleen
    - History: patient will have had antecedent nonspecific viral illness

    - Spleen is normal-sized, platelets are normal shape
    - Symptoms: usually occurs in children (especially females) < 10 years old, a few weeks after a mild viral illness
    - Physical: petechiae, bruising, bleeding (worst if purpura is in the central nervous system [CNS])
    - Treatment: 75% go into spontaneous remission
    - Treatment for chronic or persistent ITP
      - Steroids for 1–3 weeks in patients with persistent thrombocytopenia. Failure to respond to steroids may result in chronic ITP; patients most likely to respond to splenectomy are those in whom preoperative steroids have increased the platelet count (administer 100 mg hydrocortisone IV intraoperatively)
      - IV gammaglobulin (very expensive) is indicated if steroids fail
      - Anti-D immune globulin may be administered in some cases
      - Immunoglobulin G can be given to block platelet-antibody complex, resulting in a normal platelet count in 3–4 days after administration
    - Indications for splenectomy (see Splenectomy) include an acute bleeding episode (especially in the CNS or intraabdominal space; this requires an emergency splenectomy)
      - Relapse is possible following steroids
      - Steroids may also result in persistent platelets < 10,000
      - Splenectomy is curative in > 90% of patients with ITP; however, if accessory splenic tissue is missed, symptoms will recur
    - If platelet count is < 50,000, platelet transfusion should be given only until the splenic artery is ligated, at which time the platelet count will start to rise
    - If postoperative thrombocytosis occurs (platelets number > 1,000,000), prescribe aspirin
- Hyperspleenism
  - Pancytopenia (decreased white blood cells, RBCs, or

platelets) may be primary or secondary to portal hypertension, inflammatory diseases, storage disease, chronic hemolytic disease, myeloproliferative disorder, or neoplastic disease

    - Hypersplenism is associated with sickle cell crisis
    - Treat primary hypersplenism with splenectomy; however, splenectomy is not indicated for secondary hypersplenism resulting from Hodgkin disease, sarcoid, leukemia, and portal hypertension

- Wandering (ectopic) spleen
  - Symptoms: when spleen is attached only by hilar vessels, torsion may occur, leading to abdominal pain
  - Most common in male infants
  - Diagnosis: ultrasound
  - Treatment: splenopexy if the spleen is not infarcted
- Splenectomy
  - Most common indication for splenectomy is ITP
  - Preoperative preparation
    - Immunize patient with polyvalent capsular polysaccharide antigens of pneumococcal vaccine ideally administered > 3 weeks before elective splenectomy, and Hib vaccine
      - Pneumococcal vaccine is only effective against 80% of organisms (may be less effective in children < 2 y old) and provides protection for children 4–5 years old
    - Administer prophylactic antibiotics before, during, and after operation, and regularly until patient is 18 years old
      - Use ampicillin in children < 10 years old
      - Use penicillin if patient is > 10 years old
    - Give an intraoperative stress dose of steroids (100 mg hydrocortisone IV) if patient was treated with steroids immediately before the operation
  - Operative procedures
    - Place a nasogastric tube to prevent gastric distension and dislodgement of ties on the short gastric vessels
    - Make a laparoscopic, upper midline, or left subcostal incision
    - Mobilize by incising posterior, lateral peritoneal reflection

    - Divide short gastric vessels
    - Ligate and divide splenic artery
    - Avoid injury to the tail of the pancreas
    - Search for accessory spleens in gastrosplenic ligament
    - All splenic tissue must be removed for hematologic reasons or the disorder will recur
  - Postoperative considerations
    - The most serious postoperative complication is overwhelming postsplenectomy infection (see below), which is associated with a 50% rate of mortality, especially in children < 2 years old
    - Laboratory tests
      - Peripheral blood smear will show the following cytoplasmic inclusions:
        - Heinz bodies
        - Howell-Jolly bodies
        - Siderocytes
      - Increased white blood cell count
    - Thrombocytosis
      - A platelet count < 1,000,000 requires no treatment
      - Platelet count may be > 1,000,000 10 days after operation; treat with aspirin (80 mg/day)
      - Thrombotic complications (eg, portal vein thrombosis, diagnosed by ultrasound) are rare
    - Overwhelming postsplenectomy infection
      - Risk
        - Greatest in infancy, decreases with age
        - Twice as great in children < 2 years old
        - Least when splenectomy is done for trauma
        - Greatest when splenectomy is done for thalassemia and other hematological indications
        - Overall incidence ~ 5%
      - 80% occur within 2 years of splenectomy
      - Symptoms (extremely rapid in onset and progression)
        - Nausea and vomiting
        - Confusion
        - Seizures
        - Shock

  - Disseminated intravascular coagulation
  - Coma
  - Death (50%)
- Pneumococcus is the most common organism responsible, **not** hemophilus
- Prevention: polyvalent pneumococcal vaccine

Chapter 21

Genitourinary Tract

Introduction

The majority of pediatric patients with genitourinary trauma will have concomitant injuries (abdomen, thorax, spine, pelvis, femur). The management of genitourinary injuries in children is similar to that for adults; this chapter focuses primarily on the differences in management.

Trauma

- Renal injuries
    - Children are believed to be more susceptible to renal injury than adults
    - Preexisting renal anomalies (ureteropelvic junction [UPJ] obstruction, hydroureteronephrosis, horseshoe kidney) are 3–5 times more common in children undergoing evaluation for renal trauma than in adults
    - Children with preexisting renal anomalies are frequently noted to have hematuria out of proportion to the injury; however, the degree of injury is comparable to that in those without anomalies
    - Significant renal injury may be present in children without hematuria; up to 70% of children with grade 2 or higher renal injury will not have hematuria
    - Indications for renal imaging after abdominal trauma
        - Significant deceleration injury
            - High speed motor vehicle accident
            - Pedestrian struck by a car
            - Fall > 15 ft
            - Striking of flank with a foreign object
        - Associated injuries
            - Fractures of thoracic rib cage, spine, pelvis, or femur
            - Bruising of torso or perineum
            - Peritoneal signs
            - Gross hematuria

        - Microscopic hematuria with systolic blood pressure < 90 mmHg at any time
- Imaging
    - Focused assessment with sonography for trauma (FAST) examination
        - This fails to detect 5%–10% of clinically significant liver, spleen, kidney, adrenal, and small bowel injuries
        - A negative FAST examination **and** normal serial physical examinations over 24 hours rule out significant intraabdominal injury
    - Computed tomography (CT) scan
        - Stabilized patient: triphasic (precontrast, immediately following injection, and 15–20 min delayed)
        - Labile patient: single phase immediately following injection will miss ureteral injury or urinary extravasations
        - Severely unstable patients: intraoperative
        - Verify the presence of a functioning contralateral kidney prior to performing trauma nephrectomy
        - Administer a single shot intravenous (IV) pyelogram using 2 mL / kg IV contrast; perform a radiograph of the kidneys, ureters, and bladder at 10–15 minutes
- Management
    - Grade
        - 1: contusion / subcapsular hematoma
        - 2: < 1 cm laceration
        - 3: > 1 cm laceration and / or devitalized fragments
        - 4: laceration with urinary extravasation or major renovascular injury, controlled hemorrhage
        - 5: shattered kidney / hilar avulsion / major renovascular injury with uncontrolled hemorrhage
    - Indications for nonsurgical management
        - Patient is hemodynamically stable, grade 1 or 2, with or without associated abdominal injury
        - Isolated grade 3 or 4, provided the distal ureter is intact
        - A hemodynamically stable, grade 5 injury
    - Treatment

        - Monitor bed rest (urine output, vital signs) until gross hematuria has resolved
        - Perform serial physical examinations and hematocrit measurements
        - Administer antibiotics
        - 2–3 days after injury, reimage grade 3, 4, and 5 injuries that were managed nonoperatively
  - Operative intervention
    - Relative indications
      - Ongoing hemorrhage (consider embolization)
      - Urinary extravasation and progressive pain or ileus
      - Ureteral stent or percutaneous drainage of urinoma
      - No strenuous activity for 6 weeks
    - Absolute indications for operative intervention
      - Hemodynamic instability due to renal source
      - Expanding/pulsatile retroperitoneal hematoma
      - Unsuccessful attempt at angioinfarction
      - Renal exploration (operative technique equivalent to adults)
      - Coexisting abdominal injuries and grade 3 or greater renal injury
      - Unstable patient with inadequate preoperative staging and finding of retroperitoneal hematoma at exploration
    - Principles of renal exploration
      - Verify function of the contralateral kidney before exploration
      - Obtain control of the renal vessels prior to exploration
      - Repair the renal injury
      - Keep drainage separate from coexisting injuries
      - Separate intraabdominal and retroperitoneal injuries using omentum
- UPJ disruption
  - CT scan findings
    - Good renal contrast excretion with medial perirenal extravasation
    - No parenchymal laceration
    - Nonvisualization of ipsilateral ureter on delayed images

- Treatment
  - Retrograde pyelogram to evaluate continuity of the UPJ
    - If the UPJ is intact and there is a renal parenchymal or pelvic laceration, place a ureteral stent; nephrostomy may be indicated
    - If the UPJ is disrupted and the problem is diagnosed **within 5 days**, perform immediate surgical repair
      - Debride devitalized tissue
      - Spatulate and reanastomose the ureter to the renal pelvis with fine, absorbable suture over a ureteral stent (5–6 French size [Fr]) or feeding tube
      - Place an intraoperative nephrostomy tube and retroperitoneal drain
      - Mobilize the kidney for a tension-free anastomosis, if necessary
    - If the UPJ is disrupted and problem is diagnosed **after 6 days**
      - Perform nephrostomy
      - Reassess after 12 weeks
      - Perform retrograde pyelogram and functional imaging

- Ureteral injury
  - Accounts for < 4% of penetrating injuries in children
  - Mortality rate of > 30% is related to concomitant injuries
  - Two thirds of cases do not have hematuria
  - High-velocity injury produces a blast effect
  - Ureter may appear intact at exploration
  - Delayed necrosis leads to urinary extravasation
  - Presentation: urine output from surgical drains 3–5 days after injury
  - Management
    - Within 5 days of injury: perform a primary repair
      - Remove devitalized tissue
      - Spatulate and perform tensionless anastomosis over a stent with a fine, absorbable suture
      - Use renal mobilization or a bladder flap to relieve tension
    - In an unstable patient or in the presence of extensive in-

jury, occlude the ureter with a large clip at the proximal end and place a nephrostomy tube for delayed repair

- Bladder injury
  - Frequently associated with multiorgan trauma
  - Absolute indications for surgical repair
    - Gross hematuria and pelvic fracture
    - Inability to void
  - Relative indications for surgical repair
    - Clot retention
    - Perineal hematoma
  - Image using cystogram
    - Instill at least ½ estimated bladder capacity under gravity via urethral catheter (bladder capacity = [age + 2] × 30; Table 21-1)

Table 21-1. Urethral Catheter Size Estimation*

Age	Size (Fr Feeding Tube† or Foley Catheter)
Newborn	5
3 mo	8
1 y	8–10
3–6 y	10
8 y	10–12
10 y	12
12 y	12–14
Teenager	16+

*In males, use a tube that fits the meatus, the narrowest part of the male urethra.
†A French-sized feeding tube may be used if a Foley catheter is unavailable or if the Foleys available are too big.

    - Standard cystogram
      - Plain film
      - Contrast film
      - Drain film
    - CT cystogram
      - Only requires fill film
      - Dilute contrast by ¼ to ⅓
      - Must fill bladder, not just clamp catheter
  - Treatment

- Administer antibiotics until 48 hours after the catheter is removed
- Explore and repair extraperitoneal region
- If CT scan shows a bone spicule in the bladder or if there is bladder neck injury,
  - Small children, particularly boys, will need a large-caliber suprapubic tube (SPT; a small urethral catheter will not drain clots)
  - Drain 7–10 days, then reimage
- If no bone spicules are evident and bladder neck injury is ruled out, place an indwelling catheter and observe
- Intraperitoneal
  - Free intraabdominal fluid will be visible on CT scan
  - Diagnose with intraperitoneal contrast on cystogram
  - Explore and repair
- Transvesical approach
  - Identify and spare ureteral orifices
  - Use absorbable suture in 2-layer closure
  - Place a large-bore urinary catheter (SPT for boys and small girls to allow large bore) and / or Foley catheter
  - Place perivesical drain
  - Perform cystogram at 7–10 days prior to catheter removal
  - Bladder injury in children is twice as likely to involve the bladder neck than it is in adults
    - If bladder neck is not repaired, patient will likely sustain persistent urinary extravasation
    - Bladder neck injury increases incontinence risk
    - Suspect a bladder neck injury if there is contrast extravasation and an incompetent bladder neck is apparent on cystogram
- Repair of bladder neck injury
  - Open bladder at dome
  - Use care to avoid disrupting a pelvic hematoma
  - Use an intravesical closure (absorbable) suture in multiple layers with suprapubic and urethral catheter drainage
  - Perform retrograde urethrogram or cystoscopy to

assess for urethral injury
      - Place urethral and suprapubic catheters
- Urethral injury
  - Children versus adults
    - Pelvic fracture is more likely to be unstable in children than in adults, displacing the prostatic urethra
    - Complete posterior urethral disruption is more common in boys than men
    - There is a 20% incidence of both bladder and urethral injuries in children
    - Prepubertal girls are 4-fold as likely to have urethral injury with a pelvic fracture than adult women
  - Imaging
    - Indications
      - Perineal/penile hematoma
      - Blood at meatus/introitus
      - Inability to void
      - One or more pubic rami factures **or** symphyseal diastatis
      - Evidence of bladder neck injury
    - Males
      - Perform retrograde urethrogram
      - Insert a 6 Fr or 8 Fr Foley catheter, with balloon gently inflated with approximately 1 cc, in the fossa navicularis and perform retrograde instillation of 10–15 cc contrast with an oblique film, visualizing contrast into the bladder
    - Females
      - Anesthetize patient and perform vaginoscopy or cystoscopy
      - For prepubertal girls, use a nasal speculum or cystoscope
  - Urethral injury combined with pelvic fracture mandates a rectal examination
    - Blood in stool indicates a potential occult rectal injury
    - Treat the rectal injury with diversion
  - Urethral injury in girls
    - Invariably associated with a pelvic fracture
    - 75% are associated with a vaginal injury

        - 30% are concurrent with rectal injury
    - Treatment
        - Administer broad-spectrum antibiotics
        - Assess bladder neck
        - Establish urinary drainage with an urethral catheter or suprapubic tube; vesicostomy is a diversion option in infants
        - Make a small transverse incision between the pubis and the umbilicus, mobilize and open dome of the bladder, and mature stoma to rectus fascia and skin
        - Encourage gentle passage of urethral catheter (if disruption is not complete) to establish continuity; abort if passing the catheter is difficult
        - Repair small lacerations of the anterior urethra with fine, absorbable suture
- External genital injuries
    - Management of penile, scrotal, and testicular injuries is equivalent to that of adults
    - Evaluate for concomitant rectal injury in the presence of penetrating scrotal or vulvar trauma
    - Perform meticulous examination under anesthesia to assess depth and extent of wound, debridement of nonviable tissue, and evidence of concomitant injuries
    - In the presence of associated hematuria or blood on rectal examination, evaluate for urethral injury or rectal injury, respectively

Conditions of the Genitourinary Tract

- Urinary tract infection (UTI)
    - Diagnosis
        - Neonates
            - Symptoms include jaundice, failure to thrive, and fever
            - Laboratory tests: bacteriuria
        - Older children
            - Symptoms: dysuria, urgency, frequency, enuresis
    - A positive bagged urine culture should be confirmed by a specimen obtained by suprapubic aspiration
    - UTI: > 105 colonies/mL of a single bacterial species

- Accuracy
  - 80% in a bagged specimen
  - 95% in a catheterized specimen
  - 99% in a specimen obtained from suprapubic aspiration
- White blood cells in urine are suggestive of UTI
- Nitrite test: nitrate that is normally present in urine is converted to nitrite by bacteria
- Classification
  - Upper tract infection (pyelonephritis)
    - Symptoms: fever, flank pain or tenderness, increased white blood cell count
    - Treatment: IV antibiotics
  - Lower tract infection
    - Diagnosis: suprapubic aspiration, catheterized specimen
- Epidemiology
  - Neonates: occurs more frequently in males than females (due to congenital abnormalities)
  - Other ages: more common in females than males; incidence increases with age in both sexes
- Pathophysiology
  - Protective factors
    - Regular complete bladder emptying (avoid urine stasis)
    - Antimicrobial activity of urothelium (urothelial cells secrete a mucopolysaccharide coating, which traps bacteria)
    - Acid pH, high urinary osmolality
  - Potentiating factors
    - Urinary stasis
    - Vesicoureteral reflux
    - Urolithiasis
    - Obstruction
    - Periurethral colonization (usually with gut flora)
    - Phimosis
    - Bacterial factors
      - O (lipopolysaccharide), K, H antigens
      - Hemolysins
      - Urease produces alkalization of urine, resulting

in stone formation

- Laboratory findings
  - 50% of patients < 12 years old with a UTI have associated urinary tract abnormalities
  - If culture from urinary analysis (suprapubic in infants, midstream clean catch or straight catheter in older patients) is positive, proceed to ultrasound and voiding cystourethrography
- Treatment
  - Ampicillin + gentamicin for 7 days
  - Hydration

Penis

- Foreskin retractility
  - Newborn (term): usually not retractile
  - 6 months: 20%
  - 6 years: 40%
  - 13 years: 100%
- Hypospadias
  - Urethral meatus opens onto the ventral surface of the penis, proximal to the end of the glans
  - Associated anomalies include inguinal hernia and undescended testicles
  - Usually repaired in first year of life
  - Most commonly glandular (subcoronal)
  - May be associated with ventral curvature (ie, chordee)
  - Avoid circumcision to facilitate reconstruction; perform meatal advancement and glanuloplasty procedure
- Epispadias
  - Urethral meatus opens onto the dorsal surface of the penis, proximal to the end of the glans
- Phimosis
  - Physical: male foreskin cannot be fully retracted from the head of the penis (normal in infancy)
  - Etiology: congenital or acquired from recurrent infections of the foreskin (balanitis)
  - Complications include impairment or obstruction to urinary flow and paraphimosis (see page 255)
  - Treatment: circumcision

- Paraphimosis
  - Physical: the foreskin becomes trapped behind the glans penis and cannot be pulled back to its normal position
  - Complications include constriction of blood supply to the glans
  - Treatment options
    - Compress the glans and move the foreskin back to its normal position
    - Make a dorsal slit in the foreskin or perform circumcision
    - Make multiple needle punctures in the swollen foreskin and express the edema fluid using manual pressure
  - Prevention: pull the foreskin back over the glans after it has been retracted (eg, to insert a Foley catheter)
- Circumcision
  - Surgical indications for circumcision
    - Definite
      - Phimosis
      - Paraphimosis
      - Recurrent balanitis
    - Relative: recurrent UTI
  - Techniques
    - Freehand
    - PlastiBell (Hollister, Inc, Libertyville, Ill)
    - Gomco clamp
    - Mogen clamp
  - Complications
    - Bleeding
    - Infection
    - Urethral injury
    - Removal of too much/too little foreskin

Testicular and Scrotal Conditions

- Undescended testes (UDT)
  - Definitions
    - Retractile testis
      - Etiology: overactive cremasteric muscle
      - Testis can be brought into scrotum by careful manipulation

        - Usually bilateral
        - Testis remains in scrotum after onset of puberty
            - Testicle becomes heavier and larger than the external inguinal ring
            - Cremaster becomes less active
    - Cryptorchidism
        - Testis does not descend into scrotum due to inadequacy or maternal gonadotrophic hormones
        - Associated with abnormal spermatogenesis
        - The higher the position of the testis, the more abnormal
        - Most fail to reach scrotum because spermatic artery is too short
    - Ectopic
        - Testis is located in an abnormal position (thigh, groin)
        - Results from abnormally positioned gubernaculum
        - Increased risk for trauma
        - Treatment: orchidopexy by 1–2 years of age
    - Anorchism
        - Absent testis resulting from torsion or infarction during fetal life
        - Ultrasound and laparoscopy aid in diagnosis
        - Treatment involves surgical exploration; dysplastic or intraabdominal testes have a high incidence of malignant degeneration
    - Polyorchism: > 2 testes
- Embryology
    - Testicular descent through the internal ring starts at 30 weeks
    - Failure to descend can result from:
        - Inadequate gonadotrophic hormones (testosterone)
        - Failure of end organ (testis) response to testosterone
- Pathology
    - Location of UDT: anywhere from the renal hilum to the external inguinal ring
    - Smaller, softer, and more elongated than normal testes
    - 90% have an associated hernia sac
    - Testicular degeneration begins after the second year of age
    - Unilateral UDT may produce autoantibodies that injure

the other testis

- Incidence (similar to inguinal hernias)
  - Right side: 50%
  - Left side: 25%
  - Bilateral: 25%
  - 10-fold more common in premature infants
- Differential diagnosis: retractile testis
- Indications for operation
  - Spermatogenesis
    - Cryptorchid testis is exposed to increased temperature, resulting in decreased spermatogenesis
    - Determinants of degree of testicular damage
      - Length of exposure
      - Degree of nondescent
    - Unilateral: associated with approximately normal fertility if corrected before 2 years of age
    - Bilateral: usually results in sterility
    - Optimal age for repair is 1–2 years of age
  - Malignant change
    - May be more common in UDT
    - Orchidopexy has not been shown with certainty to influence the incidence of malignancy, but does permit earlier detection (average age at the time of diagnosis is 26 y old)
    - Tumor development (seminoma, teratocarcinoma, embryonal); orchiopexy makes it easier to examine for a malignant tumor
    - Children > 14 years old with unilateral UDT should undergo orchiectomy
  - Increased risk of trauma and torsion in UDT
  - Cosmetic and psychological considerations
- Treatment
  - Rationale for orchiopexy
    - Enhances fertility
    - Decreases risk of torsion
    - Repairs coexistent hernia
    - Prevents trauma
    - Makes it easier to examine for the presence of a testicular tumor, permitting earlier detection

- Surgical treatment
  - Optimal time for surgery is at 1–2 years of age
  - Technique: formation of a dartos pouch
  - Limiting factor: length of spermatic artery
  - If testis is not palpable, perform laparoscopy
  - Testis present
    - First stage Fowler-Stevens (laparoscopic): ligate (clip) the spermatic artery and vein high in the retroperitoneal space; testicular blood supply is then derived from vessels to the vas, deep epigastric collaterals, and processes vaginalis; place testicle as low as possible in the scrotum at this first operation
    - Second stage Fowler-Stevens (at 6–12 mo of age): bring testicle down into scrotum
  - Testes absent ("anorchia")
    - Diagnose by identifying a blind-ending vas and vessels (using laparoscopy)
    - Treatment: close
  - Atrophic/dystrophic testes
    - Biopsy to confirm
    - Orchiectomy if contralateral testis is normal (usually performed after onset of puberty)
  - Testis palpable in canal
    - Perform orchiopexy
    - Testosterone production will be unchanged after orchiopexy
    - Perform orchiectomy only if patient is > 14 years of age (ie, after onset of puberty)
- Results
  - Injury to vas (uncommon)
  - Injury to spermatic vessels may cause atrophy
  - Patients with uncorrected bilateral UDT are infertile
  - 70% of patients with bilateral UDT corrected < 2 years of age are fertile

- Acute conditions of the scrotum
  - Torsion
    - Most common genitourinary emergency of childhood

- Occurs in late childhood to early adolescence, predominantly before age 6, peaking at age 14
- Pathology: twisting of the testicle on its blood supply, which may result in infarction
- Differential diagnosis
  - Major
    - Torsion of testis (torsion of appendix testis)
    - Epididymitis
    - Orchitis
    - Trauma
    - Tumor
    - Hemorrhage
  - Minor
    - Idiopathic scrotal edema
    - Hernia/hydrocele
- Types
  - Extravaginal: occurs in perinatal period
  - Intravaginal: due to lack of testicular fixation in tunica ("bell-clapper anomaly"); occurs at birth
- Symptoms of torsion
  - Scrotal pain
    - Abrupt onset suggests testicular torsion; acute scrotal pain must be considered torsion of the testicle until proven otherwise
    - Gradual (12–24 h) onset suggests torsion of the appendix testis; pain radiates upward toward groin and lower abdomen
    - History: prior transient episodes of testicular pain with spontaneous resolution
    - Physical: red, painful, tender scrotum; testis is enlarged, tender, and elevated within scrotum
    - Pain is increased when scrotum is lifted
  - Associated abdominal and gastrointestinal symptoms include nausea, vomiting, and lower quadrant abdominal pain
  - Differential diagnosis: localization of tenderness to particular scrotal structures

◦ Neonatal torsion

- Pathology

        - True torsion of the spermatic cord
        - Extravaginal (outside the tunica vaginalis) torsion
    - Usually results in complete infarction, requiring orchidectomy
    - Probable etiology of "vanishing testis" syndrome (unilateral anorchia)
    - Extravaginal etiology
        - Inadequate fixation of testis, resulting in twisting of the cord structures and infarction
        - Usually occurs in neonates
    - Intravaginal or bell clapper deformity
        - Abnormally high reflection of the tunica vaginalis upward from its usual, more equatorial position about the testicle to a level of attachment to the spermatic cord itself
        - Leaves the testicle hanging (like the clapper of a bell) within the tunica vaginalis, able to spin freely around the long axis of the spermatic cord
    - Laboratory tests
        - Complete blood count
        - Urinary analysis will show increased white blood cell count
        - Use Doppler flow study to assess blood flow to testicle and differentiate ischemia (torsion) from an inflammatory process (epididymitis; see following page)
        - Use technetium-99m scan
            - Torsion will reveal a halo of increased activity around the scrotum surrounding a cold center (ischemic testicle)
            - Epididymitis and torsion of appendix testis will show markedly increased blood flow to affected side
    - Treatment
        - Sedate and attempt manual detorsion
        - Perform prompt bilateral orchidopexy
            - Use midline scrotal raphe incision
            - Suture tunica albuginea to scrotal wall using four nonabsorbable sutures

- If torsion is present for > 12 hours or is necrotic,
  - Perform orchiectomy (necrotic testes may produce autoimmune antibodies)
  - Apply testicular prosthesis at a later time (~ 6 mo of age)
- If torsion is present at birth, stabilize the baby before exploration (salvage is not possible)

- Prognosis
  - Increased risk of impaired spermatogenesis and infertility
  - < 6 hours: 90% chance of salvage
  - 6–12 hours: 75% chance of salvage
  - 12–24 hours: 50% chance of salvage
  - > 24 hours: < 10% chance of salvage

- Torsion of appendix testis
  - Physical: transillumination may reveal the "blue dot" sign
  - Treatment
    - Bed rest, scrotal support, and analgesics
    - Operative intervention if symptoms persist > 2–3 days
    - If torsion of the testis cannot be distinguished from appendix testis by physical examination or Doppler ultrasound, prompt surgical exploration is indicated
- Epididymitis
  - Etiology
    - Reflux of urine up the vas to epididymis, inciting an inflammatory response
    - Sexually transmitted disease (usually gonococcus or chlamydia)
  - Symptoms
    - Pain is decreased when scrotum is lifted (Prehn sign)
    - Urinary tract symptoms associated with epididymitis (usually seen in postpubertal boys) include urinary frequency, dysuria, and pyuria
  - Diagnosis and laboratory tests
    - Urinary analysis will revel bacteria
    - If urine culture is positive in a nonsexually active male, rule out congenital urinary tract anomaly
    - Perform renal ultrasound to rule out hydronephrosis
    - Perform voiding cystourethrography to rule out

bladder outlet obstruction

- Treatment: antibiotics for chlamydia (doxycycline), analgesics

- Orchitis
  - Etiology: usually due to a viral infection (eg, mumps)
  - Physical: scrotal skin is erythematous and edematous, white blood cell count is increased, urinary analysis is normal, ultrasound shows good blood flow to testis
  - Treatment: bed rest, observation
  - Associated with decreased fertility
- Varicocele
  - Most common on left (left spermatic vein drains into the left renal vein)
  - Etiology
    - Idiopathic: incompetent venous valves
    - Obstruction of renal vein
      - Left renal vein thrombosis
      - Retroperitoneal tumor
  - Symptoms
    - Pain
    - Testicular atrophy
    - Decreased fertility (due to increased temperature)
  - Diagnosis: ultrasound
  - Treatment
    - Measure dimensions of the testicle; atrophy and pain are the primary indications for operation
    - Perform laparoscopic, retroperitoneal ligation of the spermatic veins and artery

Tumors

- Most common testicular tumors in childhood include teratomas, yolk sac tumors, rhabdomyosarcoma, and lymphoma
  - Physical: solid scrotal mass
  - Diagnosis: radiograph, α-fetoprotein, β-human chorionic gonadotrophin
  - Treatment
    - Inguinal incision (**note: never approach through a scrotal incision!**)
    - Clamp and individually ligate cord structures at the internal ring

    - Deliver testicle
    - Perform high inguinal orchiectomy if a neoplasm is present

Vaginal Conditions

- Labial fusion (labial adhesions)
  - Etiology: chronic irritation, lack of estrogen stimulation
  - Symptoms: difficulty urinating
  - Diagnosis: labia minora are fused on physical examination
  - Treatment
    - Incision under general anesthesia
    - Topical estrogen cream once a day for 30 days
    - Gentle separation in office after application of lidocaine jelly or lidocaine/prilocaine cream
    - Prevention: maintain good hygiene
- Vaginitis
  - Etiology
    - Prepuberty: allergy/irritation due to bubble bath or laundry detergent is most common
    - Postpuberty: infections; **rule out child abuse**
    - Foreign body
  - Diagnosis: vaginoscopy
  - Treatment: removal of foreign body or irritant; antibiotics for infection
- Pelvic inflammatory disease
  - *Neisseria gonorrhoeae* is the most common cause
  - *Chlamydia trachomatis* is increasing in incidence as an etiology

Medicine

Chapter 22

Basic Fluid and Electrolytes

Introduction

Infants and young children have a greater need for water and are more vulnerable to alterations in fluid and electrolyte imbalances than adults. Water and electrolyte imbalances occur more frequently and more rapidly in children, and children adjust less promptly to those disturbances. Infants and children also have a greater proportional amount of extracellular fluid volume.

Normal Distribution of Body Water and Electrolytes

Total body water (TBW) varies with an individual's age and amount of muscle mass and body fat; the more fat an individual has, the smaller the proportion of body weight attributed to body water

- 80%–85% of a premature infant's body weight is attributed to water
- About 70% of a full-term infant's body weight is attributed to water
- Body weight attributed to water in young adults differs between males and females:
  - Males: ~ 65% total body weight
  - Females: ~ 52% of total body weight

During infancy, a larger proportion of body water is extracellular; about half an infant's extracellular fluid is exchanged daily

Changes in Fluid Composition and Distribution During Critical Illness

Critically ill infants and children tend to retain fluids because of increased secretion of antidiuretic hormone (ADH) and aldosterone

- Catecholamine release, hypotension, fright, and pain stimulate the release of ADH, renin, and aldosterone
- ADH release is also stimulated by any condition that reduces left atrial pressure (eg, hemorrhage, positive-pressure ventila-

tion, or severe pulmonary hypertension), general anesthetics, morphine, and barbiturates

- Critically ill pediatric patients often exhibit decreased urine volume and increased urine concentration in the presence of hemodilution
- A newborn's kidney has a limited ability to concentrate urine; a neonate may have decreased urine volume and only moderate urine concentration

Administering Maintenance Fluid

Fluid administration must be tailored to prevent fluid overload or sodium balance (Tables 22-1 and 22-2)

- Fluid and electrolyte losses in urine most closely resemble 0.45 normal saline (½NS); insensible losses are more similar to 0.2 NS

Table 22-1. Pediatric Daily Fluid Requirements

Age/Weight	Fluid Goal	Calories (kcal/kg)	Dextrose*
Infants (> 1 mo)	100–120 mL/kg	~ 120	5%–10%
< 10 kg	100 mL/kg	~ 110	5%
10–20 kg	1,000 mL + 50 mL/kg > 10 kg	~ 80	5%
> 20 kg	1,500 mL + 20 mL/kg > 20 kg	≥ 45	5%

*Percent of dextrose in water.

- ½NS is usually administered with 5% or 10% glucose immediately postoperatively to replace insensible and urine losses
- Excessive gastrointestinal losses are generally replaced with ½NS
- All infusions should be connected to a constant infusion pump
    - Specific electrolyte needs and therapies require different concentrations
        - Generally use D_{10}¼NS for neonates; D_5½NS for other infants and children
        - Add potassium (20 mEq/L) if urine output is documented or after evaluating serum electrolytes

Table 22-2. Pediatric Daily Electrolyte Requirements*

Age	Sodium	Potassium	Magnesium†	Calcium†	Phosphorus†
Infants/children	3.0 mEq/kg‡	2.0 mEq/kg	0.25 mEq/kg	1.0 mEq/kg	0.50 mEq/kg
Adolescents	2.0 mEq/kg	1.0 mEq/kg	0.25 mEq/kg	0.25 mEq/kg	0.25 mEq/kg

*A standard pediatric fluid is D_5½NS with 20 mEq of KCl/L.
†Consider adding if using intravenous fluids for more than 3–5 days.
‡1 mEq potassium phosphate = 0.68 mmol phosphorus (1 mEq sodium phosphate = 0.75 mmol phosphorus).

Table 22-3. Differentiating Sources of Sodium Disturbances

Condition	Intravascular Volume Status	Serum Sodium	Urine Volume	Urine Sodium	Net Sodium Status
Hyponatremic dehydration	↓	↓	↓	↓	↓
SIADH	Normal or ↑	↓	↓	↑	Normal
CSW	↓	↓	↑	↑	↓

↓: decreased
↑: increased
CSW: cerebral salt wasting
SIADH: syndrome of inappropriate antidiuretic hormone

- Monitor urine volume closely, using a Foley if necessary
  - Should average > 1 mL/kg/h if fluid volume is adequate
  - If fluid is severely restricted, urine volume may average 0.5–1 mL/kg/h

Electrolyte Management

- Hypokalemia
  - Encountered most commonly following use of loop and thiazide diuretics
  - Also found following vomiting, diarrhea, intestinal fistulas, ileostomy drainage, or gastric suctioning
  - Excessive renal excretion of potassium is associated with metabolic alkalosis, renal tubular acidosis, and diabetic ketoacidosis
  - Cardiac dysrhythmias occur infrequently unless the hypokalemia is severe
  - Electrocardiogram (ECG) findings include low voltage, flattened T waves, and prolonged QT interval
  - **Management**
    - Use intravenous (IV) potassium replacement if the child is nauseated and vomiting; continuous replacement is preferred over potassium chloride bolus therapy
      - Potassium chloride infusions should not exceed 1 mEq/kg and should not be delivered faster than over 60–90 minutes (maximum 25 mEq KCl)
      - Patient should be observed closely on a monitor
      - Peripheral veins will routinely tolerate up to 40–60 mEq KCl/L in IV fluids
    - Consider potassium chloride supplements to enteral feeds in the absence of vomiting
      - Administer 1 mEq/kg/dose 3–4 times daily, depending on the degree of hypokalemia
      - Do not exceed 1 mEq/oz of enteral formula during tube feeds
- Hyperkalemia
  - Etiologies include excessive potassium administration, significant cell destruction, and reduced renal excretion of potassium

  - Common signs include generalized muscle weakness and flaccidity
  - ECG findings include tall, peaked T wave on ECG initially, followed by widened QRS, ST segment depression, and increasing R wave amplitude
  - As serum potassium level rises, PR interval prolongs
  - Ventricular fibrillation may occur
  - Management includes frequent reassessments, careful monitoring of "ins and outs" (ie, fluids in and urine and drainage out)
    - Reexpand intravascular volume with NS 10–20 mL/kg
    - Administer calcium gluconate 100 mg/kg over 5 minutes (maximum dose is 2 g). Give IV calcium through central line, if available; calcium preparations can cause skin burns if peripheral IV is infiltrated
    - Use sodium bicarbonate (1 mEq/kg over 5 min) in the presence of metabolic acidosis
    - Glucose and insulin therapy are very effective in children; give 0.5 g/kg of glucose (5 cc/kg of 10% dextrose in water) and 0.1 unit/kg of insulin over 30 minutes
    - Administer sodium polystyrene sulfonate 1 g/kg/dose diluted in 3–4 mL of water every 6 hours orally, nasogastrically or rectally
    - Consider giving an albuterol treatment, which will begin to lower the serum potassium level in 30 minutes
- Hyponatremia
  - Common etiologies for hyponatremia include hyponatremic dehydration due to excessive sodium loss or diuretic use; syndrome of inappropriate antidiuretic hormone (SIADH) and cerebral salt wasting can be seen with major head trauma or meningitis (Table 22-3)
  - Hyponatremic dehydration can be corrected over 24 hours, with half the deficit replaced in the first 8 hours
    - The sodium (Na^+) deficit can be calculated as follows:

$$Na^+ \text{ deficit} = (140 - \text{serum } Na^+) \times \text{weight (kg)} \times 0.6$$

    - Add the deficit sodium and water to the daily maintenance sodium and water to derive the most appropriate fluid (usually at least ½NS)

- The serum sodium should rise no more than 0.5 mEq/L/h
- Potassium chloride (20 mEq/L) may be added when patient voids

  - Managing SIADH involves relative fluid and free water restriction; use NS to avoid giving free water
  - Managing cerebral salt wasting involves aggressively replacing ongoing salt and water loss
    - Check urine electrolytes if possible
    - Replace sodium deficit with a combination of NS and 3% hypertonic saline, ideally through a central line; maximum infusion rate 2 mL/kg/h (1 mEq/kg/h)
- Hypernatremia ($Na^+ > 165$)
  - Etiologies include hypernatremic/hypertonic dehydration and diabetes insipidus
  - Management of hypernatremic dehydration, like all severe hypertonic states (eg, diabetic ketoacidosis) requires a slower correction, usually over 48–72 hours, depending on the duration and severity of the hypernatremia (eg, a 10-day-old breast-fed infant whose serum sodium rose to 165 mEq/dL over many days)
  - Calculating the sodium deficit can be complex; if all volume lost is assumed to be isotonic saline 140 mEq/L, the most likely calculation error will be avoided
    - For severe hypernatremic dehydration ($Na^+ \geq 165$), do not use anything less tonic than NS for at least the first 12 hours
    - The sodium level should fall no more than 0.5 mEq/L/h

Chapter 23

Nursing Assessment

Growth and Development

- **Infant (0–12 mo)**
  - Developmental progression
    - Infants develop vertically, then horizontally
    - Body control begins with head control at 2 months, followed by chest control at 4 months, sitting at 6 months, crawling (arm and knee control) at 8 months, standing (cruising) at 10 months, and walking at 12 months
    - By 1 year of age, children learn to feed themselves and talk using a few words
  - Physical development
    - Infants are totally dependent on their caregivers
    - They manifest separation anxiety and loss of control with crying and rage; they expect that crying will bring an immediate response when they are otherwise unable to express their needs or understand a situation
    - Immobility leads to irritability
    - Infants respond to pain by crying or withdrawing
  - When examining an infant, assess vitals (see Chapter 2, Anesthesia, Table 2-2 for normal vital signs by age)
    - Infants and children have the same normal ranges for temperature and oxygen saturation as adults
    - Infants should exhibit the following characteristics:
      - Ability to make eye contact, orient preferentially to faces, and track brightly colored objects
      - Ability to move all extremities spontaneously
      - Irritability or high-pitched, weak crying (these characteristics are concerning)
        - Deterioration manifests as a weak, flaccid, and unresponsive examination
      - An open anterior fontanelle until around 16 months
- **Toddlers (1–3 y)**
  - Developmental progression

- Toddlers begin to eat regular foods
- They have around 10 teeth
- They talk using one or two words
- They begin to toilet train, bowel first and bladder second (daytime first, nighttime last)

◦ Physical needs are more independent; toddler can walk and grasp
  - Toddlers will often regress to "baby" behavior when ill or stressed
  - They may return to earlier, dependent behaviors like clinging, bed wetting, or wanting bottle, breast, or pacifier

◦ Toddlers fear the unknown and abandonment; upon separation, they may protest loudly or cry monotonously

◦ Denial or saying "no" is common toddler behavior

◦ Toddlers are very ritualistic; disruption in routine leads to a feeling of loss of control

◦ Forced immobility as a result of illness or injury may interfere with motor and language development

◦ Toddlers may fear intrusive procedures and often become emotionally distraught before and during bedside procedures

◦ When examining a toddler, assess vitals (see Chapter 2, Anesthesia, Table 2-2)

◦ Toddlers should exhibit the following characteristics:
  - Bulging abdomen
  - Numerous "do not like" considerations, which may challenge the bedside nurse
  - Resistance to being touched, separated from their caregivers, having their clothing removed, and donning masks (eg, oxygen)
  - Dislike of needles and pain
  - Belief that injury and illness may be a form of punishment
  - Protest vigorously if separated from parents (lack of protest when parent or caregiver departs may signify a clinical deterioration)

- **Young children (3–6 y)**
  - Developmental progression
    - Talk in full sentences

        - Better fine motor movement (eg, can use scissors)
        - Toilet trained
        - Behavior regression is common
    - Physically, the child can run, jump, and skip
    - Separation may be viewed as punishment
    - Exhibit more subtle responses to stress than toddlers (eg, loss of appetite or sleep)
    - Active imagination may lead to exaggeration and fear, or fantasies may take over
        - This may lead to confusion between reality and fantasy
        - A young child may worry over body integrity (eg, wonder if a body part under a cast is actually missing)
    - Understand when a pain event is coming and may try to escape
    - Immobility as a result of illness or injury leads to a sense of helplessness
    - When examining a young child, assess vitals (see Chapter 2, Anesthesia, Table 2-2)
    - Young children:
        - Think concretely and interpret literally what they hear
        - Have vivid imaginations and tend to dramatize events
        - Believe that injury and illness are their own fault and view them as punishment
        - Are aware of death and are afraid of pain, blood, and permanent injuries
        - Fear loss of body integrity, which may lead to mistrust of hospital personnel
        - Are curious about equipment and tasks
        - Can localize pain
        - Like games
- **Older children (6–12 y)**
    - Children of this age are in school, are very concerned about privacy, and are interested in a lot of things
    - Physically, these children's vital signs are within adult parameters; they are typically agile and in good physical shape
    - Separation from family and friends is better tolerated
    - Immobility as a result of illness or injury leads to a sense of frustration or agitation

    - May be anxious about death
    - Illness or injury affects sense of self worth or achievement
    - Children this age are stoic
        - They avoid letting others see them lose control
        - They may lie rigid, with their eyes shut and teeth and fists clenched
    - Pain perception and reporting is influenced by cultural variables; some children are afraid to cry even when in pain
    - When examining an older child, assess vitals (see Chapter 2, Anesthesia, Table 2-2)
    - The following are some characteristics of older children:
        - Honesty is important to children this age; avoid talking down to them
        - They should be able to cooperate with procedures and answer questions about health, symptoms, and activities
        - They are self-conscious about physical examinations
        - Critically ill children are initially more irritable and uncooperative
- **Adolescents (12–18 y)**
    - Children this age are moody and want to spend most of their time with friends
    - Puberty and secondary growth occur, changing breasts and the scrotum area; underarm hair develops
    - Other than bone growth, children this age are physically very similar to adults, undergoing puberty and developing secondary sexual characteristics
    - Adolescents fear loss of control and enforced dependence
    - Vital signs are similar to those of adults; children this age:
        - Are concrete thinkers and are learning to think in the abstract
        - Believe that nothing bad can happen to them
        - Fear disability and disfigurement may cause them to be different and not "fit in"
        - Appreciate honesty
        - Are concerned about privacy and modesty

Communicating with Children

- Understand the stages of development
- Explain procedures to children and their parents; plan on having to repeat explanations

- Talk in a quiet, gentle tone
- Be reassuring to children and parents
- Provide a security object
- Keep your hands visible
- Use appropriate terminology
- Assign the child a task if possible (eg, "keep your eyes on the purple cow in your bed")
- Explain monitoring noises
- Use the child's name

Nursing Tips

- **Pediatric intubation**: Have monitors, suction, ventilator, airway, intravenous (IV) access, and medications ready
- **Pediatric medications**: Have emergency medications specific to the child's age and weight listed at the bedside
- **Pediatric diets**: Have nipples, 60-cc graduate feeders, pacifiers, and oral electrolyte solution in stock
- **Pediatric catheters**: Feeding tubes (5 and 8 Fr) can be used as Foley catheters if needed in infants 6 months old and younger
    - Connect the tube to an urometer using a syringe without a plunger
    - An inline burette can also be used as a collection device
- **Arm boards**: Use tongue blades or cut down larger arm boards; cover the board with disposable washcloths and apply
- **IV access**: Have plenty of people around to help place an IV
    - Make sure the extremity is well restricted
    - It is not unusual to have 4–5 people hold a toddler down for blood work or an IV
    - Butterflies are **not** acceptable to use as IVs; use pore tape to secure (do not use paper tape)
- **Blood samples**: If the laboratory processing the blood work cannot handle pediatric blood amounts, use adult amounts or a handheld blood analyzer (it is better to stick for blood once for a larger amount than to repeat several sticks for a laboratory that cannot process a small amount); note all blood in output
- **Tubes** are often flimsy in children and will occlude
    - Consider using a stiffer tube as a stent outside the primary tube

  - Smaller tubes also frequently occlude from the inside
  - Endotracheal (ET) tubes need to be suctioned at least every 2–3 hours
  - Foleys can often get plugged; irrigation is necessary if there is concern over decreasing urine output or if a nasogastric (NG) tube is being used
    - NG tubes: to record small amounts of drainage, hook the NG tube up to a Lukens trap, then to suction so hourly outputs can be accurately measured
    - Tracheal and ET tubes: always have an extra at the bedside for emergencies; use cloth tape to secure ET tubes
- **Nasal samples**
  - Get a 19-gauge butterfly and cut off the needle
  - Attach the tubing to a 10-cc syringe with 3 cc of normal saline
  - Place cut-off tubing into nose and push in 1 cc of normal saline, then pull back
  - Look for mucus in the syringe
- **Temperature measurement**
  - Routine rectal temperature measurement in neonates and young infants should be avoided due to the risk of rectal perforation
  - Ear, oral, and bladder methods are all more accurate than axillary temperatures
  - Hypothermia is a temperature < 36°C
  - Fever is a temperature > 38°C

Chapter 24

Respiratory Emergencies

Introduction

Breathing should be effortless, and individuals should exhibit respiratory rates and tidal volumes appropriate for their ages (normally 5 mL/kg in spontaneously ventilating infants and children; Table 24-1). A comprehensive equipment table inside the front cover contains weight-based recommendations for all respiratory equipment.

Table 24-1. Pediatric Respiratory Rates

Age (y)	Respiratory Rate (breaths per min)
< 1	30–60
1–3	24–40
4–5	22–34
6–12	18–30
> 12	12–16

Work of Breathing

- Evidence of increased work of breathing in a child may include the following:
  - Tachypnea
  - Retractions (intercostal, subcostal, or suprasternal)
  - Use of accessory muscles
  - Head bobbing
  - Open-mouth breathing
  - Nasal flaring
  - Grunting (**ominous sign!**)
- Appropriate tidal volume should be judged by thoughtful analysis during auscultation. Does the breath sound normal, small, or excessive?
  - Stridor is an abnormal breath sound that signifies upper-airway obstruction

    - Causes: foreign body, infection, congenital airway anomalies, upper-airway edema, mass effect on airway
  - Grunting is a short, low-pitched sound during exhalation and is a **late and ominous sign**
    - Child's attempt to create positive end-expiratory pressure (PEEP), which helps maintain airway and alveolar patency (functional residual capacity), thereby improving oxygenation and ventilation
    - May be present in a variety of conditions, including pneumonia, pulmonary contusion, and acute respiratory distress syndrome, and requires immediate intervention (possibly intubation)
- Wheezing is typically a musical expiratory sound associated with lower-airway obstructive disorders
  - Asthma and bronchiolitis typically manifest with polyphonic wheezing, signifying the closure of many airways at different times
  - Central airway collapse disorders, such as tracheomalacia or bronchomalacia, typically manifest with monophonic wheezing (the same noise can be heard throughout the chest)
- Crackles/rales are inspiratory sounds typically associated with airway or alveolar disease and collapse (pneumonia, atelectasis, pulmonary edema)
- Pulse oximetry
  - $\geq 94\%$ is normal for a child
  - $< 90\%$ despite 100% oxygen via a nonrebreather is **ominous**
  - Must be checked on warm, well-perfused extremity
  - Consider previously undiagnosed congenital cyanotic heart disease in infants and children who present with minimal respiratory distress and cyanosis that does not improve, despite oxygen

Status Asthmaticus

- Characterized by respiratory distress due to airway obstruction from bronchospasm, excess mucous production, and airway inflammation
- The following plan can be used for all acutely symptomatic asthma exacerbations (Tables 24-2–24-4):
  - Rapidly categorize severity based on presenting signs and

Table 24-2. Acute Asthma Severity

Signs and Symptoms	Category: Mild	Moderate	Severe	Imminent Respiratory Failure
Respiratory rate	30% above mean	30%–50% above mean	> 50% above mean	> 50% above mean, or very slow
Alertness	Normal	Usually agitated	Agitated	Drowsy, confused
Dyspnea	Mild	Moderate	Severe	Severe
Color	Good	Pale	May be cyanotic	Cyanotic
Accessory muscle use	Mild	Moderate	Severe	Paradoxical thoracoabdominal movements
Auscultation	End-expiratory wheeze	Inspiratory and expiratory wheezing	Inaudible wheezing	Inaudible wheezing, minimal breath sounds
PEFR (% of predicted)	70%–90%	50%–70%	< 50%	< 20%
Air movement	Good	Fair	Poor	Poor/absent
$PaCO_2$	< 35 mmHg	< 40 mmHg	> 40 mmHg	> 40 mmHg

PEFR: peak expiratory flow rate
$PaCO_2$: partial pressure of carbon dioxide in arterial blood
Adapted from: National Institutes of Health, National Heart, Lung, and Blood Institute. *Guidelines for the Diagnosis and Management of Asthma*. Bethesda, Md: NIH; 1991.

symptoms
  - Use time-based management, depending on severity
  - Evaluate disposition based on response to prompt therapy
- Admit the patient to the hospital if the patient cannot take medications or fluids orally, cannot maintain saturation ≥ 94% on room air, requires bronchodilators more often than every 3–4 hours, or if the patient is rapidly deteriorating (Table 24-5)
- Watch for toxicities and side effects of medications used (Table 24-6)
  - For example, extreme tachycardia can be seen when al-

Table 24-3. Acute Asthma Treatment for Mild to Moderate Attacks

Time Frame	Treatment
Presentation	Check vitals and pulse oximetry; take brief Hx and perform PE, administer supplemental oxygen for sat ≤ 90%, preferably keeping sats ≥ 94%
10–20 min	Administer an immediate β-agonist (eg, albuterol): • MDI with spacer 4–8 puffs **OR** • Albuterol (nebulized) 2.5–5 mg Reassess and repeat q10–20min; consider adding ipratropium to subsequent nebulizer 0.25–0.5 mg
30 min	Consider steroids: • Oral prednisone 2 mg/kg if tolerating PO **OR** • Methylprednisolone sodium succinate (IV or IM) 2 mg/kg if unable to tolerate PO
60 min	Consider $MgSO_4$: 40 mg/kg over 20 min and reassess (maximum single dose 2 g)
120–240 min	Patient may be discharged if clinically improved with sat ≥ 94% and reliable follow-up established

Hx: history
IM: intramuscular
IV: intravenous
PE: physical examination
PO: per os (by mouth)
MDI: metered-dose inhaler
$MgSO_4$: magnesium sulfate
sat: saturation
SQ: subcutaneous

buterol, ipratropium inhalation, and terbutaline are used in combination
- An infant or toddler will tolerate a heart rate of 180 beats per minute, but an adolescent will not

Managing Chronic Asthma

- Optimal long-term management of asthma leads to fewer acute exacerbations, minimal use of medications (short-acting β-agonists and oral corticosteroids), fewer restrictions on activity, and preservation of lung function. The following steps provide a framework for long-term asthma management:
  - Classify asthma severity
    - Although spirometry provides an objective means for evaluating lung function, it is unlikely to be available
    - Classifying asthma severity using an age-based table

Table 24-4. Acute Asthma Treatment for Severe Attacks

Time Frame	Treatment
Presentation	Check vitals and pulse oximetry; take brief Hx and perform PE, administer supplemental oxygen for sat ≤ 90%, preferably keeping sats ≥ 94%
10–20 min	Administer an immediate β-agonist: • Albuterol (nebulized) 2.5–5 mg. Reassess and repeat q10–20min **OR** • Terbutaline or epinephrine (1:1,000) .01 mg/kg (SQ) if unresponsive to albuterol or not moving air; may repeat in 15 min; max dose 0.3 mg Add ipratropium to subsequent nebulizer 0.25–0.5 mg
30 min	Steroids: Methylprednisolone sodium succinate 2–4 mg/kg IV and reassess
60 min	$MgSO_4$ 40 mg/kg over 20 min and reassess (max single dose 2 g) Continue nebulizer as necessary
120–240 min	Admit if not improved (ward or PICU)

Hx: history
IV: intravenous
PE: physical examination
PICU: pediatric intensive care unit
$MgSO_4$: magnesium sulfate
sat: saturation
SQ: subcutaneous

can help guide initial management (Table 24-7)

- Control precipitating factors and comorbid conditions
  - Identification and avoidance of known triggers, along with aggressive use of rescue medications, can help minimize symptoms
    - Common triggers include upper respiratory infections, inhaled allergens (eg, pollen, dust mites), and irritants (eg, tobacco smoke)
  - Comorbid conditions, such as rhinitis, reflux, obesity, and stress, are known to worsen or attenuate asthma symptoms and should be treated
- Provide asthma education
  - Education should focus on appropriate use of medications (proper use of inhaler, chamber, and spacer), avoiding environmental exposures, recognizing worsening symptoms and adjusting medications, and seeking appropriate medical care when needed
  - A written asthma action plan is a validated

Table 24-5. Asthma Inpatient Management Plan

Ward	Pediatric Intensive Care Unit
If O_2 sat ≥ 94% on ≤ 50% FiO_2, requires ≤ q2–3h **albuterol** prn (MDI with spacer or nebulized)	If patient remains in distress, use **albuterol** continuously (.5 mg/kg/h, range 10–40 mg/h) with O_2 to keep O_2 sat ≥ 94% (always use humidified O_2)
Use **prednisone** 2 mg/kg/day or **methylprednisolone sodium succinate** 2–4 mg/kg/day ÷ q6h	Use **terbutaline** drip as adjunct, bolus with 10 µg/kg over 10 min, then run drip .1 µg/kg/min, titrating q15–30min, up to max of 4 µg/kg/min
Consider **ipratropium** neb 0.25–0.5 mg q4–6h	Use **methylprednisolone sodium succinate** 4 mg/kg/day ÷ q6h
Consider $MgSO_4$ 40 mg/kg IV q6h (if not already given)	**Ipratropium** neb 0.25–0.5 mg q4-6h
Consider temporary NPO status with maintenance IVFs if in distress	Consider repeating $MgSO_4$ 25–50 mg/kg IV q6h
Discharge patient to home if clinically improved with O_2 sat ≥ 94%, and reliable follow-up established	Consider temporary NPO status with maintenance IVFs if in distress, especially if intubation a possibility
	Other options include: **Heliox** 70:30 Consider **theophylline** 6–7mg/kg bolus, followed by drip Must follow levels 30 min after bolus and 12–24 h after initiation of drip **Ketamine** sedation 0.5–1 mg/kg/dose for agitation out of proportion to respiratory distress. **CAUTION**: may cause respiratory depression **Inhaled anesthetics**

FiO_2: fraction of inspired oxygen
IV: intravenous
IVF: intravenous fluid
MDI: metered dose inhaler
$MgSO_4$: magnesium sulfate
neb: nebulized
NPO: nil per os (nothing by mouth)
prn: pro re nata (as needed)
sat: saturation

educational tool

Other Common Respiratory Emergencies

- Anaphylaxis
  - Generalized, potentially fatal allergic reaction
    - Symptoms usually develop seconds to minutes after contact with the offending agent

Table 24-6. Asthma Medication Toxicity Profile

Medication	Toxicity
Albuterol	Tachycardia, hypokalemia, tremors
Ipratropium	Dry mouth, tachycardia, dry secretions
Terbutaline	Tachycardia, arrhythmias, hypokalemia, muscle twitching, increased muscle CPK
Steroids	Hyperglycemia, gastritis, CNS stimulation, hypertension, immune suppression
Magnesium	Hypotension, weakness, nausea, flushing
Theophylline	Tachycardia, nausea, ventricular dysrhythmias, tremors, seizures
Ketamine	Potent sialogogue, respiratory depression, emergence phenomena, tachyphylaxis
Heliox	Theoretical risk of atelectasis
Inhaled anesthetics	Hypotension, apnea, myocardial depression

CNS: central nervous system
CPK: creatine phosphokinase

Table 24-7. Chronic Asthma Severity and Suggested Treatment

Severity	Intermittent	Mild	Moderate	Severe
Frequency of symptoms	< 2/wk	> 2/wk (not daily)	Daily	Throughout day
Nighttime awakenings	None	1–2/mo	3–4/mo	> 1/wk
Impairment	None	Minor limitation	Some limitation	Extremely limited
Treatment (alternate)	Albuterol (as needed) corticosteroid	Low-dose inhaled corticosteroid or leukotriene receptor antagonist	Low- or medium-dose and albuterol or leukotriene receptor antagonist	Medium-or high-dose corticosteroid and albuterol; consider oral corticosteroids

- Several organ systems may be involved, including the skin, respiratory tract, cardiovascular system, and gas-

trointestinal tract
    - If not recognized and promptly treated, anaphylaxis may lead to death from respiratory or cardiovascular collapse
- Causes can include foods, drugs, and hymenoptera venom
    - **Foods**: peanuts, tree nuts, milk, eggs, fish, shellfish, fruits, grains
    - **Drugs**: penicillins, cephalosporins, sulfonamides, nonsteroidal antiinflammatory medicines, opiates, insulin, local anesthetics
    - **Hymenoptera venom**: honeybee, yellow jacket, wasp, hornet, and fire ant venom
    - **Other**: latex, exercise, vaccinations
- Evaluation
    - History should include investigations into interaction with anaphylaxis-associated allergens via contact, ingestion, inhalation, or medication administration; inquiries into previous history of anaphylaxis; and past medical history
    - Review of symptoms and physical examination should check for the following:
        - Dermatologic: urticaria, angioedema, pruritus, flushing, or warmth
        - Oropharynx: swelling of the lips, tongue, or mouth
        - Throat: hoarseness, cough
        - Pulmonary: dyspnea, wheeze
        - Gastrointestinal: nausea, vomiting, diarrhea, or abdominal pain
        - Cardiovascular: hypotension, dizziness, syncope, or cardiovascular collapse
- Treatment
    - **Immediate**
        - Check airway, breathing, and circulation (ABCs)
        - Administer epinephrine 0.01 mg/kg (1:1,000) intramuscular (IM)
            - Maximum single dose: 0.3 mg
            - Repeat every 15 minutes as needed
        - Auto injectors: epinephrine 0.15 mg (0–25 kg) or epinephrine 0.3 mg (> 25 kg)

        - Obtain intravenous (IV) access, administer 100% oxygen, observe cardiac monitor and pulse oximetry
        - Bolus normal saline (NS) 20 cc/kg, repeat as needed for hypotension
    - **Therapy after epinephrine**
        - H1 antagonist (diphenhydramine 1–2 mg/kg PO/IM/IV)
        - Corticosteroids (prednisone 1 mg/kg PO or methylprednisolone 2 mg/kg IV)
        - Consider nebulized albuterol 1.25–2.5 mg every 20 minutes for bronchospasm
        - Consider H2 antagonist (ranitidine 2 mg/kg PO or IV)
    - **Disposition**
        - Following initial stabilization, observe at least 4 hours (may have biphasic response)
        - Discharge with 72 hours of antihistamine and corticosteroids (albuterol if bronchospasm present)
        - Prescribe epinephrine auto injector (use age-based dosing)
        - Educate on anaphylaxis trigger avoidance and proper use of epinephrine auto injector

- **Bronchiolitis**
    - Acute, infectious, inflammatory disease of the upper and lower respiratory tracts; major cause of respiratory disease worldwide
        - Obstruction of bronchioles from inflammation, edema, and debris leads to hyperinflation (evident on chest radiograph), increased airway resistance, and atelectasis
        - Although wheezing is common, bronchoconstriction is not
        - Most cases are mild and self-limiting; however, inpatient mortality can be as high as 5%
    - Causes
        - Bronchiolitis is most often caused by respiratory syncytial virus (RSV), but parainfluenza, adenovirus, human metapneumovirus and *Mycoplasma* have been implicated
        - Common in infants and during the winter or rainy season (may be year-round near the equator)

   - Infants are affected most often because of their small airways
     - Premature, chronically ill, or malnourished infants are at higher risk for severe disease
- Evaluation
   - A clinical diagnosis is based on age, season (winter), and presentation with a low-grade fever, nasal congestion that can progress to lower tract symptoms with cough, dyspnea, wheezing, and feeding difficulties
   - Severe cases can manifest with respiratory distress, tachypnea, nasal flaring, retractions, irritability, and cyanosis
   - Common auscultory findings include biphasic wheezing and crackles
   - Hypoxemia on pulse oximetry is the best predictor of severe illness and correlates with a respiratory rate > 50 breaths per minute
   - Consider hospitalization for respiratory distress, room air saturation values < 92%, dehydration, apnea, or hypothermia
   - Bronchiolitis, particularly RSV, can present with otitis media, myocarditis, dysrhythmias, and syndrome of inappropriate antidiuretic hormone (SIADH)
   - A significant number of young or premature infants will have apnea
   - Radiograph, if available, will show hyperexpansion, diffuse bilateral perihilar peribronchial cuffing
- Treatment
   - Therapy is supportive, using oxygen and IV fluids in infants who are hypoxemic and cannot take oral liquids
   - Excess fluid administration may exacerbate pulmonary edema
   - Although studies do not support the routine use of nebulized albuterol or racemic epinephrine, some infants may experience short-term symptom relief with these agents
   - Mild nasal decongestants or bulb suctioning are more likely to be of symptomatic benefit
   - If mechanical ventilation becomes necessary, use syn-

chronized intermittent mechanical ventilation with pressure support and PEEP, ventilating at relatively slow rates to allow adequate exhalation time

- Croup
  - Laryngotracheobronchitis is an infection of the upper airway characterized by inspiratory stridor, cough, wheezing and hoarseness
  - Causes
    - The etiology is predominately viral infection (parainfluenza, RSV, adenovirus)
    - Often occurs during winter or cooler months
    - Measles can be a cause in unimmunized populations
  - Evaluation
    - Children ages 3–36 months typically present with gradual symptoms, including barky cough, hoarse voice, inspiratory stridor, tachypnea, and retractions (usually worse at night)
    - Significant hypoxia, biphasic stridor, change in mental status, poor air movement, or apparent fatigue may suggest impending respiratory failure and require urgent management
    - Chest radiograph will demonstrate laryngeal narrowing or "steeple sign"
  - Treatment
    - Urgent treatment includes rapid-acting nebulized racemic epinephrine (0.05 mL/kg, maximum dose of 0.5 mL) of 2.25% solution diluted to 3.0 cc with NS, repeated as needed
      - Rapid onset, short duration (about 2 h)
      - Patients should be monitored closely for rebound symptoms 2 hours after nebulized treatment, and may tachyphylax with repeated dosing
      - If racemic epinephrine is unavailable, use L-epinephrine (0.5 mg/kg, maximum dose 5 mL of 1:1,000 solution)
    - Corticosteroids are the mainstay of treatment to decrease airway edema
      - Onset of action is around 6 hours
      - Dexamethasone: 0.6 mg/kg IV/IM/PO (IV formula-

tions can be given orally)
- Prednisolone: 2 mg/kg/day IV divided bid for 2 days
- Prednisone: 4 mg/kg PO (equivalent to 0.6 mg/kg dexamethasone)

- Management includes supplemental oxygen and supportive measures, including IV fluids and humidified air

- Epiglottitis (see also Chapter 13, Face and Neck)
  - Epiglottitis is a rapidly progressive bacterial infection of the epiglottis, aryepiglottic folds, and surrounding tissues that leads to edema, airway compromise, and respiratory failure
  - Causes
    - More common in unimmunized populations due to *Haemophilus influenzae* type b
    - Rare causes in immunized populations include: *Pneumococcus, Staphylococcus aureus*, group A β-hemolytic streptococci (GABHS), and nontypeable *H influenzae*
  - Evaluation
    - Children ages 1–5 years old can present with a rapid progression from minimal symptoms to fever, sore throat/dysphagia, inability to manage secretions, and toxic appearance
    - Airway compromise appears rapidly with respiratory distress and a muffled "hot-potato" voice, and patient may exhibit abnormal positioning (tripoding or leaning forward with mouth open) to maintain maximum airway patency
    - Hoarseness and stridor are typically absent or mild
    - Work of breathing is normal to minimally elevated
    - Clinical diagnosis is based on high index of suspicion; cherry-red epiglottis may be seen on passive visualization
    - Aggressive attempts to visualize the airway should be avoided until skilled personnel are present (ie, an anesthesia professional and a surgeon capable of emergent pediatric tracheostomy) and prepared to intervene
    - Lateral neck radiographs should be obtained with caution in children with airway concerns; however, the enlarged epiglottis can be visualized (it appears as the so-called "thumb sign" on the lateral neck)

- Treatment
  - Total airway obstruction may occur due to massively enlarged epiglottis
  - Management includes intubation by the most experienced provider, with an endotracheal (ET) tube 0.5–1.0 size smaller than that routinely used for a child of that age and size
  - Simple bag-valve mask ventilation may be successful if absolutely necessary
  - Once the child is intubated, it is critical to secure the ET tube and sedate the child sufficiently to avoid a potentially catastrophic self-extubation
  - Treatment includes broad-spectrum IV antibiotics
    - Oxacillin or nafcillin (150–200 mg/kg/day divided qid),

      OR
    - Cefazolin (75–100 mg/kg/day divided tid),

      OR
    - Clindamycin (30–40 mg/kg/day divided tid)

      PLUS
    - Third-generation cephalosporin (ceftriaxone 75–100 mg/kg/day divided bid)
    - Cover for methicillin-resistant *S aureus* in endemic area

- **Bacterial Tracheitis**
  - Symptoms: similar to epiglottitis but with copious purulent tracheal secretions
    - Often complicates viral croup
  - Etiology: usually *S aureus*, also GABHS, Hib, or *S pneumoniae*
  - Diagnosis: clinical; trachea may appear "shaggy" on radiograph
  - Treatment
    - Intubate for 5–7 days (usually needed for pulmonary toilet)
    - Nafcillin, cefazolin, cefuroxime or ampicillin/sulbactam, all IV
    - Cover for methicillin-resistant *S aureus* in endemic area

Chapter 25

Status Epilepticus and Epilepsy

Status Epilepticus

- Defined as protracted or recurrent seizures causing prolonged changes in sensorium and other neurological impairment
- Often due to missed doses of daily seizure prevention medication
  - May result from noncompliance, illness, or vomiting
  - Caregivers should always have emergency seizure medications on hand
- Convulsive status epilepticus
  - Characterized by continuous seizures lasting > 15 minutes, or a series of seizures lasting > 30 minutes without a return to baseline consciousness
  - Can occur in patients with epilepsy (4% incidence overall); more common in children < 5 years old
  - More common in "bad syndromes" (eg, Lennox-Gastaut, cerebral dysplasias, etc)
  - Also seen in acute or chronic brain disease (eg, trauma, hypoxic ischemic encephalopathy, infection, neurodegeneration, toxic or metabolic disease, neoplasm)
  - Complications
    - Pediatric mortality rate is around 5%
    - Other complications include hypoxia, oropharyngeal obstruction, aspiration, hypotension, pulmonary edema, cardiac arrhythmia, hyperkalemia, acidosis, hypoglycemia, hyponatremia, fractures, oral injuries, rhabdomyolysis, hyperthermia, primary neuronal injury, sudden unexplained death
  - Emergency management can be simplified into a series of sequential interventions using the memory aid **AAP** (Table 25-1)
  - Computed tomography (CT) scan of the head is indicated in the following cases:
    - Head trauma
    - Evidence of increased intracranial pressure (ICP)
    - Focal neurologic deficits

Table 25-1. Status Epilepticus Emergency Management

Time (min)	Mnemonic	Intervention
0–5	A	**ABCs**, **ample** Hx (allergies, medications, past medical Hx, last meal, preceding events), **adjuncts** (glucose, Na^+, Ca^{2+}, ABG, anticonvulsant levels)
5–10	A	**Ativan*** 0.1 mg/kg IV (2 mg maximum single dose in a child); can cause respiratory depression and decreased BP; consider IO if IV unavailable
10–20	P	**Phosphenytoin** 20 mg/kg IV (2–3 mg/kg/min; can cause respiratory depression, decreased BP, and arrhythmias)
	A	**ABCs**
	A	Repeat **Ativan** 0.1 mg/kg IV
20–30	P	**Phenobarbital** 20 mg/kg IV over 5–10 min (can cause respiratory depression and decreased BP)
	A	**ABCs**; anticipate intubation; volume bolus may be needed
> 30	A	Repeat **Ativan** 0.1 mg/kg IV
40–60	P	Repeat **phenobarbital** 10 mg/kg aliquots × 2 (will cause respiratory depression and decrease BP)
	A	**ABCs**, intubate
	A	Consider **arterial** line for BP monitoring and central line for possible dopamine administration
	P	Take patient to **PICU** for pentobarbital or versed drips; consider continuous EEG, especially if neuromuscular blockade is needed (goal is burst suppression)

ABC: airway, breathing, and circulation
ABG: arterial blood gas
BP: blood pressure
EEG: electroencephalogram
Hx: history
IO: intraosseous
IV: intravenous
PICU: pediatric intensive care unit
*Ativan (lorazepam) is manufactured by Biovail Corporation (Mississauga, Ontario, Canada).

        - Focal seizure activity
    - Lumbar puncture is contraindicated in the following cases:
        - Suspected increased ICP
        - Focal neurologic deficits
        - Cardiopulmonary instability
        - Severe coagulopathy or thrombocytopenia
    - If status epilepticus persists, consider inducing coma with electroencephalogram (EEG) monitoring
        - Titrate EEG to seizure suppression, burst suppression pattern, or flat line
        - Administer midazolam (versed) infusion
            - 0.2 mg/kg (range 0.05–0.2 mg/kg bolus), repeat every 5 minutes as needed, to total 3 mg/kg
            - 0.1 (range 0.05-1.1) mg/kg/h

OR

        - Pentobarbital infusion
            - 5 (3–15) mg/kg bolus, repeat as needed
            - 1–3 mg/kg/h
        - Alternatively, consider:
            - Rectal diazepam (helpful if IV is unavailable)
                - 2–5 years old: 0.5 mg/kg/dose
                - 6–11 years old: 0.3 mg/kg/dose
                - 12 years and older: 0.2 mg/kg/dose
            - Buccal diazepam
            - Thiopental: 1–3 mg/kg IV bolus, (3–5 mg/kg/h infusion)
            - Ketamine: 1–2 mg/kg (1–2 mg/kg/h)
            - Isoflurane: titrate to burst suppression on EEG

Posttraumatic Seizures

- These require treatment in the acute setting, especially in the presence of increased ICP
    - Phenobarbital is the preferred antiepileptic agent in patients < 2 years old
    - Treat older children with phenytoin sodium or fosphenytoin (see Chapter 10, Neurosurgery)
- Seizures within the first week of trauma need to be treated

acutely; however, there is a low risk of long-term epilepsy
- Patients who develop seizures after the first week following trauma are more likely to have posttraumatic epilepsy

Evaluation of First-Time, Nonfebrile Seizure in Children
- Laboratory studies
  - Based on and directed at individual clinical circumstances
  - History: record clinical findings such as vomiting, diarrhea, dehydration, and failure to return to baseline alertness
  - Chemistry: check serum glucose and calcium in infants with seizures and in older children whose histories indicate the possibility of a metabolic disturbance
    - Consider hyponatremia if history suggests fluid imbalance
    - Screen toxicology or specific drug levels if drug exposure or substance abuse is possible
- Lumbar puncture
  - Of limited value unless meningitis or encephalitis is possible
  - Consider in infants who have sustained their first seizure
- EEG (if available) does not need to be emergent, although it may provide more information if obtained within 24 hours following seizure
- Neuroimaging
  - Perform emergent imaging (CT scan) in the following cases:
    - Presence of focal deficit (eg, Todd paralysis) that does not quickly resolve
    - Patient has not returned to baseline within several hours after the seizure
    - At-risk patients with abnormal neurological examination, history of malignancy, sickle cell disease, bleeding disorder, closed head injury, or travel to an area endemic for cysticercosis
    - Focal seizures
  - Magnetic resonance imaging (MRI) is preferred, but frequently unavailable

Febrile Seizures
- Simple febrile seizure
  - Single, brief, generalized seizure that occurs with fever (sei-

zure may occur while the fever is rising or may be present before the fever is discovered)
  - Patient looks normal after the seizure (no obtundation or mental status change)
  - A third of infants with one simple febrile seizure have a second; half of these have a third
    - Half of recurrences are experienced within a year of the first
    - 90% develop within 2 years
    - There is no evidence that a second or third simple febrile seizure, even if prolonged, causes epilepsy or brain damage
- Febrile seizures not related to infection or other definable cause
  - Occur in 4% of children; 2% of those with a first seizure associated with fever have nonfebrile seizures (epilepsy) by age 7
  - Most important predictor of epilepsy is abnormal neurological or developmental state
- Complex febrile seizures (prolonged, focal, or multiple seizures) as well as family history of epilepsy, slightly increase the probability of epilepsy in a patient
- Evaluation
  - Lumbar puncture
    - Perform only if concerned about nervous system infection (age < 12 mo, focal seizure, abnormal neurological examination)
    - Unnecessary after a brief, generalized seizure from which infant recovers rapidly and completely, especially if fever subsides spontaneously or is otherwise explained
  - Check complete blood count (CBC), electrolytes and/or urinary analysis (UA), depending on clinical circumstances
- Treatment
  - Unnecessary in low-risk children who have had a single, brief, generalized seizure
  - Antipyretics given at the time of another febrile episode do not prevent recurrence
  - Prophylactic antiepileptic drugs may be considered when the patient has:

   - An abnormal neurological examination or developmental delay
   - A family history of epilepsy with an initial complex febrile seizure
- Consider phenobarbital or valproic acid daily for 1–2 years
   - Decreases the risk of recurrence, but has severe side effects
   - Blood levels need to be monitored
   - If there is an adverse drug reaction (ADR), change to oral or rectal diazepam 0.5 mg/kg/day at the onset of subsequent fevers

Epilepsy

- Recurrent convulsive or nonconvulsive seizures caused by partial or generalized discharges in the cerebrum
- Two or more seizures not precipitated by a known cause
- Treatment
   - Goal: eradicating seizures or decreasing them so that they no longer interfere with physical and social well being
   - Consider treatment:
      - After a first unprovoked seizure (treatment in this case is rarely warranted)
      - After a second seizure or first seizure with ancillary evidence (family history, abnormal EEG, or MRI) indicating increased recurrence risk
   - **Consult a neurologist for help managing specific epilepsy syndromes**
   - Treatment by seizure type (drugs available in the US Army Central Command formulary)
      - Partial: simple, complex, and secondary generalized
         - Carbamazepine
         - Valproate (second choice)
         - Phenobarbital
      - Partial and generalized
         - Valproate
         - Topiramate
      - Myoclonic seizures
         - Valproate
         - Topiramate
         - **Caution** carbamazepine and phenobarbital can make

myoclonic seizures worse

Drugs, Doses, and Adverse Reactions in Pediatric Patients

- Carbamazepine: 5 mg/kg/day PO divided bid
    - Increase by 5 mg/kg/day every 3–5 days up to 15–20 mg/day divided bid or qid
    - Maximum adult dose is 2,400 mg/day, which can be as high as 35 mg/kg
    - If patient is taking more than 400 mg/day, convert to extended release carbamazepine (same dose, divided bid), if available
    - Levels 4–12 μg/mL therapeutic (toxic serum level ≥ 15 μg/mL)
    - Monitor CBC, blood chemistry (sodium, blood urea nitrogen), serum iron, lipid panel, liver function tests (LFTs), UA, and thyroid function tests at 1 week, 1 month, 3 months, 6 months–1 year, then yearly
    - ADRs include hepatitis, neutropenia, aplastic anemia, diplopia, ataxia, rash, and syndrome of inappropriate antidiuretic hormone
- Clonazepam: 0.01–0.03 mg/kg/day PO divided qd–tid
    - Increase by 0.025 to 0.05 mg every 3–7 days until condition is controlled
    - Maximum: 0.1–0.2 mg/kg (adult 20 mg)
    - Levels (none)
    - Monitor LFTs
    - ADRs include rebound insomnia, anxiety, dysphoria, disinhibition, tremor, headache, confusion, dysarthria, and syncope (tolerance may develop to ADRs and drug)
- Diazepam: 0.2–0.3 mg/kg/dose IV; 0.5–0.75 mg/kg/day rectal
    - Levels (none)
    - Monitor CBC and LFTs
    - ADRs include sedation and disinhibition
- Gabapentin: 5 mg/kg/day PO
    - Not preferred for seizures; has minimal interactions with other medications
    - Increase by 5 mg/kg/day every 3 days to 15–20 mg/kg/day divided tid
        - Usual dose is 30–40 mg/kg/day divided tid

    - Maximum: 45–60 mg/kg/day
  - Levels: < 5
  - Monitor white blood cell count
  - ADRs include irritability, tremor, neuropsychosis, sedation, headaches, fatigue, weight gain, and ataxia
- Lorazepam: 0.025–0.10 mg/kg PO (usually 0.05 mg/kg due to respiratory suppression)
  - Maximum: 10 mg/dose
  - Levels: not established
  - ADRs include sedation, dizziness, and disinhibition
- Phenobarbital (luminal)
  - Used mostly in newborns and infants 2–12 months old
  - Associated with cognitive slowing in older patients
  - Interacts with several other drugs and increases the metabolism of many drugs
  - Not recommended for woman of childbearing age; decreases oral contraceptive effectiveness
  - Dosing
    - Oral load 4 mg/kg bid × 2 days
    - Maintenance 4 mg/kg/day divided qd–bid
    - Faster oral 4 mg/kg/d every 4–6 hours × 4
    - IV load 20 mg/kg/dose
  - Levels: 15–40 μg/mL (check after 2–5 days); toxic: 40 μg/mL
    - Slowness, ataxia, nystagmus 35–80 μg/mL
    - Coma with reflexes 65–117 μg/mL
    - Coma without reflexes > 100 mg/mL
  - Monitor CBC and LFTs
  - ADRs include rash, Stevens Johnson Syndrome, serum sickness, depression, and rickets
- Phenytoin
  - Oral (PO) load 6 mg/kg/dose every 8 hours × 3 doses
    - Maintenance 5 mg/kg/day divided bid or tid
    - Maximum: 10 mg/kg/day (adult 500 mg/day)
  - IV load 18–20 mg/kg once, then 10 mg/kg × 2 (check levels at 2 h)
    - Fosphenytoin preferred in children: 18 mg/kg/dose phenytoin equivalent
    - Then 5–6 mg/kg/day divided bid
  - Levels 10–20 (free 0.1–2)

    - Toxic > 30; lethal > 100
    - Zero order kinetics; can become toxic quickly; must monitor levels closely
  - ADRs
    - IV: hypotension, bradycardia, arrhythmia, venous irritation
    - PO: gingival hypertrophy, coarsening facial features, hirsutism, rash, hepatitis, rickets, folic acid deficiency, peripheral neuropathy, lupus, vision problems, dizziness, fatigue, alterations in mood
- Topiramate: 0.5–1 mg/kg/day divided once or bid; increase 0.5–1 mg/kg every 2 weeks × 2, then weekly
  - Usual dose 5–8 mg/kg/day PO divided once or bid
  - Maximum: 15 mg/kg/day (25 mg/kg for infantile spasms)
  - Levels not established (10–35)
  - Monitor electrolytes occasionally (however, medication is often not decreased because of acidosis)
  - ADRs include renal stones, anhydrosis, low bicarbonate levels, metabolic acidosis, dehydration, anorexia, encephalopathy, somnolence, nausea, ataxia, confusion, dysarthria
    - Also decreases appetite and the effectiveness of oral contraceptives
    - Keep the patient hydrated
- Valproic acid
  - Good anticonvulsant; limited by ADRs
  - Regular release and delayed release varieties are usually divided bid or qid; extended release is usually given once a day
  - When moving to extended release, might need to increase daily dose 8%–20% for same serum concentrations
  - IV/PO doses are equivalent
    - PO: 5–10 mg/kg/day divided once or bid; increase by 5–10 mg/kg/day divided bid every 3–5 days to 15–25 mg/kg/day divided bid or tid
    - IV: load 20 mg/kg/dose (maximum < 20 mg/min)
      - Give oral dose with IV load
      - IV maintenance equals total daily dose divided every 6 hours
      - Maximum: 60–70 mg/kg/day

- Levels 40–140 μg/mL
- Monitor LFTs and CBC before starting, then at 1 week, 1 month, and 3 months, then every 6 months; if lethargy or mental status changes, check prothrombin time, partial thromboplastin time, and serum ammonia
- The following conditions increase risk for hepatotoxicity:
  - Underlying liver disorder in a child < 2 years of age
  - Taking multiple antiepileptic drugs
- Carnitine can be used for hepatoprotection
- ADRs
  - Not recommended for women of childbearing age
  - Slows metabolism of other drugs
  - Can cause hepatitis, thrombocytopenia, pancreatitis, alopecia, weight gain, nausea, polycystic ovaries, somnolence, headaches, and tremor

Chapter 26

Care of the Newborn

Routine Resuscitation

- When called to the delivery of a newborn, first learn the basic maternal history (time permitting), including the following:
  - The infant's gestational age (term vs preterm)
  - If prenatal care was obtained. If possible, gather laboratory information, including the ultrasound, infant weight, etc
  - Complications, if any, leading to delivery (eg, bleeding, change in fetal movements, etc)
  - Maternal medications (during pregnancy and in the last 24 hours of pregnancy)
  - Maternal health status (eg, medical conditions, immunizations, etc)
- Gather the proper equipment needed for resuscitating a newborn
  - Warm towels
  - A heat source to keep the infant warm
    - Use radiant warmers, if available
    - If a radiant warmer or other appropriate heat source is not available, skin-to-skin contact with the mother can be used to keep the baby warm
  - A bulb syringe
  - A suction device, such as wall suction, that can be used with a suction catheter
  - Oxygen source
  - Self-inflating bag or flow-inflating bag that can provide positive pressure ventilation
  - Mask, size 0 or 1, that can fit over the mouth and nose of an infant
  - A minute–second timer (though not essential, this helps mark 1 and 5 min and is useful if positive pressure ventilation is needed)
- Attempt to have a neonatal resuscitation provider available;

larger medical commands should identify people with this experience, even in the deployed environment

- Resuscitation
  - First 60 seconds following birth:
    - Ensure the obstetrical provider securely clamps the umbilical cord before passing the infant to the pediatric team; start the minute–second timer
    - All infants need to be warm, dry, suctioned, and stimulated; in the delivery room, this takes place within a period of 30 seconds
      - Dry the infant with the warm towels, discarding damp ones; it is typical to use two or three towels within the first 30 seconds
      - Rubbing the infant's back and chest while drying is stimulating; if further stimulation is necessary, flicking or slapping the soles of the infant's feet may help
      - Position the infant's head at the foot of the bed or radiant warmer
      - Manage the patient's airway and position the head in the sniffing position, allowing for slight hyperextension of the neck (this is usually done by the person closest to the patient's head)
      - Suction the mouth and nares with the bulb syringe or suction catheter to clear amniotic fluid that could occlude the airway
    - Monitor the infant's heart rate by gently palpating the base of the umbilical cord to feel for a pulse, or by listening to the heart with a stethoscope
      - If the newborn is active and crying, the heart rate should be above 100 beats per minute (bpm)
        - A "vigorous" infant has good muscle tone, a heart rate > 100 bpm, and is crying
        - If the baby is vigorous, stop resuscitation and allow the infant to transition (transitioning from the intrauterine environment to the outside world takes 2–4 h)
    - Further care is described in Routine Care of the Newborn

- All infants are born with a hue ranging from blue to pink; if healthy, they will transition to pink with adequate heart rate and ventilation
  - Sometimes an infant's hands and feet stay blue even when the rest of the body is pink (acrocyanosis)
    - Assess for central cyanosis by examining the color of the lips, gums, and central trunk
    - A brief period of free-flowing oxygen is beneficial to infants with adequate ventilation and heart rate who remain centrally blue
    - An infant requiring persistent oxygen needs more than typical resuscitation
- Every infant is assigned an Apgar score (activity, pulse, grimace, appearance, and respiration; Table 26-1) at 1 minute and 5 minutes of life
  - The score ranges from 0–10, with 10 being given to healthy, vigorous infants
  - Properly assigning an Apgar score requires training, but knowledge of the components will help providers unfamiliar with scoring know what is important when assessing a newborn during resuscitation, and will facilitate communication with a consulting specialist

Special Circumstances Requiring Advanced Resuscitation

- The term infant is not vigorous after warming, drying, suctioning, and stimulating
  - If an infant is apneic, has a heart rate < 100 bpm, or has

Table 26-1. Apgar Evaluation of Newborn Infants

Sign	0	1	2
Heart rate	Absent	Below 100	Over 100
Respiratory effort	Absent	Slow, irregular	Good, crying
Muscle tone	Limp	Some flexion of extremities	Active motion
Response to catheter in nostril*	No response	Grimace	Cough or sneeze
Color	Blue, pale	Body pink, extremities blue	Completely pink

*Tested after oropharynx is clear.

persistent central cyanosis despite free-flowing oxygen, further intervention is required

- Ventilation is the most important step in the resuscitation of infants that are not vigorous
- The two standard ways of providing ventilation are the self-inflating bag and flow-inflating bag
- Various mask sizes are needed, depending on the gestational age of the infant
  - Mask should cover the mouth and nose and provide a good seal
  - Most term newborns will use a size 1 infant mask
  - Preterm infants or infants that are small for their gestational age may need a size 0 newborn mask
- Use 100% oxygen when giving positive pressure ventilation
- Suction the mouth and nose again
- Place the mask over the infant's face
  - Hold the mask with your thumb and index finger; use your other three fingers to lift the jaw into the mask
  - Ensure there is an airtight seal
- Begin delivering breaths at a rate of 40–60 breaths per minute; use a manometer if available
- Pressures should be sufficient to provide adequate chest rise and fall
  - The first few breaths can require pressures in excess of 25 cm H_2O, but it is rare to need pressures in excess of 40–60 cm H_2O
  - Using excessive pressure can cause a pneumothorax
  - It takes experience to achieve the correct balance of pressure
    - Novices typically make one of two mistakes: they do not use sufficient pressure to provide adequate chest rise and fall, or they give breaths at a rate exceeding 60 breaths per minute
    - Using the minute–second timer can alleviate the frequency problem (give a breath every second)

    - If positive pressure ventilation is adequate, heart rate will improve to over 100 bpm, color will improve, and the infant will start spontaneous respiration; gradually stop giving positive pressure ventilation
    - If there is no improvement, check that the face mask is sealed adequately, reposition the head, and suction out the mouth
    - If problems persist, reevaluate the pressure being administered; if it is adequate but there is still no improvement, the infant needs to be intubated
- The term infant needs to be intubated
  - Depending on the location and resources, intubating and ventilating a newborn infant may be impossible. When working in austere environments, it is reasonable and ethical to decide ahead of time the limits of the providers' resuscitative efforts
  - There are five main differences between the neonatal and adult airway:
    - The infant's head and tongue are proportionally larger than the adult's
    - The infant's larynx is more anterior and cephalad
    - The infant's epiglottis is long, narrow, and floppy (making it easier to use a Miller [straight] blade instead of a Macintosh blade)
    - The infant's vocal cords are slanted anteriorly
    - The cricoid cartilage is the narrowest part of an infant's larynx, not the vocal cords
  - A term infant is generally intubated with a 3.5 or 4.0 uncuffed endotracheal tube (ETT), using a Miller size 1 blade
  - Confirm ETT placement by observing one or more of the following:
    - Equal chest rise
    - Breath sounds over the lungs and not the stomach
    - Misting inside of the ETT
    - Positive color change using a pediatric-size disposable colorimetric carbon dioxide detector (fast, accurate)
    - Chest radiograph
    - Clinical improvement in ventilation and perfusion

  - Upon successful intubation, continue providing positive pressure ventilation with enough pressure to ensure adequate chest rise at a rate of 40–60 breaths per minute
  - In the rare case when an infant does not improve with establishing an airway and providing adequate ventilation, start chest compressions and establish intravenous access to give epinephrine and volume resuscitation, if necessary
- The infant develops a **tension** pneumothorax
  - Pneumothorax occurs in a small percentage of all newborns, rarely causing respiratory distress and need for rapid evacuation
  - There are cases when an infant develops a tension pneumothorax, especially those infants receiving excessive positive pressure ventilation
    - The infant will be in respiratory distress (with grunting or nasal flaring or retracting)
    - There are decreased breath sounds on the ipsilateral side, with tracheal deviation toward the contralateral side
    - Transilluminating the chest with a light source may show lucency over the side with the tension pneumothorax (chest radiograph confirms the presence of a pneumothorax, but is not usually available before intervention is required)
  - Treatment of a pneumothorax is accomplished using the same technique in any age group, except that a provider will use a smaller-gauge needle and the volume of air evacuated will be less in an infant
    - Use a needle attached to a three-way stopcock, with one end closed to air and the other open to a syringe
    - Insert the needle in the second intercostal space, at the mid-clavicular line
      - While inserting the needle, apply gentle retraction to the syringe
      - When the tip of the needle is in the correct place, you will hear a "whoosh" sound and will be able to rapidly pull back on the syringe
    - Draw off the air, turning the stopcock off to the patient and on to evacuate the air in the syringe, and repeat

until no further air is evacuated from the lungs
  - Infants with rapidly reaccumulating air require placement of a chest tube, which is beyond the scope of this chapter
- The amniotic fluid is meconium stained
  - Infants who are stressed prior to birth or are late in gestation (more than 41 weeks) are at increased risk to pass stool in the amniotic fluid prior to birth
    - When the mother's membranes rupture, the amniotic fluid is stained various shades of dark green
    - This places the infant at risk for aspiration of meconium fluid, which can lead to respiratory compromise (called meconium aspiration syndrome)
  - Obstetrical inventions reduce the risk of aspiration and include amniotic fluid infusion, bulb suctioning of the nares and mouth on presentation of the head (prior to delivery of the body), and not stimulating the infant at birth
  - The infant should not be stimulated when passed to the neonatal resuscitation team
    - If the infant is not vigorous, a provider experienced in intubating newborns should place an appropriately sized ETT, attach a meconium aspirator, and suction any meconium from below the vocal cords
    - The vigorous infant only requires routine resuscitation; if intubation and airway suctioning are impossible, the basics of resuscitation should be provided (warming, drying, stimulation, and suctioning, with the focus being on suctioning the oral pharynx)
  - Infants who develop signs of respiratory distress following delivery in meconium-stained fluid most likely aspirated meconium
    - These infants need to be cared for in a facility equipped to care for sick newborns
    - Consultation with a neonatologist is indicated
- The infant is preterm
  - An infant born at < 37 weeks is preterm (the age of viability is 24 gestational weeks; however, this may differ in other countries depending on their neonatal resuscitation resources)
  - Know the available hospital resources in the local area and

Table 26-2. Infant Endotracheal Tube Sizes

Tube Size	Depth (cm)	Birth Weight (g)	Gestational Age (wk)
2.5	7	< 1,000	25–29
3.0	7–8	1,000–2,000	30–34
3.5	8–9	2,000–3,000	35–37
3.5–4.0	9–10	> 3,000	> 37

consult a pediatrician or neonatologist when delivering and resuscitating a preterm infant

- Remember the basics
  - For infants born in the third trimester (> 28 wk), basic resuscitation (see Routine Resuscitation) may be all that is needed
  - If positive pressure ventilation is indicated, a size 0 neonatal mask is typically used
  - Intubation is achieved using 2.5–3.5 ETT to a depth of 7–10 cm, depending on the age and size of the infant (Table 26-2)
  - Intubation of the preterm infant requires prior experience in the intubation of children and newborns
- Following successful resuscitation, infants born at < 35 weeks or weighing < 2 kg will typically be admitted to a neonatal intensive care unit; infants older than this may be allowed to stay with their mothers, provided they can be watched closely
  - Resuscitated infants need to be kept warm and are easily susceptible to cold intolerance
  - Blood glucose levels should be checked shortly after birth and then every 3–5 hours before feeds until feeding is well established, especially in newborns that weigh < 10% of normal for their gestational age (Table 26-3)
    - Infants who are too young to begin oral feeds should be started on dextrose 10% in water ($D_{10}W$) at 3.3–5 mL/kg/h (80–120 mL/kg/day; consult a pediatric provider to determine exact rates)
  - Vital signs should be checked at least every 4 hours (Table 26-4)

Table 26-3. Expected Newborn Weight by Gestational Age

Gestational Age (wk)	Mass (g)
25	650
26	750
27	880
28	1,000
29	1,150
30	1,325
31	1,500
32	1,700
33	1,900
34	2,150
35	2,375
36	2,600
37	2,860
38	3,075
39	3,300
40	3,460
41	3,600
42	3,690

    ▹ Abnormal vital signs, temperature intolerance, hypoglycemia (blood glucose < 40), or poor feeding, regardless of gestational age, should prompt consultation with a neonatologist and transport to a hospital equipped to care for a sick neonate
    ▹ Consultation with a neonatologist regarding a preterm newborn is always strongly encouraged
- The infant does not appear normal
    - Few abnormalities require urgent recognition and management in the delivery room (see below). In austere environ-

Table 26-4. Normal Infant Vital Signs

Respiratory rate	30–60 breaths/min
Heart rate*	120–160 beats/min
Temperature (axillary)	36.1°C–37°C

*Some healthy, term infants may have a resting heart rate as low as 90 beats per minute while asleep. A heart rate that remains this low in an awake, crying infant is not normal.

ments management may be limited to recognition and supportive care without the ability to refer to a neonatal center.

- **Abdominal wall defect**. It is rare for an infant's abdominal contents to develop outside the abdomen. In gastroschisis, the abdominal wall defect is typically to the right side of the umbilical cord. In omphalocele, the defect is through the umbilical cord insertion. In either case, the same steps should be followed
  - Immediately place the infant in a clear, sterile, plastic bag up to the neck to reduce insensible water losses and minimize exposure of the open bowel; if this is impossible, consider using plastic wrap or warm saturated gauze
  - Use an oral gastric tube to decompress the intestine (a Replogle tube is preferred); if the infant requires advanced resuscitation, limit positive pressure ventilation delivered using a bag-valve mask
  - Contact a surgeon
    - Rarely, dusky blue to black bowel requires urgent reduction to prevent ischemia and bowel death
  - These patients may require initial intense fluid management and attention to acidosis status
    - Begin $D_{10}W$ at 3.3–5 mL/kg/h (80–120 mL/kg/day)
    - Hypotension, poor perfusion, or acidosis should prompt a fluid bolus of 10 mL/kg given over 20–30 minutes
    - Transport to a tertiary care facility
- **Neural tube defect**. Protrusion of the spinal cord or the meninges outside the spinal canal is also rare
  - Place the infant prone on the infant warmer
  - Cover the protruding mass in warm, sterile gauze
  - Contact a neurosurgeon and arrange for transport to a tertiary care facility
- **Upper airway anomaly**. Infants are obligate nose breathers
  - Infants with small jaws, large tongues, and cleft lips

may have Pierre-Robin sequence and difficulty keeping their upper airways open. These patients may benefit from being placed in the prone position, and some require placement of an oral airway. Severe cases need bag-mask ventilation and intubation
            - Infants born with upper airway stenosis, such as choanal atresia, may also need an oral airway to breathe
            - Typically, infants with only cleft lips or palates do not have respiratory issues, but may have difficulty feeding, which can be addressed by a pediatric care provider
    - Most other cases of infants appearing abnormal can wait for further evaluation until after initial stabilization
- The term infant appears ill
    - When an infant appears ill, it is important to ensure that the infant is not septic. Infection in infants can present with soft signs and progress to death within hours. Maternal risk factors for neonatal infection include:
        - Intrapartum temperature 100.4°F (38.5°C)
        - Amniotic membrane rupture > 18 hours before delivery
        - Chorioamnionitis
        - Maternal group B streptococcus positive or unknown and without maternal intrapartum antibiotic prophylaxis
    - Draw a complete blood count with differential and blood culture
        - An experienced provider should perform a lumbar puncture to obtain cultures and Gram stain, cell count, and glucose and protein levels
        - For infants < 48 hours old, a urine culture is typically not helpful
    - Empiric antibiotic treatment often consists of administering ampicillin and an aminoglycoside (usually gentamicin) or ampicillin and a broad-spectrum, third-generation cephalosporin, such as cefotaxime
    - The ill-appearing infant needs transfer to a tertiary care facility

    - Consult a pediatric provider
    - If the term infant is < 48 hours old, start $D_{10}W$ at 2.5 mL/kg/h (60 mL/kg/day)
    - Infants > 2 days old require some electrolytes; consult a pediatric provider to determine the appropriate fluids (see recommendation in Chapter 22, Basic Fluid and Electrolytes)
  - Observe vital signs
    - Warm hypothermic infants
    - Check blood glucose
    - Hypoglycemia can mimic infection; infants that appear ill and are hypoglycemic (blood glucose < 40) should receive a $D_{10}W$ bolus (2 mL/kg), then be started on intravenous fluids (see above)
  - Infants with evidence of respiratory distress or persistent cyanosis require evaluation by a specialist
    - Obtain an arterial blood gas reading by drawing blood from the radial artery
    - Place a pulse oximeter on the infant's right hand and left foot to help monitor preductal and postductal saturations
    - If possible, deliver either positive pressure ventilation via bag mask or intubation, or continuous positive pressure using 100% oxygen
    - Obtain a chest radiograph and discuss the results with a specialist
    - Begin a sepsis evaluation (see previous page)
- The infant is large or small for gestational age
  - Infants that are large or small for their gestational age are at risk for hypoglycemia
    - Check blood glucose once every few hours (for a total of three times) until patient is stable

Routine Care of the Newborn

- Feeding
  - Breast-feeding is the recommended method for feeding a newborn, and may be all that is available
    - Breast-feeding should occur on demand (ie, when the infant is showing interest in feeding), 8–10 times in a

    24-hour period, for 10–20 minutes on each breast
  - In the stable, vigorous newborn, initiate breast-feeding immediately after birth; it takes priority over the newborn examination, delivery of vitamin K, and administration of eye drops
  - Most medications are safe to use during breast-feeding
    - Exceptions include chemotherapeutic agents, radioactive isotopes, and antimetabolites
    - LactMed (http://toxnet.nlm.nih.gov/cgi-bin/sis/htmlgen?LACT) is an online Web site that can be used to determine a medication's safety during breast-feeding; it is available though the National Library of Medicine and is accessible through PubMed by selecting TOXNET, then the LactMed database
- Infants fed formula may start with only a half ounce per feed, but quickly increase to 2 ounces or more per feed over the next few days

- Newborn prophylaxis
  - After the first breast-feeding attempt has been accomplished, give 1 mg of vitamin K (phytonadione), if available, intramuscularly in the thigh to prevent hemorrhagic disease
  - Administer 1% silver nitrate eye drops or erythromycin (0.5%) and tetracycline (1.0%) sterile ophthalmic ointment, if available, for prevention of gonococcal eye infection
- General care
  - Infants should be dressed or blanketed in one or two layers more than what everyone else is wearing
    - Excessive wrapping and layering can lead to hyperthermia
    - Place wrapped infants in a crib in the supine position
  - Infants are typically given a sponge bath at birth to remove the vernix
  - Infants typically void once the first day, twice the second day, then more frequently after that
    - Most infants will stool at least once in the first 24–48 hours
    - The stool will be meconium (dark and tarry) for the first few days

- If voiding or stooling is delayed, consultation is recommended

- Most infants stay 2 days in the hospital
  - A weight loss of up to 10% of the birth weight can be expected, especially in breast-fed infants
  - Weight loss in excess of 10% should prompt further evaluation and consultation with a specialist
  - During this time, vitals should be checked at least every 8–12 hours
  - The newborn should be assessed for jaundice
    - Infants with yellowing skin should be evaluated for hyperbilirubinemia or an elevated indirect bilirubin
    - Normal values for a newborn are significantly higher than adult values and vary based on the age (in hours) of the infant (see American Academy of Pediatrics Subcommittee on Hyperbilirubinemia. Management of hyperbilirubinemia in the newborn infant 35 or more weeks of gestation. *Pediatrics*. 2004;114:297–316). An indirect bilirubin of > 10 after the first week of life in a term infant, or persistent elevation of the direct bilirubin fraction require further diagnostic investigation

Chapter 27

Cardiology

History

- In newborns, exercise tolerance is approximated by asking caregivers about feeding difficulties, specifically tachypnea, cyanosis, and diaphoresis during feeding
- In infants, failure to thrive (gain weight at an appropriate rate) warrants consideration of congenital heart disease
- Children with other congenital anomalies are more likely to have congenital heart disease
  - Particularly defects along the midline or involving other solid organs
  - Family history should focus on family members with heart disease (congenital or acquired), sudden unexplained deaths, and arrhythmias

Examination

- Blood pressure should be measured in both arms and one leg to evaluate for coarctation of the aorta
- Murmurs: more than 90% of all children are noted to have a murmur at some time in their lives
  - Most murmurs are harmless
  - Characteristics concerning for a pathologic murmur include associated cardiac symptoms, a loud or harsh-sounding systolic murmur (>3/6 or with a palpable thrill), a diastolic murmur, abnormal heart sounds, presence of a click, and weak or absent peripheral pulses
- Electrocardiograms (ECGs) are helpful if available (consult *The Harriet Lane Handbook* for help interpreting an ECG)

Evaluating the Cyanotic Newborn, Infant, and Child

- Central cyanosis is universally consistent with hypoxemia and is best appreciated in the oral mucosa, conjunctivae, and the tip of the tongue

- The most common cause of cyanosis in newborns, infants, and children is respiratory compromise from a host of pulmonary diseases
- Cyanosis from congenital heart disease is typically due to a right-to-left intracardiac shunt and persists beyond the newborn period
- Evaluation
  - Initial evaluation should include pulse oximetry and measurement of the partial pressure of oxygen in arterial blood (PaO_2) by blood gas to confirm hypoxemia
    - The PaO_2 in a normal, 1-day-old newborn may be as low as 60 mmHg
  - Primary pulmonary processes are associated with tachypnea and dyspnea; congenital cyanotic heart defects are generally associated with effortless tachypnea often described as "comfortable tachypnea"
    - If a cyanotic heart defect is suspected, perform chest radiograph, ECG (if available), and a hyperoxitest
    - Ultimately, the diagnosis of congenital cyanotic heart disease is made by echocardiography
    - The hyperoxitest compares PaO_2 and pulse oximetry values after a 100% oxygen challenge as a means of differentiating pulmonary from cardiac causes of hypoxemia
      - Arterial blood gas samples should be taken from the right upper extremity
      - PaO_2 and pulse oximetry values are taken while the newborn is breathing fraction of inspired oxygen (FiO_2) = 0.21, and after FiO_2 is increased to 1.00 for 10 minutes
      - Care should be taken to get the FiO_2 as close as possible to 1.00
        - Pulmonary disease: an increase in PaO_2 > 150 and pulse oximetry = 100%, with FiO_2 = 1.00
        - Cardiac disease: PaO_2 < 150 and pulse oximetry < 90%, with FiO_2 = 1.00
- Treatment
  - Although some children with cyanotic heart defects can survive past infancy (eg, most commonly those with mild

forms of Tetralogy of Fallot), definitive treatment of cyanotic heart defects requires surgical correction

- In the newborn period, if surgical intervention is a feasible option, a prostaglandin E_1 intravenous (IV) infusion can be started to maintain patency of the ductus arteriosus
    - The starting dose of prostaglandin E_1 is 0.05–0.1 μg/kg/min
    - Common side effects include flushing, apnea, hypotension, and fever

Arrhythmias

- Bradycardia
    - Most common cause of true bradycardia in infants and children is hypoxia, usually due to respiratory compromise
    - Sinus bradycardia can be normal in adolescents and athletes
    - Can also be caused by increased vagal tone, increased intracranial pressure, hyperkalemia, hypercalcemia, hypothyroidism, hypothermia, long QT syndrome, and drugs (eg, digoxin, β-blockers)
    - In newborns, physiological stresses (eg, hypoxia, cold, hypoglycemia) often manifest as bradycardia (manifest as tachycardia in older children and adults)
    - Bradycardia can also occur as a result of heart block
    - Management
        - Treat the underlying cause
        - A hemodynamically unstable patient with underlying bradycardia requires emergent attention
        - Begin with effective oxygenation and ventilation via bag-valve mask if necessary
        - Epinephrine is the drug of choice after oxygen; dose 0.01 mg/kg (0.1 mL/kg) of 1:10,000
        - Atropine should be considered a second-line agent, unless vagal stimulation is thought to be the source of the bradycardia
            - Dose 0.02 mg/kg (minimum dose 0.1 mg)
- Tachycardia
    - Most common cause of tachycardia in pediatric patients is sinus tachycardia

    - This can be caused by hypovolemia, hemorrhage, hypoxia, anemia, fever, sepsis, shock, congestive heart failure, myocardial disease, anxiety, and drugs (eg, β-agonists, atropine)
  - Management requires distinguishing sinus tachycardia from supraventricular tachycardia (typically narrow QRS complex) and ventricular tachycardias (wide QRS complex)
    - Sinus tachycardia is almost always accompanied by a history that explains it (ie, volume loss, fever, hemorrhage, etc)
    - Maximum heart rates for infants and children can be surprising
      - Infants: up to 200 beats per minute (bpm)
      - Children: 180 bpm
      - Adolescents: 160 bpm
    - Treatment involves correcting the underlying causes
  - Supraventricular tachycardia is the most common tachyarrhythmia seen in children with increased ventricular rates (infants > 230 bpm, children > 180 bpm)
    - P waves, if visible, are usually abnormal
    - Heart rate is regular, rapid, and monotonous, with minimal variation
    - Narrow QRS complexes are typical
    - Can be associated with congenital heart disease (eg, Ebstein's anomaly, transposition) and preexcitation syndromes, like Wolff-Parkinson-White syndrome
    - Most often idiopathic
    - Treatment includes vagal maneuvers and adenosine (initially 0.1 mg/kg/dose) IV administered quickly, followed immediately by a flush of 5–10 cc normal saline, given its short half-life
    - If patient is unstable, perform synchronized cardioversion (0.5–1 J/kg)
- Atrial flutter
  - Less common and usually associated with a narrow complex tachycardia (unlike in adults) secondary to excellent conduction through the atrioventricular node
  - Treatment includes digoxin, synchronized cardioversion, or overdrive pacing; short-acting β-blockers may be used

to control the ventricular rate
  - Treat the underlying etiology when possible
- Atrial fibrillation
  - Less common in pediatric patients than in adults
  - Defined as an irregular-appearing and fast atrial rate (350–600 bpm), narrow QRS complexes, and an irregular ventricular response rate of 110–150 bpm
  - Causes and treatment are similar to atrial flutter
  - Anticoagulation may be necessary if present for more than 48 hours and pharmacologic or electrical cardioversion can be postponed
- Ventricular dysrhythmias
  - Premature ventricular contraction (PVC)
    - Typically benign; multifocal PVCs are more concerning
    - Causes include myocarditis, cardiomyopathy, congenital and acquired heart disease, long QT syndrome, hypokalemia, hypoxemia, hypomagnesemia, anxiety, and drugs (eg, digitalis, catecholamines, caffeine, and anesthetics)
    - Treatment is only necessary if the PVCs are associated with symptoms, hemodynamic changes, or underlying heart disease, or are made worse with exercise
    - Treatment can include lidocaine, β-blockers, and other antiarrhythmic drugs
- Ventricular tachycardia (VT) and ventricular fibrillation (VF)
  - Uncommon in children
  - Represent the initial arrest rhythm in only 10% of pediatric cardiopulmonary arrests, but will appear during up to 25% of all pediatric codes
  - For stable VT, consider a slow load of amiodarone 5 mg/kg, but be prepared to cardiovert or defibrillate if necessary
  - For pulseless VT and VF, treat with immediate cardiopulmonary resuscitation, defibrillate 2–4 J/kg, and administer either lidocaine (1 mg/kg) IV or amiodarone (5 mg/kg) IV bolus

Congestive Heart Failure

- Congestive heart failure (CHF) can be caused by a variety of congenital or acquired medical conditions

- By far, the most common cause of CHF in infancy is congenital heart disease
  - Volume overload lesions, such as ventricular septal defect, patent ductus arteriosus, and endocardial cushion defects are most common
  - Tachyarrhythmias and heart block can cause heart failure at any age, including in utero
  - Acquired heart diseases become more common as children get older
    - These conditions include myocarditis, acute rheumatic carditis, rheumatic valvular diseases with significant mitral or aortic regurgitation, dilated cardiomyopathy, metabolic abnormalities, endocrinopathies, and severe anemia
- Diagnosis
  - Historically, infants present with poor feeding, tachypnea that worsens during feeding, poor weight gain, and diaphoresis, particularly with feeding
  - Older children report dyspnea (particularly with activity), orthopnea, easy fatigability, and swelling of the eyelids, feet, and hands
  - Like in adults, the following are common physical examination findings consistent with but not specific to CHF:
    - Wheezing or crackles
    - Tachycardia
    - Gallop rhythm
    - Displaced point of maximal impulse
    - Weak pulses
    - Hepatomegaly
    - Extremity and eyelid edema
  - Unlike in adults, jugular venous distention is not a common finding
  - Cardiomegaly is almost always seen on a chest radiograph
- Management
  - Address the underlying etiology, provide support, and control underlying heart failure state
  - Supportive measures include providing adequate calories given fluid restrictions (for infants, as much as 150–169 kcal/kg/day)

  - Medical management includes a combination of inotropic agents, diuretics, and afterload-reducing agents

Acquired Heart Disease

- Rheumatic heart disease
  - Acute rheumatic fever is a common cause of heart disease in underdeveloped countries
  - Pathophysiology includes a postinflammatory reaction affecting the whole body
    - Believed to be immunologically mediated following a group A streptococcal infection of the pharynx
    - Other streptococcal infections, like impetigo, do not cause acute rheumatic fever
  - Most cases occur in children between 6–15 years old (peak incidence at 8 y) following a history (1–5 w) of streptococcal pharyngitis with nonspecific symptoms of malaise, fatigue, abdominal pain, and pallor; there is often a positive family history of rheumatic fever
  - The diagnosis is ultimately made using the revised Jones Criteria and requires two major manifestations or one major and two minor manifestations, in addition to evidence of an antecedent streptococcal pharyngitis by either throat culture or serology
  - Treatment includes administering benzathine penicillin G (0.6–1.2 million units intramuscular [IM]) followed by penicillin prophylaxis, relative bed rest, and antiinflammatory therapy
    - Supportive care measures include diuretics, digoxin, morphine, sodium and fluid restriction, and prednisone for severe carditis
    - Preventing recurrence includes administering benzathine penicillin G (1.2 million units IM every 28 days)
      - Alternatively, use penicillin VK 250 mg by mouth (PO) bid or erythromycin 250 mg PO bid for penicillin-allergic patients
      - Prophylaxis should continue until age 21–25 years
- Kawasaki disease
  - Kawasaki disease is an acute, febrile vasculitis of unknown etiology with a predilection for the coronary arteries

- Most common cause of acquired heart disease in developed countries and seen almost exclusively in children < 8 years old
- Diagnosis is clinical and based on a history of high fever lasting 5 days or more, plus four of the following five criteria:
    - Bilateral bulbar conjunctivitis without exudates
    - Erythema of the mouth and pharynx, strawberry tongue, or red and cracked lips
    - Polymorphous exanthema
    - Swelling of the hands and feet, with erythema of the palms and soles
    - Cervical lymphadenopathy (> 1.5 cm), usually single or unilateral
- Additional associated features include extreme irritability, abdominal pain, vomiting, diarrhea, and skin changes (particularly desquamation of the hands, feet, and perineal region), usually after the fever ends
- Laboratory findings include elevated erythrocyte sedimentation rate (ESR) and C-reactive protein (CRP), leukocytosis with left shift, normocytic or normochromic anemia, thrombocytosis, sterile pyuria, and elevated liver enzymes
- If left untreated, there is a 15%–25% risk of coronary artery aneurysm and subsequent coronary artery thrombosis and stenosis, although aneurysms can develop elsewhere in the body
- Rarer complications include carditis, valve regurgitation, pericardial effusion, and CHF
- Treatment
    - One dose of IV immunoglobulin (IVIG; 2 g / kg over 12 h)
    - High-dose aspirin (80–100 mg / kg / day divided qid) PO until the fever resolves, followed by 3–5 mg / kg / day of aspirin PO divided once a day for 6–8 weeks, or until the ESR and platelet count return to normal

Infective Endocarditis Prophylaxis

- The use of antibiotic prophylaxis to prevent bacterial endocarditis was greatly changed in 2007. Under current guidelines, prophylaxis is recommended for only the following procedures:

  - Dental procedures that involve manipulation of gingival tissues, the periapical region of teeth, or perforation of oral mucosa
  - Procedures on the respiratory tract involving incision of the respiratory tract mucosa
  - Procedures on infected skin, skin structures, or musculoskeletal tissue
  - Cardiac conditions associated with the highest risk of adverse outcome from endocarditis, including:
    - Prosthetic cardiac valve
    - Unrepaired congenital heart disease, including palliative shunts and conduits
    - Congenital heart defects completely repaired with a prosthetic material or device (placed surgically or by catheter) during the first 6 months after the procedure
    - Repaired congenital heart defects with residual defects at the site or adjacent to the site of a prosthetic patch or prosthetic device
    - Cardiac transplantation recipients with cardiac valvulopathy
    - Previous infective endocarditis
    - Prophylaxis is no longer recommended for procedures involving the gastrointestinal or genitourinary tracts
- Medication and dosing
  - Amoxicillin: 50 mg/kg PO initially (do not exceed maximum adult dose of 3 g), then 25 mg/kg in 6 hours (do not exceed 1.5 g)
  - Ampicillin: 50 mg/kg IV initially, then 25 mg/kg
  - Clindamycin: 10 mg/kg IV initially, then 5 mg/kg
  - Erythromycin ethylsuccinate and stearate: 20 mg/kg PO initially, then 10 mg/kg
  - Gentamicin: 1.5 mg/kg IV initially, then 1 mg/kg
  - Vancomycin: 20 mg/kg IV initially, then 10 mg/kg

Cardiac Syncope

- Although syncope is more frequently the result of vasovagal and orthostatic mechanisms, cardiac causes of syncope include:
  - Obstructive heart lesions
    - Aortic stenosis

- Pulmonary stenosis
- Hypertrophic obstructive cardiomyopathy
- Coronary artery abnormalities
- Arrhythmias

- Red flags during the evaluation of syncope include:
  - Exercise-induced syncope
  - Preceding chest pain
  - Associated seizure-like activity
  - Atypical history
  - Recurrent or progressive syncope
  - Physical examination suggestive of cardiac disease
  - Abnormal ECG
  - Family history of unexplained death

Chest Pain and Myocardial Infarction

- Chest pain is a frequent chief complaint among children and adolescents, but it is rarely due to any underlying cardiovascular cause. The most common etiologies of chest pain among pediatric patients are:
  - Chest wall pathology
    - Muscle strain
    - Trauma
    - Costrochondritis
  - Respiratory conditions
    - Pneumonia
    - Cough
    - Asthma
  - Gastrointestinal disease, specifically esophagitis related to gastroesophageal reflux disease
  - Psychogenic (anxiety)
- Red flags for underlying cardiovascular disease include:
  - Pain that radiates down the left arm or up the neck, jaw, or back
  - Associated presyncope or syncope
  - Palpitations
  - Dyspnea
  - Dull, squeezing, or heavy chest pain (as opposed to sharp or pinpoint pain that is often reproducible and worse on palpation)

- Cardiac causes of chest pain include:
  - Obstructive congenital heart conditions that put additional strain on the myocardium, such as aortic stenosis, subaortic stenosis, coarctation of the aorta, and pulmonary stenosis
  - Mitral valve prolapse
  - Cardiomyopathy
  - Coronary artery abnormalities
  - Aortic dissection or aneurysm
  - Pericarditis
  - Myocarditis
  - Arrhythmias

Myocardial Infarction

- Rare in children
- Predisposing conditions include history of Kawasaki disease, anomalous origin of a left coronary artery, congenital heart disease, and dilated cardiomyopathy
- Diagnosis and management are similar to that used in adults

Further Reading

1. Robertson J, Shilkofski N. *The Harriet Lane Handbook: A Manual for Pediatric House Officers*. 17th ed. Philadelphia, Pa: Elsevier Mosby; 2005.

2. Park MK. *Pediatric Cardiology for Practitioners*. 4th ed. St Louis, Mo: Mosby; 2002.

3. Keane JF, Lock JE, Fyler DC. *Nadas' Pediatric Cardiology*. 2nd ed. Philadelphia, Pa: Saunders Elsevier; 2006.

Chapter 28

Gastroenterology

Intestinal Infection

- **Acute** gastroenteritis is the most common cause of infant mortality worldwide
- **Viral** gastroenteritis is usually associated with small bowel disease, presenting with 5–10 watery, large-volume episodes per day
  - Rotavirus: lasts 5–7 days; symptoms include fever, vomiting, and profuse diarrhea
  - Adenovirus: milder than rotavirus, but lasts 8–12 days
  - Norovirus, calicivirus, and astrovirus: mildest, lasting 1–3 days
- **Bacterial** gastroenteritis usually starts watery; may become colitis or dysentery
  - Symptoms include frequent episodes (10–20/day); mucousy, bloody stools; positive hemoccult test
  - Species include *Salmonella, Shigella, Escherichia coli* (enterohemorrhagic or enteroinvasive), *Campylobacter, Yersinia,* and *Clostridium difficile*
  - Enterotoxigenic *E coli* and cholera only cause watery diarrhea
- **Protozoal** can be dysenteric (*Entamoeba histolytica*) or consist of more chronic loose stools (*Giardia, Cryptosporidium,* etc)

Osmotic Diarrhea

- Osmotic diarrhea usually indicates an injury to the small bowel mucosa and can be seen transiently in postinfectious diarrhea
- Treat with soy or other lactose-free formula until healed
  - Rice formula is not recommended because it mainly consists of carbohydrates and lacks the protein and fat that the bowel needs to promote rapid healing and epithelial cell growth
  - Juice is not recommended

Allergic Colitis

- Allergic colitis is seen mostly in infants
  - Usually presents at age 6–8 weeks
  - Often diagnosed after clinical presentation of blood-tinged, mucousy diarrhea
  - Babies usually outgrow typical allergic colitis by 12 months of age
- Children with allergic colitis often appear well otherwise, but can present with malnutrition, protein-losing enteropathy, or anemia
- Skin manifestations are typically absent, especially in younger infants, because the colitis is frequently due to an immunoglobulin G-mediated allergy (rather than an immunoglobulin E-mediated one)
- To treat: remove all cow's milk protein from the patient's diet
  - If the baby is not severely ill, try feeding with soy formula
  - If the baby is severely ill, treat with semielemental formula (eg, Nutramigen or Pregestamil [Mead Johnson Nutrition, Glenview, Ill] or Alimentum [Abbott Laboratories, New York, NY]) or amino acid-based formula
  - If the infant's mother can breast-feed, continue breastfeeding, but remove all cow's milk from the mother's diet

Malabsorption

- Malabsorption disorders in infants are usually manifestations of chronic duodenal infection, such as occurs with parasites
- May also be caused by genetic disorders that lead to fat malabsorption (cystic fibrosis is the common etiology for fat malabsorption in the first year of life)
- In the second year of life, infection is still likely, but celiac disease also becomes more prevalent
  - Celiac disease is an autoimmune disorder that requires gluten, a byproduct of wheat-containing foods, to manifest itself (thus, it is less common in certain areas of the world)
  - Treatment is a gluten-free diet for the patient's lifetime
- In older children showing evidence of malabsorption, infection and inflammatory bowel disease are the two most likely causes
  - Inflammatory bowel disease is an autoimmune disorder

that is rarely seen in underdeveloped countries
- Protein-losing enteropathy presents with diarrhea and edema and has many etiologies
  - Begin by ruling out allergic colitis, infection, and other inflammatory conditions
  - In remote locations, the diagnosis can be made by evidence of protein malnutrition, low serum albumin, and a urinalysis that is clear of protein
  - The differential also includes primary protein malnutrition from deficient dietary protein; a dietary history is essential in any child with diarrhea
  - Treatment of protein malabsorption requires determining the etiology
    - In the meantime, use an amino acid-based formula or a formula that is as elemental as possible (eg, breast milk from a mother who has removed dairy from her diet)
    - Some children need total parenteral nutrition for nutritional rehabilitation if feeding exacerbates the symptoms

Constipation
- Functional constipation usually begins at age 1½–2 years old, when toilet training begins
- It manifests as infrequent, large, hard stools, sometimes predisposing to anal fissures
- Encopresis (overflow of bowel movement into the underwear) or intermittent overflow diarrhea can occur in severe cases
  - Treatment: clean out (typically administered over 2–3 days) is usually required first because megarectum tends to develop following chronic retention
  - Administer enema once a day for 2 days, followed by bisacodyl (5 mg tablet orally [PO] or 10 mg suppository every day for 1–2 days)
    - When used in an enema or child dose, halve the adult size (60 cc of phosphosoda)
    - **Never give an infant with rectal outlet obstruction an electrolyte solution,** such as phosphosoda enemas or polyethylene glycol 3350 electrolyte solution; this type of treatment has been reported to cause severe electrolyte disturbances and death in infants

- Mineral oil enemas are sometimes effective (1–2 cc/kg as single dose)
- Recommended daily medications are as follows:
  - Polyethylene glycol at a dose of 1 capful mixed with water, juice, or poured on soft food, given 1–3 times per day; this treatment has largely replaced the other daily medications listed below and should be tried first
  - Milk of magnesia: 1–2 cc/kg/day
  - Mineral oil: 1–2 cc/kg/day
  - Lactulose: 1–2 cc/kg/day

- Organic disorders that cause constipation
  - Hirschsprung disease: usually presents with obstructive symptoms and no bowel movement in the first 24 hours of life, but can also present later in infancy
    - Take abdominal films prior to rectal examination, flat plate then prone, cross-table lateral with hips slightly flexed (ie, "butt up")
      - These show distended loops of bowel, but also the absence of air in the area that should be the rectal vault
      - Because rectal air will be expelled with a digital rectal examination, films must be taken first
    - Bowel movements are usually explosive and watery, which can be documented on a digital rectal examination (in which forceful expulsion of soft stool occurs on extraction of the examiner's finger)
    - The physical examination reveals a long, tight sphincter canal
    - Follow this with a contrast enema to rule out etiologies besides Hirschsprung's, such as microcolon and imperforate anus
    - Confirmatory diagnosis is only made by rectal biopsy
    - Treatment is surgical, but can be temporized by frequent rectal washings with normal saline (5–10 cc every 3 h) via a rectal tube (10–12 Fr red rubber catheter inserted a few centimeters from the anus)
  - When a newborn does not stool in the first 24 hours of life, obstructive lesions are possible, but also consider meconium plug syndrome
    - Usually benign

    - Symptoms are relieved after contrast enema or serial rectal washings
    - May indicate cystic fibrosis, but is not pathognomonic
- Anatomical defects
  - Some anatomical defects that can result in constipation include:
    - Anorectal malformations, such as imperforate anus, rectal stenosis, and anterior displaced anus
    - Microcolon (especially in infants of diabetic mothers)
    - Obstructive intestinal lesions, such as ileal atresia
    - Neurological disorders, such as caudal regression syndrome
  - Treat first with oral hyperosmotic agents, such as lactulose or milk of magnesia; eventually administer enemas as needed (patients with these conditions do not have adequate sensation to have a bowel movement)

Vomiting and Gastroesophageal Reflux

- If vomiting is bilious, an upper gastrointestinal (GI) series is imperative to rule out malrotation with volvulus, duodenal atresia, or atresia of the small intestine
- For nonbilious vomiting in an infant 4–6 weeks old, consider hypertrophic pyloric stenosis
- If vomiting is chronic, consider gastroesophageal reflux disease
  - Gastroesophageal reflux in children may present as respiratory disease (either apnea and bradycardia in infants, or asthma in older children)
  - Severe vomiting with failure to thrive, lethargy, or delayed development can be a sign of metabolic disease in infancy
- Another etiology of chronic vomiting in infants and children is peptic ulcer disease (especially if accompanied with abdominal pain), with or without *Helicobacter pylori;* and urinary tract infection, especially with hydronephrosis
- Laboratory evaluation for chronic vomiting or vomiting causing chronic problems (such as failure to thrive, abdominal pain, etc) includes:
  - Complete blood count (CBC)
  - Erythrocyte sedimentation rate complete metabolic panel

- Amylase
- Lipase
- Urinalysis and culture
- If possible, an upper GI series can also rule out malrotation in the presence of chronic vomiting

- Treatment
  - Treat gastroesophageal reflux disease in children using any of the following:
    - Ranitidine: 1–2 mg / kg bid
    - Omeprazole: 0.7–3 mg / kg / day (capsule can be emptied into yogurt or applesauce to encourage ingestion)
    - Over-the-counter antacids, such as aluminum hydroxide with magnesium hydroxide (1–2 cc / kg given frequently through the day with feeds; watch for changes in bowel movements)
    - Metoclopramide (0.1–0.2 mg / kg 3–4 times per day prior to a meal) may be helpful for infants as well
      - If possible, rule out malrotation with severe gastroesophageal reflux before adding this medication (and definitely if the emesis is bilious)
  - If *H pylori* is expected, the suggested antibiotics are similar to those recommended for adults, including the following:
    - Amoxicillin: 80 mg / kg / day divided bid
    - Clarithromycin: 15 mg / kg / day divided bid
    - Metronidazole: 15 mg / kg / day divided tid
    - Proton pump inhibitors: 1–2 mg / kg / day at weight-appropriate doses for 2 weeks
    - The usual choices are amoxicillin, clarithromycin, and omeprazole, but that can be altered if the patient is allergic to amoxicillin

Gastrointestinal Bleeding

- To treat GI bleeding, first check ABCs (airway, breathing, and circulation) and perform hemodynamic stabilization if bleeding is severe
- Take a patient history and perform a physical examination to determine etiology or source of the bleeding and ongoing losses

- Potential laboratory examinations include CBC, prothrombin time or activated partial thromboplastin time, liver function panel, disseminated intravascular coagulation panel, electrolyte panel with blood urea nitrogen/creatinine, blood type and cross-match, and stool guaiac
- If the patient has bloody diarrhea, send a stool sample for fecal leukocytes test and culture
- Consider blood transfusion
- Perform gastric lavage if upper GI bleeding is evident
- Etiologies are based on age
    - Toddlers to children of early school age: painless rectal bleeding (either hematochezia or melena) in large quantity that drops hemoglobin levels is likely Meckel's diverticulum
        - If this is suspected, admit the patient and observe by frequently checking hemoglobin levels
        - Radiologic diagnosis is made by Meckel's scan
        - Treat with surgical resection of the Meckel's diverticulum
    - In older children, significant upper GI bleeding is usually peptic disease, gastritis, or esophagitis
        - Occult liver disease can present as upper GI bleeding from esophageal varices in children
        - The other "at-risk" population includes patients who had omphalitis or umbilical cord catheterization complicated by portal vein thrombosis, causing portal hypertension
    - Another relatively common presentation of rectal bleeding is allergic colitis in an infant 1–2 months old
- The most common cause of lower GI bleeding in the first year of age is anal fissure. Treat using warm soaks and stool softeners

Chronic Abdominal Pain

- Warning signs of organic disease include frequent vomiting, diarrhea, GI bleeding, weight loss or failure to gain weight normally, associated systemic symptoms, nocturnal wakening symptoms, localized pain, poor appetite, and early satiety
- *H pylori* may cause vomiting associated with upper abdominal pain
- Intussusception presents with severe abdominal pain that

manifests as colicky pain, followed by bowel movement that may be appear as melena or bright red blood
- The classic appearance of the stool in the late stages is described as the "currant jelly stool" due to bowel wall ischemia
- In younger infants and children, subjective localized pain will be absent
  - On physical examination, tenderness can often be localized in the right lower quadrant
  - This presentation usually occurs in children 6 months–2 years old and is ileocolic
- A kidney, ureter, and bladder (KUB) radiograph will show paucity of bowel gas in the right lower quadrant, and a barium enema can be diagnostic and therapeutic
  - The risk of bowel perforation is higher during the diagnostic and therapeutic contrast enema if there has been a delay from the time of onset of symptoms; exercise caution
  - Admit and observe the patient; there is significant risk of recurrence in the first 24 hours, and fluids and electrolytes must be managed
  - If the enema does not reduce the intussusception, surgery will be needed for manual reduction
  - If it occurs in an older child or occurs in a less typical location, such as ileal-ileal, be wary of other types of lead points, such as polyp disease or cancer lesions (as in lymphoma)

Acute Abdominal Pain

- Omental cysts
  - May cause abdominal pain
  - May be difficult to diagnose on physical examination because of the large size and fluidity of the structure
  - Readily noticeable on ultrasound and computed tomography (CT) scan of the abdomen
  - Treatment is surgical resection
- Intraabdominal masses and tumors
  - Cause abdominal pain
  - Ultrasound and CT scan of the abdomen are sufficient for diagnosis

- Sometimes evident on a KUB radiograph
- Peptic disease, celiac disease, esophagitis, and colitis cause abdominal pain
- Nephrolithiasis and hydronephrosis, with or without urinary tract infection, can cause severe flank pain
- Cholelithiasis and cholecystitis
  - Uncommon in children; however, children may have congenital lesions that predispose them to these diseases
  - Sickle cell and cystic fibrosis patients are also prone to these problems

Tube Feedings

- Tube feeding may be necessary for nutritional rehabilitation
  - Can be useful in the acute setting of a child with dehydration
  - Also useful for enteral drip fluid and electrolyte replacement when IV placement is impossible
- Usually the feeding tube is placed nasogastrically, but transpyloric feeds can be used in children if severe vomiting continues with a nasogastric (NG) tube
  - To encourage transpyloric stool passage, allow slack on the tube and add metoclopramide (0.1–0.2 mg/kg PO/IV)
  - Appropriate tube size depends on the patient's age (verify using Broselow tape):
    - Infants and toddlers: use an infant-sized tube or one measuring at most 6 Fr
    - Child 2–12 years old: 8 Fr; weighted tubes are easier to keep in place
    - Child > 12 years old: 10 Fr
  - Tube should be soft and changed periodically (approximately every 4–6 wk) if use is long term
- Feeding with a continuous drip is helpful in vomiting patients because more calories can be delivered with less vomiting
  - In the case of a transpyloric tube, continuous feeding is imperative; however, bolus feeds can also be given via the NG route
  - The appropriate fluids through an NG tube are formulas or electrolyte solution, not pureed foods

Chapter 29

Infectious Diseases

Ocular Infections (see also Chapter 11, Ophthalmology)

Neonatal Conjunctivitis

- Symptoms: significant findings may be either profuse purulence or hemorrhage in the conjunctiva
- Etiology: *Neisseria gonorrhoeae, Chlamydia trachomatis*, herpes simplex virus (HSV)
- Diagnosis
  - Gonococcal: perform deoxyribonucleic acid (DNA) probe if available, Gram stain, and culture on Thayer-Martin or chocolate agar
  - Chlamydia: perform a Giemsa stain for intracytoplasmic inclusions (low sensitivity)
  - HSV: take a viral culture; in neonates, rule out disseminated HSV by checking cerebrospinal fluid and liver transaminases
- Treatment
  - Gonococcus
    - Administer ceftriaxone (50 mg/kg intramuscular [IM] or intravenous [IV] × 1 dose) or cefotaxime bid for 7 days if neonate is hyperbilirubinemic
    - Irrigate every 2–3 hours with saline
    - Topical antibiotics are not recommended
  - Chlamydia
    - Administer oral (PO) erythromycin (50 mg/kg/day in 4 divided doses) for 14 days, or azithromycin 20 mg/kg as single dose or over 3 days
  - HSV
    - Apply topical trifluridine or vidarabine for 7–10 days
    - Consult an ophthalmologist if possible
    - In severe cases or if infection has disseminated, administer IV acyclovir 20 mg/kg/dose tid for 14–21 days
- **Neonatal prophylaxis**: apply topical 1% silver nitrate, 1% tetracycline, or 0.5% erythromycin ointment

Trachoma

- Symptoms
  - Chronic, mucopurulent drainage
  - Follicular inflammation on the upper eyelid
  - Trichiasis (scarring with lashes turned inward)
- Etiology
  - *C trachomatis* serovars A–C
  - Endemic in developing parts of world
  - Major cause of blindness worldwide
- Diagnosis: clinical
- Treatment
  - PO azithromycin (20 mg/kg × 1; 1 g maximum dose)

OR

  - Erythromycin or tetracycline ophthalmic drops bid for 2 months

Periorbital Cellulitis

- Symptoms: erythema and edema surrounding eye
- Etiology
  - Inoculation from trauma or insect bite (*Staphylococcus aureus* or group A streptococcus) or bacteremic seeding (*Haemophilus influenzae* type B [Hib] or *Streptococcus pneumoniae*)
- Diagnosis
  - Clinically assess for normal globe movement, lack of proptosis, and lack of pain with extraocular muscle use
  - Obtain blood cultures
- Treatment
  - Administer third-generation cephalosporin
  - Add an antistaphylococcal drug if trauma is suspected or skin is broken
  - Perform lumbar puncture if Hib is suspected or if there is evidence of meningitis

Orbital Cellulitis

- Symptoms
  - Periorbital edema and erythema
  - Proptosis, severe eye pain, vision loss; limitation of extraocular movement in more severe cases
- Etiology

- Underlying bacterial sinusitis
- *S pneumoniae*
- *Streptococcus pyogenes*
- *S aureus*
- *H influenzae* (nontypable)
- *Moraxella catarrhalis*
- Anaerobes in older children

- Diagnosis
  - Clinical
  - Computed tomography (CT) scan, if available, to assess for abscess
- Treatment
  - IV ceftriaxone and clindamycin; or ampicillin (AMP)/sulbactam as alternative
  - Consider surgical intervention if condition continues to progress 24–48 hours after treatment, or if there is evidence of subperiosteal abscess

Disease of the Face and Neck

Buccal Cellulitis

- Symptoms
  - Acute cheek edema and erythema anterior to parotid, associated with fever
- Etiology
  - *H influenzae*
  - Oral flora will be present if the condition is an extension of odontogenic infection
- Diagnosis
  - Clinical
  - Blood culture
- Treatment: IV third-generation cephalosporin or AMP/sulbactam

Epiglottitis (see Chapter 24, Respiratory Emergencies)

Bacterial Tracheitis (see Chapter 24, Respiratory Emergencies)

Parotitis, Sialadenitis, and Mumps

- Symptoms
  - Painful swelling of the salivary glands (parotid, sublingual,

  or submandibular)
  - Fever and toxicity with bacterial infection
- Etiology
  - Viral (usually mumps, human immunodeficiency virus [HIV], or enteroviruses)
  - Bacterial (*S aureus*, gram-negative bacilli, *S pyogenes, S pneumoniae*)
- Diagnosis
  - Clinical
  - Bacterial infection manifests with purulent drainage from Stensen's duct
  - Perform Gram stain and culture
- Treatment
  - Bacterial: hydration and parenteral antibiotics (eg, ceftriaxone, AMP / sulbactam, or other broad-spectrum varieties); cannulate duct or perform surgical drainage in severe or refractory cases
  - Viral: supportive

Parapharyngeal Abscess

- Symptoms
  - Preceding adenitis, tonsillitis, or dental infection, in children ≥ 5 years old
  - Trismus
  - Parotid-area swelling extending below mandible
- Etiology
  - *S pneumoniae*
  - *S aureus*
  - Group A β-hemolytic streptococci
  - Anaerobes
- Diagnosis
  - Retropharyngeal abscess may have bulging posterior pharyngeal wall on plain film
  - Prevertebral soft tissue swelling of greater than 7 mm at the level of the second cervical vertebra, or greater than 14 mm at the level of the sixth cervical vertebra, is suggestive
  - Reversal of the normal cervical curvature may be present. Imaging with CT or magnetic resonance is required for definitive diagnosis
- Treatment: surgical drainage and appropriate IV antibiotic therapy

for primary infection (usually ceftriaxone and clindamycin)

Skin, Soft Tissue, Bone, and Joint Infections
In areas with a high prevalence of community-acquired methicillin-resistant *S aureus*, consider using clindamycin, trimethoprim-sulfamethoxazole (TMP/SMX), or vancomycin (IV only) when initiating empiric therapy for staphylococcal infections.

Cellulitis and Lymphangitis
- Symptoms
  - Erythema
  - Induration
  - Warmth
  - Tenderness
  - Lymphangitic spread (streaks)
- Etiology: most commonly *S aureus*, group A streptococcus, and *H influenzae* in unimmunized toddlers
- Diagnosis
  - Clinical
  - Positive blood culture in < 10%
  - Positive aspirate culture in 50%
- Treatment
  - Oral or IV antibiotics for *S aureus* and group A streptococcus (first-generation cephalosporin, antistaphylococcal penicillin, clindamycin)
  - Rapid progression may indicate infection in deeper tissue planes, such as necrotizing fasciitis

Cutaneous Candidiasis/Yeast Infections
- Symptoms: painful or itchy erythematous rash, usually concentrated in skin folds or covered areas (eg, diaper rash)
- Etiology: *Candida* species (usually *Candida albicans*)
- Diagnosis
  - Clinical appearance
  - Erythema with sharp borders and smaller satellite lesions are frequently seen around the rash border
- Treatment
  - One dose of fluconazole (6–12 mg/kg; maximum dose of 400 mg),

OR

  - Topical antifungals, such as nystatin, terbinafine, econazole, miconazole, etc

Lymphadenitis

- Symptoms: swollen lymph nodes often associated with erythema, warmth, and tenderness
- Etiology
  - *S aureus*, group A streptococcus, mycobacterial species, toxoplasmosis, and many viruses
  - Consider plague in endemic areas
- Diagnosis
  - Clinical appearance
  - Depending on location, consider throat culture, complete blood count, monospot, and Gram stain and culture of drainage
- Treatment
  - Empiric antibiotics against *aureus* and group A streptococcus
  - Surgical drainage of abscess if needed
  - If not improving, consider tuberculosis (TB), chronic viral infection (eg, HIV), and atypical mycobacteria

Septic Arthritis

- Symptoms: pain, swelling, erythema, warmth, and tenderness of the joint
- Etiology
  - Most common is *S aureus*
  - *N gonorrhoeae* if patient is sexually active
  - Others include group A streptococcus, *S pneumoniae*, *Brucella* (especially hip or sacrum), *H influenzae*, and other gram negatives
- Diagnosis
  - Elevated white blood cell (WBC) count
  - Erythrocyte sedimentation rate (ESR)
  - C-reactive protein (CRP)
  - Ultrasound may reveal fluid in joints
  - Perform Gram stain and culture of joint aspirate
- Treatment
  - Joint drainage is mandatory for hip joints; it may be indicated for other joints
  - Empiric IV antibiotics should cover *S aureus* (first- or second-generation cephalosporin, antistaphylococcal peni-

cillin; alternatively, use vancomycin and clindamycin) and Hib in unimmunized population (AMP, second- or third-generation cephalosporin)
  - Administer ceftriaxone for *N gonorrhoeae*
  - Differential diagnosis in children includes toxic synovitis (reaction to viral infection, especially in the hips), reactive arthritis, and juvenile rheumatoid arthritis

Osteomyelitis

- Symptoms
  - Pain
  - Tenderness over bone (with or without swelling)
  - Overlying erythema
  - Warmth
  - Fever
- Etiology
  - Most commonly *S aureus*
  - Others include group A streptococcus, *H influenzae, Kingella, Brucella,* and mycobacteria species (including TB)
- Diagnosis: patient will have elevated WBC count, ESR, and CRP; take radiographs of the suspected bones
- Treatment
  - Use empiric IV antibiotics against *S aureus* (first-generation cephalosporin, antistaphylococcal penicillin; alternatively, use vancomycin, or clindamycin)
  - If patient initially presents with a high fever or appears very ill, or for patients with sickle cell disease, cover for gram negatives with ceftriaxone (or similar)
  - Complete 3–6 weeks of antibiotics (switch to PO after 1 week or when CRP is normal)
  - Surgical debridement may be necessary if condition is severe or patient fails to respond
  - Chronic osteomyelitis requires long-term therapy (months to years)
  - If the patient fails to respond to antistaphylococcal medication, broaden coverage to include gram negatives

Pulmonary Infections

Croup (laryngotracheitis / laryngotracheobronchitis; see Chapter

24, Respiratory Emergencies)

Bronchiolitis (see Chapter 24, Respiratory Emergencies)

Pneumonia

- Symptoms: fever, tachypnea, retractions, and focal lung findings
- Etiology
  - **Bacterial:** *S pneumoniae, H influenzae, S aureus, Mycoplasma pneumoniae, Chlamydia pneumoniae, Bordetella pertussis, Mycobacterium tuberculosis, Chlamydia trachomatis* (infants), group B streptococcus (infants)
  - **Viral:** respiratory syncytial virus, influenza, parainfluenza, adenovirus, measles
  - **Parasitic/fungal:** *Pneumocystis carinii/jiroveci* (if the patient has HIV or is immunosuppressed or malnourished)
- Epidemiology
  - All ages, all seasons, high morbidity and mortality in children < 5 years old
  - Risk factors include poverty, crowding, environmental exposures, prematurity, malnutrition, immunosuppression, lack of breast-feeding
- Diagnosis
  - Clinical
  - Radiological: chest radiograph (if available)
  - Laboratory: cultures, bronchoscopy (if indicated and available)
- Treatment
  - Supportive care (eg, IV fluids, oxygen)
  - Consider TB skin test in all children
  - Duration: 5–10 days for uncomplicated infection, 2–4 weeks for complicated or severe infection
  - Antibiotics
    - < 2 months old: IV penicillin + gentamicin; **OR** penicillin + cefotaxime
    - > 2 months old: IV ceftriaxone or penicillin alone; PO TMP / SMX
    - If HIV is suspected or patient is severely malnourished, consider TMP / SMX
    - If nosocomial or immunosuppressed, consider vanco-

    mycin, antifungals, or TMP/SMX
    - If aspiration is the etiology, provide anaerobic coverage (clindamycin or AMP/sulbactam)
- Complications
  - Suspect complications in cases of severe pneumonia with prolonged fever, septic appearance, slow response to antibiotics, and clinical deterioration
  - Abscess
    - Obtain a CT scan, if possible
    - Include anaerobic coverage
    - Extend treatment to 3–4 weeks or more
  - Effusion/empyema
    - Suspect in patients with dyspnea and pleuritic pain
    - Patients will exhibit dullness to percussion and decreased breath sounds
    - Take decubitus films, CT scan, and ultrasound, if available
    - Use a chest tube rather than thoracentesis to address large effusions, if possible

Whooping Cough/Pertussis

- Symptoms
  - Suspect if patient exhibits paroxysmal cough, facial petechiae, or posttussive emesis, or if patient's face turns red or blue with cough
    - Catarrhal: mild symptoms of upper respiratory infection (URI), antibiotics may ameliorate disease and limit spread; neonates may present with apnea
    - Paroxysmal: paroxysms of cough with inspiratory whoop, with or without posttussive emesis
    - Convalescent: symptoms wane gradually over weeks to months (usually afebrile); can last 6–10 weeks or longer
  - Most severe in children < 6 months old, who may present with apnea or elevated WBC count with lymphocytosis
- Epidemiology
  - *B pertussis, Bordetella parapertussis*
  - Humans are the only hosts
  - Transmitted via aerosolized droplets
  - Adolescents and adults are important infectious sources;

incidence is increased in conditions of close contact

- Diagnosis: clinical (culture or polymerase chain reaction, if available)
- Treatment
  - Macrolides (azithromycin, erythromycin, clarithromycin)
    - Alternatively, use TMP/SMX (in children > 2 mo old)
    - Do not use erythromycin in infants < 2 months old; it may cause pyloric stenosis
  - Supportive (eg, IV fluids, rest, oxygen)
  - Prophylaxis and control
    - Immunization
    - Postexposure prophylaxis (same dose and duration as treatment)
      - Erythromycin: 40–50 mg/kg/day, qid for 14 days (maximum 2 g/day; estolate salt is better tolerated)
      - Azithromycin: 10–12 mg/kg once daily for 5 days (**do not step down doses on days 2–5**; maximum of 600 mg/day)
      - Clarithromycin: 15–20 mg/kg/day, bid for 7 days (maximum 1 g/day)
      - TMP/SMX: if patient cannot tolerate erythromycin, give 8 mg/kg/day TMP component, bid for 14 days

Tuberculosis

- Symptoms: fever, weight loss/failure to thrive, cough, night sweats, chills
  - Extrapulmonary findings may include meningitis, lymphadenitis, and involvement of bones, joints, skin, and middle ear or mastoid
- Epidemiology
  - *M tuberculosis*
  - Increased in populations with high HIV rates
- Diagnosis
  - A positive TB skin test in children is defined as:
    - 5–9 mm induration, if the child:
      - Shows clinical or radiological evidence of TB
      - Has had close contact with an adult with active pulmonary TB

        - Is on immunosuppressive drugs or is immunosuppressed
    - 10–14 mm induration if the child:
        - Is < 4 years old
        - Has other serious medical conditions
        - Is born in a high-prevalence area
        - Has been exposed to adults with HIV
        - Is homeless
    - > 15 mm induration in a child ≥ 4 years old with no risk factors
  - Use chest radiograph to evaluate for evidence of active disease
- Treatment
  - Active disease
    - Pulmonary / extrapulmonary (except meningitis):
        - 2 months of isoniazid + rifampin + pyrazinamide **followed by**
        - 4 months of isoniazid and rifampin (see drug dosages below)
    - If resistance is a concern due to location, history, or presentation, add:
        - Ethambutol or streptomycin for the first 2 months until susceptibilities are available
        - Ethambutol can cause optic neuritis, so avoid use in young children unless they can cooperate with tests for visual acuity and color blindness
    - For meningitis:
        - 2 months of isoniazid, rifampin, pyrazinamide, and an aminoglycoside or ethambutol once a day, followed by 7–10 months of isoniazid and rifampin once a day or twice weekly for 9–12 months total
    - In active pulmonary disease, patient should get a follow-up chest radiograph after 2 months for response evaluation
    - Drug dosages:
        - Isoniazid: 10–15 mg/kg/day (maximum 300 mg/day) **OR** 20–30 mg/kg twice weekly
        - Rifampin: 10–15 mg/kg/day (maximum 600 mg/day) **OR** 10–20 mg/kg twice weekly

            - Pyrazinamide: 30–40 mg/kg/day (maximum 2 g/day) **OR** 50 mg/kg twice weekly
            - Ethambutol: 15–25 mg/kg/day (maximum 2.5 g/day) **OR** 50 mg/kg twice weekly
            - Streptomycin: 20–40 mg/kg/day (IM or IV), maximum of 1 g
    - Children with TB likely acquired it from an adult, so investigate all who have had contact with the infected child, looking for the index case as well as other infected children
        - Children and adolescents exposed to a contagious case of TB should have a TB skin test, physical examination, and chest radiograph
        - Children < 4 years old or whose immune systems are impaired should receive 9 months of isoniazid prophylaxis, regardless of TB skin test results
            - In immunocompetent patients with negative TB skin tests, continue isoniazid and recheck TB skin test in 12 weeks
            - If skin test is still negative, discontinue medication
    - Latent TB infection
        - 9 months of isoniazid once a day for 9 months, or 6 months of rifampin once a day if patient is isoniazid resistant
        - Routine laboratory checks are unnecessary; monitor transaminases in children with severe active disease or risk factors for hepatitis
        - Provide B_6 (pyridoxine) supplementation for adults or malnourished children to prevent isoniazid-induced neuritis

Diarrhea in a Humanitarian-Assistance Setting

- Symptoms
    - Three or more loose or watery stools per day
    - Acute diarrhea starts suddenly and is generally self-limited after several days
    - Persistent diarrhea starts like acute diarrhea but lasts 14 days or more
- Etiology
    - Major cause of morbidity and mortality among children worldwide

- The World Health Organization (WHO) recognizes acute watery diarrhea and dysentery as the two basic types of acute diarrhea
  - Acute watery diarrhea may be caused by rotavirus, cholera, *Campylobacter, Escherichia coli, Salmonella,* or *Yersinia*; when patient presents with a high volume of watery stools with flecks of mucous (rice water stools), rule out cholera
  - Dysentery is defined as bloody, mucoid diarrhea, and is usually caused by gram-negative bacteria (*Shigella, Salmonella* species, or *E coli*), *Entamoeba histolytica,* and rarely, *Clostridium difficile*
- Almost all these agents are transmitted by ingestion of contaminated food or water and by person-to-person spread; contact precautions are encouraged

- Diagnosis
  - Use clinical diagnosis and empiric treatment for most cases
  - Most cases in infants are of viral etiology (rotavirus)
  - Confirm initial cases of cholera and bacillary dysentery microbiologically, if possible
  - WHO case definitions for cholera:
    - Person ≥ 5 years old with severe dehydration or death due to watery diarrhea
    - Person ≥ 2 years old with watery diarrhea in an area with a cholera outbreak
- Treatment (derived from WHO guidelines; assumes limited resources and limited or no laboratory support)
  - Assess dehydration (ie, none, some, severe)
  - Prevent dehydration by increasing fluid intake (use oral rehydration solution [ORS] or breast milk)
  - Treat dehydration
  - Provide nutritional support and encourage feeding; support breast-feeding
  - Use antibiotics selectively
  - Avoid use of antimotility agents
  - Empiric treatment
    - No dehydration: increase fluid intake to more than usual amount
    - Some dehydration: give ORS until skin turgor normal-

izes and thirst abates; start with 75 mL/kg in first 4 hours

- Severe dehydration: use IV fluid therapy
  - Use a nasogastric tube if unable to place an IV within 30 minutes
  - Start ORS as soon as the patient can tolerate it
  - Give 30 mL/kg bolus, then another 70 mL/kg over next 4–6 hours
- Zinc supplementation for 10–14 days will mitigate current illness and decrease incidence of subsequent episodes (10 mg a day for children < 6 mo old, 20 mg a day for those > 6 mo old; check the available zinc salt preparation for zinc content)
- Treat with an antibiotic if dysentery is likely (know local resistance patterns if possible)
- WHO guidelines for empiric therapy:
  - Ciprofloxacin: 500 mg PO bid for 3 days (adults), 15 mg/kg PO bid for 3 days (off-label use for pediatric patients)
  - Azithromycin 10 mg/kg PO for 3 days is an alternative
  - Resistance rates to TMP/SMX and AMP make them poor empiric choices
- Antibiotics will shorten duration of cholera symptoms
  - In large outbreaks, reserve for severe cases
  - Administer one dose of doxycycline (300 mg PO; WHO guidelines recommend this as off-label use for all patients)
- For patients with persistent diarrhea in the absence of a confirmed parasitological diagnosis, provide two courses of antibiotics for dysentery; if symptoms persist, treat for giardia and amoeba
- Amebiasis
  - Symptoms
    - Abdominal pain
    - Fever
    - Diarrhea, usually bloody or mucoid
    - Right upper quadrant abdominal pain may represent amebic abscess
  - Etiology: *Entamoeba histolytica*
  - Diagnosis

        - Identify trophozoites or cysts on stool sample
        - Rapid antigen tests may be available
      - Treatment
        - Give metronidazole for dysentery and abscesses
        - Administer diloxanide furoate, iodoquinol, or paromomycin to eradicate cysts from stool
    - For endemic population, eradicating cysts from stools is not indicated. Chlorinating water will not kill *Entamoeba*; boil water for 1 minute

Systemic Conditions

Sepsis and Meningitis

- Symptoms
  - The clinical case definition of meningitis is sudden onset of fever (> 38°C axillary) and one of the following:
    - Neck stiffness
    - Altered consciousness
    - Other meningeal sign, such as:
      - Kernig sign: flex the patient's knees and the neck bends in response
      - Brudzinski sign: flex the patient's neck and the knees bend in response
    - Petechial or purpural rash
    - In patients < 1 year old, meningitis is suspected when fever is accompanied by a bulging fontanel
    - *Neisseria meningitidis* also causes meningococcal septicemia
      - Severe disease with signs of acute fever, purpura/petechiae, and shock
      - Though less common, the case fatality rate is high
- Etiology: *N meningitidis*, *S pneumoniae*, and *H influenzae* account for > 80% of all cases of bacterial meningitis and sepsis in unimmunized populations
- Diagnosis
  - Blood culture
  - Lumbar puncture should be done as soon as meningitis is suspected and before starting antimicrobial treatment
    - In bacterial meningitis, cerebrospinal fluid is usually

    - cloudy or purulent (but may be clear or bloody)
    - In malaria-endemic areas, thick and thin smears of blood should be made to differentiate meningitis from cerebral malaria
- Treatment
  - If bacterial meningitis is suspected, antibiotic treatment should be started immediately after a lumbar puncture without waiting for the results; treatment should not be delayed if lumbar puncture cannot be performed in a timely manner (Table 29-1)
  - Viral meningitis is rarely serious and requires supportive care, but a lumbar puncture is necessary to differentiate it from bacterial meningitis
  - During large epidemics among refugees or displaced populations, a single-dose regimen of oily chloramphenicol (100 mg/kg, maximum 3 g; IM) can be used if resources or circumstances do not permit a full course of standard treatment
    - Oral chloramphenicol also effectively penetrates the central nervous system
    - Single-dose ceftriaxone IM or IV (100 mg/kg, maximum 4 g) was equivalent to the single dose of oily chloramphenicol in one study
  - Chemoprophylaxis of local civilian contacts is often not recommended in emergency situations; however, exposed healthcare workers should receive prophylaxis if meningococcus is suspected or confirmed. Administer:
    - Rifampin: 20 mg/kg, maximum 1,200 mg, every 12 hours for 2 days
    - Ceftriaxone: single dose, 125 mg IM for those ≤ 14 years old, 250 mg for those ≥ 15 years old
    - Ciprofloxacin: single dose, 500 mg PO for those ≥ 18 years old

Acute Rheumatic Fever

- Symptoms: most commonly presents with arthritis or carditis
- Etiology: inflammatory process occurring after pharyngitis due to certain group A β-hemolytic streptococci types; however, fewer than two thirds of patients remember having a sore throat in the months before presenting

Table 29–1. Empiric Therapy for Bacterial Meningitis and Sepsis in Developing Countries

Patient Group	Likely Etiology	Treatment	Duration of Therapy
Immunocompetent children < 2 mo old	Group B streptococcus *Escherichia coli* *Listeria* *Salmonella* spp	Ampicillin 200–300 mg/kg/day ≤ 7days ÷ q8h; > 7 days ÷ q6h **PLUS** Gentamicin 2.5 mg/kg q12h **OR ADD** Cefotaxime 50 mg/kg q8h	3 wk
Immunocompetent children 2 mo–18 y old	*Haemophilus influenzae* *Streptococcus pneumoniae* *Neisseria meningitidis* *Salmonella* spp	Ceftriaxone 100 mg/kg q24h (if resistant *Streptococcus pneumoniae* is present,add vancomycin 40 mg/kg/day, divided q6–8h)	*Haemophilus influenzae*: 10 days *Streptococcus pneumoniae*: 10–14 days *Neisseria meningitidis*: 7 days *Salmonella* spp: 21 days
Neurosurgical problems and head trauma	*Staphylococcus aureus* *Staphylococcus epidermidis* Gram-negative organisms *Streptococcus pneumoniae*	Vancomycin and a third-generation cephalosporin	Minimum 3 wk

  - No specific diagnostic test exists
  - Common among children aged 6–15 years, rare in infants and preschool-aged children, may occur in adults
- Diagnosis
  - Evidence of recent streptococcal infection is required (positive throat culture or rapid streptococcal test), recent scarlet fever, or positive antibodies (antistreptolysin O or deoxyribonuclease B)
  - Must also have 2 major criteria **OR** 1 major and 2 minor criteria (chorea and recurrent acute rheumatic fever do not require minor criteria for diagnosis)
    - Major criteria
      - Carditis: congestive heart failure, pericarditis with rub, new murmur
      - Arthritis: migrates from one joint to another, usually large joints
      - Sydenham chorea ("St Vitus' Dance"): uncontrolled proximal limb movements, associated with emotional lability
      - Erythema marginatum: begins as macules on the trunk or proximal extremities, spreads outward to form a snakelike ring with clearing in the middle
      - Subcutaneous nodules: painless, firm, on the back of wrists, outside elbows, and front of knees
    - Minor criteria
      - Arthralgia
      - Fever
      - Elevated ESR, CRP, or leukocytosis
      - Prolonged PR interval on electrocardiogram (ECG)
- Treatment
  - Penicillin V 250 mg PO bid for 10 days
  - Aspirin (initially 80–100 mg/kg/day in four doses, decreased to 10–15 mg/kg/dose when afebrile) or naproxen (15–20 mg/kg/day in two doses)
  - Benzathine penicillin G 25,000 units/kg IM every 3–4 weeks (maximum of 1.2 million units/dose)

Urinary Tract Infections and Pyelonephritis

- Symptoms
  - Fever, irritability, foul-smelling or discolored urine, urinary

frequency and urgency, dysuria, emesis, diarrhea
  - Urinary tract infection (UTI) should be considered in any child < 2 years old with unexplained fever
- Etiology: Gram-negative enteric organisms, especially *E coli*
- Diagnosis
  - Culture
  - Specimens obtained by bag are useful for urinalysis, but not for culture because of skin contamination
  - If culture is not available, use urine dipstick or microscopy
    - Leukocyte esterase test on a urine dipstick is sensitive, but not specific
    - Nitrite is specific for UTI, but not sensitive
    - > 10 white blood cells per high-powered field on microscopy
    - Bacteria is also noted
- Treatment
  - Standard first-line therapies in the nontoxic child (7-day course):
    - Amoxicillin (40 mg/kg/day)
    - Amoxicillin-clavulanic acid (40 mg/kg/day)
    - Ciprofloxacin (20 mg/kg/day)
    - TMP/SMX (10 mg/kg/day of TMP)
  - Reevaluate in 1–2 days
  - If the child is toxic, IV or IM third-generation cephalosporin or an aminoglycoside are preferred
- Follow-up and prophylaxis
  - If possible, evaluate anatomy and the presence of reflux
  - If it is a recurrent infection, administer prophylactic antibiotics (consider amoxicillin or TMP/SMX at half the usual daily dose, given at bedtime)

Miscellaneous Tropical Diseases

Dengue and Dengue Hemorrhagic Fever

- Symptoms of dengue
  - Acute onset fever lasting 3–4 days
  - Intense headache
  - Retrobulbar eye pain
  - Myalgias
  - Arthralgias

- Anorexia
- Rash
- Symptoms of dengue hemorrhagic fever (high mortality rate)
  - All of the above

PLUS

  - Severe sepsis
  - Multiorgan system failure
  - Anemia
  - Thrombocytopenia
  - Disseminated intravascular coagulation (DIC)
  - Shock
- Diagnosis
  - Clinical suspicion
  - Positive tourniquet test
    - Inflate a blood pressure cuff on the upper arm to a point midway between the systolic and diastolic pressures for 5 minutes
    - A test is considered positive when 10 or more petechiae per 2.5 cm^2 (1 $in.^2$) are observed after the cuff pressure has been released for 2 minutes
    - The test may be negative or mildly positive during the phase of profound shock
    - It usually becomes positive, sometimes strongly positive, if the test is conducted after recovery from shock
    - Serology, if available
- Treatment
  - Give aggressive isotonic fluids
  - Give blood products only if there is severe bleeding

Diphtheria

- Symptoms range from a moderately sore throat to toxic, life-threatening diphtheria of the larynx or of the lower and upper respiratory tracts
  - Throat may be covered by a grey membrane and the patient may have a "bull neck" appearance from local edema of the neck
  - Nasal mucosa is generally markedly inflamed
  - Often complicated by myocarditis (rhythm disturbance due

to toxin) and neuritis (toxic damage to peripheral nerves)
- Can be fatal; 5%–10% of diphtheria patients die, even if properly treated (untreated patients die in greater numbers)
- Untreated patients are infectious for 2–3 weeks

- Etiology
  - *Corynebacterium diphtheriae*
  - In several developing countries (particularly Eastern Europe and Asia), diphtheria is the leading cause of pharyngitis in unimmunized children during an outbreak
- Diagnosis
  - Clinical and culture
  - Probable case definition according to WHO:
    - Recent (within 2 wk) contact with an individual confirmed contaminated
    - Diphtheria endemic to region
    - Stridor
    - Swelling/edema of the neck
    - Submucosal or skin petechiae
    - Toxic circulatory collapse
    - Acute renal insufficiency
    - Myocarditis and motor paralysis 1–6 weeks after onset
- Treatment
  - Equine diphtheria antitoxin (20,000–100,000 units); penicillin or macrolide
  - Obtain cultures before giving antibiotics
- Transmitted by spread of large droplets
  - Monitor contacts closely for development of disease
  - Provide prophylaxis via 600,000 units penicillin (IM) in those < 6 years old, 1.2 million units (IM) in those ≥ 6 years old

Human Immunodeficiency Virus and Acquired Immunodeficiency Syndrome

In deployment settings, there is no way to properly administer antiretroviral therapy. In underdeveloped countries, the rates of HIV may be very high, and the provider should always be suspicious that an ill or malnourished patient is infected.

- Symptoms
  - Often severe pneumonia in infancy (*Pneumocystic carinii*

  - pneumonia)
  - Generalized lymphadenopathy
  - Enlarged, nontender parotitis
  - Failure to thrive
  - Mucocutaneous candidiasis
  - Recurrent sepsis
- Diagnosis
  - Serology
  - Viral load
  - Clinical appearance
- Treatment is supportive; assume pneumonia is caused by TB or *P carinii* pneumonia until proven otherwise

Polio

- Symptoms
  - > 95% are asymptomatic
  - Others have nonspecific URI
  - A small percentage has aseptic meningitis
  - 0.1%–2% will develop flaccid paralysis
- Etiology: Poliovirus (enterovirus) types 1, 2, and 3; still endemic in parts of Africa and Asia, recent epidemics in Afghanistan
- Diagnosis
  - Viral culture of stool (best), urine, pharynx, or cerebrospinal fluid
  - Best if done within 14 days of onset of illness
  - Serology
- Treatment: supportive
- Prophylaxis and control
  - Vaccinate susceptible individuals
  - Identify all known cases and contacts for outbreak control

Japanese Encephalitis

- Symptoms
  - Headache
  - Fever
  - Meningeal signs
  - Stupor
  - Disorientation

  - Coma
  - Tremors
  - Paresis (generalized)
  - Hypertonia
  - Loss of coordination
    - ▸ Cannot be distinguished clinically from other central nervous system infections
    - ▸ Severe infections are marked by acute onset, headache, high fever, meningeal signs, and coma
- Etiology: acute, inflammatory, mosquito-borne disease involving the brain, spinal cord, and meninges
  - Common and usually asymptomatic
  - Case fatality rate among individuals with clinical disease is 25%–50%
  - Infants and the elderly are most susceptible to severe disease
  - Occurs in east, southeast, and southern Asia
  - Especially associated with rice-growing areas and pigs
- Diagnosis: demonstration of specific immunoglobulin M in acute-phase serum or cerebrospinal fluid
- Treatment: supportive
- Prophylaxis and control
  - Use protective clothing and repellents to avoid exposure to mosquitoes
  - Screen sleeping and living quarters
  - House pigs away from living quarters
  - Vaccines are available

Malaria

- Symptoms
  - *Plasmodium falciparum*
    - ▸ Anemia may be severe (hemoglobin < 5 gm/dL), particularly in nonimmune and pregnant patients
    - ▸ Hyperparasitemia (> 5% of red blood cells infected on smear)
    - ▸ Hyperthermia (body temperature > 41°C)
    - ▸ Hypoglycemia and acidosis
    - ▸ Cerebral malaria, marked by seizures or coma (more common in children, with mortality rate of 15%–30%)

- Renal failure
- Pulmonary edema
- Diarrhea is a common presenting sign in children

- *Plasmodium vivax*
  - Cyclic fevers and chills
  - Splenic rupture (late manifestation)
- *Plasmodium malariae* and *Plasmodium ovale*
  - Few complications due to low-level parasitemia
  - *P malariae* has been associated with immune complex glomerulonephritis

- Diagnosis: The presence of fever in an endemic area; confirm using laboratory methods
  - Microscopy
    - Thick smears are sensitive for diagnosis
    - Thin smears are needed for determining what species is causing the infection
    - Multiple smears must be examined to rule out malaria
  - Rapid test is useful for *P falciparum* and *P vivax*
- Treatment
  - Treatment medications are the same as for adults, and are based on the infecting species, possible drug resistance, and severity of disease (use IV therapy only for severe disease)
  - IV therapy
    - Quinidine gluconate: 10 mg/kg loading dose (maximum 600 mg) by IV infusion over period of 1–2 hours. Give the first 2 mg/kg as a test dose with continuous ECG monitoring for idiosyncratic prolongation of QRS or arrhythmias. Watch for hypoglycemia and hypotension. Follow loading dose with continuous infusion of 0.02 mg/kg/min to keep levels at 3–7 mg/L until parasitemia is < 1% or patient is able to take oral medication
    - Artesunate: 2.4 mg/kg/dose IV at 0, 12, 24, and 48 hours
  - Oral therapy
    - *Plasmodium* with no resistance noted:
      - Chloroquine phosphate: 10 mg base/kg (PO; maximum 600 mg base) initially, then 5 mg base/kg (PO; maximum 300 mg base) at 24 and 48 hours
    - *Plasmodium* with known chloroquine resistance noted:

    - Quinine sulfate: 25 mg/kg/day (PO; maximum 2,000 mg), divided tid for 3–7 days

AND one of the following:

  - Tetracycline: 20 mg/kg/day (PO; maximum 750 mg) divided qid for 7 days for children > 8 years old,

OR

  - Clindamycin: 30 mg/kg/day PO divided tid for 5 days,

OR

  - Pyrimethamine/sulfadoxine: single dose on the last day of quinine therapy
    - < 1 year old: ¼ tablet
    - 1–3 years old: ½ tablet
    - 4–8 years old: 1 tablet
    - 9–14 years old: 2 tablets
    - > 14 years old: 3 tablets,

OR

  - Atovaquone/proguanil or mefloquine can also be used
- If PO medications cannot be taken (eg, in the case of a newborn), begin with the IV dosage of quinidine gluconate as noted above
- Consider exchange transfusion at ≥ 10% parasitemia

- Prophylaxis
  - Chloroquine-sensitive areas: chloroquine 5 mg/kg base, maximum 300 mg
  - Chloroquine-resistant areas:
    - Mefloquine
      - < 15 kg: 5 mg/kg/wk
      - 15–19 kg: ¼ tablet/wk
      - 20–30 kg: ½ tablet/wk
      - 31–45 kg: ¾ tablet/wk
      - 45 kg: 1 tablet/wk
    - Doxycycline for those > 8 years old: 2 mg/kg
    - Malarone:
      - 11–20 kg: 1 pediatric tablet/day
      - 21–30 kg: 2 pediatric tablets/day
      - 31–40 kg: 3 pediatric tablets/day
      - 40 kg: 1 adult tablet/day
  - Eliminate standing bodies of water that serve as mosquito

breeding sites (eg, old tires, mud puddles, etc)
  - Use permethrin-treated bed nets

Measles

Measles (rubeola) has played a significant role in all situations involving displaced persons. It can lead to high mortality in unimmunized individuals, particularly those who are malnourished and very young

- Symptoms
  - Fever
  - Cough
  - Coryza
  - Conjunctivitis
  - Koplik spots
  - Cephalocaudal progressive rash
- Treatment
  - Recognition of the clinical disease spectrum, immunization, and treatment
  - Immunization should target malnourished children in displacement situations and those between 6 months and 5 years old, with an emphasis on the youngest children
  - Rubeola will often unmask vitamin A deficiency; prophylactic supplementation should occur as follows:
    - < 12 months old: 100,000 IU (PO)
    - > 12 months old: 200,000 IU (PO)
- Complications and associated findings
  - Cervical adenitis
  - Mesenteric: abdominal pain, appendicitis
  - Upper respiratory tract: otitis media, mastoiditis, oral ulcers
  - Lower respiratory tract: croup, bronchiolitis, pneumonia
  - Bacterial superinfection
  - Central nervous system: encephalitis
  - Malabsorption / malnutrition (significant cause of mortality)
  - Ocular: xerophthalmia / ulcerating keratomalacia in those who are vitamin A deficient
    - Individuals with these complications should receive a second dose of vitamin A on day 2
    - If ocular manifestations are present, a third dose should be given at 1–4 weeks

- Treat malnutrition and pyogenic complications with antibiotics

Humanitarian Issues

Children make up a large portion of the people involved in refugee and displacement situations. Common illnesses, such as diarrheal and respiratory illnesses, may proliferate. Limited numbers of trained medical personnel cannot care for hundreds or thousands of refugees on an individual basis. It is the goal in these settings for medical personnel to give hands-on training to volunteers from within the refugee population. Volunteers should be trained in vitamin A administration, preparation and delivery of WHO rehydration formulas, and the administration of vaccines to prevent disease within the camp. They should be given limited training in triage so they can determine who should actually receive care from the medical professionals. Medical professionals should limit their care to those most in need of trained providers. Some treatment recommendations may differ slightly in this chapter from other opinions in this text because in a refugee situation, resources are often extremely limited.

- Diarrheal disease
  - Much of the morbidity and mortality from diarrheal disease is due to dehydration
  - With these illnesses, poor hygiene and public health management may lead to outbreaks; consultation with preventive medicine specialists is important
  - For specific etiologies and treatment, see Diarrhea in a Humanitarian-Assistance Setting
- Respiratory tract infections
  - The majority of cases will be of a viral source and will **not** require antibiotic therapy
  - Antibiotics should be used for most complicated URIs and all suspected acute lower respiratory tract infections (many drugs have multiple doses depending on indication—please refer to Chapter 39, Pharmacotherapeutics, for specific guidance)
    - Complicated URIs are defined as otitis media or sinusitis with fever, or mastoiditis
      - Acute otitis media and sinusitis: give oral antibiotics

for 5–10 days

- Mastoiditis: give IV / IM antibiotics for 5–10 days
- Acute lower respiratory tract infections are defined by the presence of fever, cough, and tachypnea
  - Treat with antibiotics (TMP / SMX at 5 mg / kg / dose q12h for 5 days) respiratory rates are the following:
    - 0 months old: > 60 breaths / min
    - 2–12 months old: > 50 breaths / min
    - 1–5 years old: > 40 breaths / min
- **Danger signs**: nasal flaring, retractions, cyanosis, and persistent vomiting
  - Hospitalization is required
  - Give IV cefriaxone 100 mg / kg / day

Further Reading

1. Cashat-Cruz M, Morales-Aguirre JJ, Mendoza-Azpiri M. Respiratory tract infections in children in developing countries. *Semin Pediatr Infect Dis*. 2005;16:84–92.

2. Pickering LK, ed. *The Red Book: 2009 Report of the Committee on Infectious Diseases*. Elk Grove, Ill: American Academy of Pediatrics; 2009.

3. Connelly MA, ed. *Communicable Disease Control in Emergencies: A Field Manual*. Geneva, Switzerland: World Health Organization; 2005.

4. Robertson J, Shilkofski N, eds. *The Harriet Lane Handbook: A Manual for Pediatric House Officers*. 17th ed. Baltimore, Md: Mosby; 2005.

5. World Health Organization. Division of Child Health and Development. Antimicrobial and Support Therapy for Bacterial Meningitis in Children: Report of the Meeting of 18–20 June 1997, Geneva, Switzerland. Geneva, Switzerland: WHO; 1998.

6. Rakel RE, Bope ET, eds. *Conn's Current Therapy*. 58th ed. Philadelphia, Pa: Saunders Elsevier; 2006.

7. Long SS, Pickering LK, Prober CG, eds. *Principles and Practice of Pediatric Infectious Diseases*. 2nd ed. New York, NY: Churchill Livingstone; 2003.

Chapter 30

Endocrinology

Introduction

This chapter provides a basic approach to endocrine issues in an austere or combat environment. The emphasis is on signs and symptoms and an index of suspicion for serious, potentially life-threatening situations. Hormone dosing is best determined using accurate height and weight to allow exact calculation of body surface area.

$$\textbf{Surface area (m}^2\textbf{)} = \sqrt{\frac{\text{Ht (cm)} \times \text{Wt (kg)}}{3{,}600}}$$

When this information is not available, use the estimates obtained from a Broselow tape.

Diabetes Mellitus

- Diabetes is defined as follows:
  - Fasting blood sugar > 126 mg/dL
  - Random blood sugar > 200 mg/dL in association with symptoms of diabetes
  - Blood sugar > 200 mg/dL 2 hours after an oral glucose tolerance test
- Symptoms of diabetes mellitus include polyuria, nocturia, polydipsia, and polyphagia
- Weight loss will often occur with diabetes mellitus type 1 (DM1), but can occur with diabetes mellitus type 2 (DM2)
  - Children with the above symptoms who are not overweight should be suspected of having DM1 if their blood sugar is elevated
  - Management of DM2 depends on the presentation at the time of diagnosis
    - Random blood sugar < 200 mg/dL without marked elevations 1–2 hours after meals can often be managed by diet, exercise, and weight loss without the initiation of medications

- Random blood sugar > 200 mg/dL will require medication
  - Use caution when initiating antidiabetic medication regimens in austere environments with limited laboratory or clinical follow-up
  - Consider the risk of hypoglycemia
  - For an overweight, newly diagnosed patient with DM2 with random blood sugar between 200 and 300 mg/dL, administer metformin 500–1,000 mg once or twice a day
  - Insulin should be strongly considered in a hyperglycemic, nonacute patient with random blood sugar > 300 mg/dL, although oral therapy may be safer (see below)

Diabetic Ketoacidosis

- Diabetic ketoacidosis (DKA) is diagnosed when a patient has:
  D: high glucose
  K: ketones in the blood
  A: acidosis
- Perform a brief history and physical examination to assess for shock and degree of volume depletion (Table 30-1)

Table 30-1. Assessing Dehydration in the Pediatric Patient with Diabetes

Parameter	Mild	Moderate	Severe
Estimated volume deficit (%)	3	6	10
Clinical signs			
Perfusion	Normal	Normal or ↓	↓
Heart rate	Normal	↑	↑
Blood pressure	Normal	Normal or ↓	Normal or ↓
Labs			
HCO_3	Normal	10–20	< 10
pH	Normal	> 7.20	< 7.20
Glucose	300–400	400–600	> 600
BUN	< 20	< 30	> 25

BUN: blood urea nitrogen
HCO_3: bicarbonate

- Physicians frequently overestimate the degree of fluid depletion
- The best data are the patient's actual weight loss (use outpatient records if available)

- Obtain results from the following laboratory tests:
  - Chemistry panels, including calcium, magnesium, and phosphorous, if available
  - Arterial blood gas (ABG) or venous blood gas (VBG) analysis
  - Serum ketones test
  - Urinary analysis
  - C peptide test
  - Consider looking for an infectious trigger via complete blood count with differential, urine culture, etc
- Obtain intravenous (IV) access and begin correcting deficit slowly, unless patient is in shock
  - Give normal saline (NS) 10–20 mL/kg over 1 hour
  - The rest of the deficit should be replaced over 48 hours to avoid dropping serum osmoles too quickly and precipitating cerebral edema
  - Placing two large IVs allows treatment through one and sampling through the other
- Insulin therapy need not be viewed as emergent therapy, but should be initiated as soon as possible
  - Use regular insulin (100 units in 100 mL NS) with insulin drip at 0.05–0.1 units/kg/h
  - **Do not bolus with insulin**! It can precipitously drop glucose levels and serum osmolarity, exacerbating risk of cerebral edema
  - The goal of therapy should be a drop in serum glucose of 50–100 mg/dL/h (start on the low end of the range and increase over time)
  - Plastic tubing binds insulin; run insulin through before using
  - Blood sugar checks should be done every hour
  - In mild DKA, especially in the austere environment, if no IV access is available, intramuscular insulin can be given every 3 hours, rather than using an insulin drip
    - The dose of IM regular insulin is 0.1–0.3 units/kg
    - Start at the low end and increase over time to avoid in-

advertently administering excessive amounts of insulin

- Preferred fluid choice is ½ NS with potassium
  - Use potassium chloride and potassium phosphate to administer 40 mEq/L (even though the patient is hyperkalemic, the total-body potassium is low)
  - **Add glucose when blood sugar drops into the 250–300 mg/dL range**
    - Always anticipate the next bag needed and order it ahead of time from the pharmacy (ie, $D_5 > D_{10} > D_{12.5}$)
- Cerebral edema is a major concern; perform neurological checks hourly
  - When faced with a deteriorating mental status, consider performing a computed tomography (CT) scan of the head to look for cerebral edema
  - Administer mannitol (dose 0.25 g/kg) for progressive neurological deterioration or focal neurological examination
  - There is a high risk for cerebral edema when fluids are administered at > 4,000 mL/m^2/day
- Check glucose hourly, VBG or ABG tests and chemistry panels every 4 hours, and urinary analysis every void (or more frequently when necessary)
- Do not reduce insulin prematurely if glucose is falling—give more glucose!
  - Giving enough glucose ($D_5 > D_{10} > D_{12.5}$) allows room to provide enough insulin to correct the acidosis
- Transition to subcutaneous (SQ) insulin from insulin drip when patient is expressing hunger, the acidosis is mostly gone, and there is food immediately available
  - Turn off the drip, administer the SQ insulin, and wait 30 minutes before feeding
  - Typically, rehydration without glucose will need to be continued once the patient is eating

Diabetes Management

- Dietary management is generally the same in DM1 and DM2
  - Dietary treatment of diabetes consists of a well-balanced diet, low in refined and simple sugars
  - The diet should be approximately 55% carbohydrate, 30% fat, and 15% protein

- Carbohydrate intake should favor complex carbohydrates
  - In general, infants and toddlers (0–3 y) will need 30–45 g carbohydrate per meal
  - Older children (4–12 y) need 45–60 g carbohydrate per meal
  - Teenagers (13–18 y) need 75–90 g carbohydrate per meal
- Insulin therapy
  - Insulin therapy and timing depends on the type of insulin available (Table 30-2)

Table 30–2. Types and Action Times of Insulin

Type of insulin	Onset	Peak (h)	Duration (h)
Lispro/aspart	10–15 min	1–2	2–4
Regular	30–60 min	2–4	6–9
NPH	1–2 h	3–8	12–15
Lente	1–2 h	3–14	18–20
Ultralente	2–4 h	6–14	18–20
Glargine	1–2 h	2–22	24

NPH: Neutral Protamine Hagedorn

  - In theater, it is likely that only Neutral Protamine Hagedorn (NPH) and regular insulin are available
  - Start with a total daily dose of 0.6 units/kg/day if the initial glucose at diagnosis is < 500 mg/dL
    - **Initial glucose at diagnosis > 500 mg/dL and <u>no</u> acidosis**: use a total daily dose of 0.8 units/kg/day
    - **Initial glucose at diagnosis > 500 mg/dL and acidosis present**: use a total daily dose of 1.0 unit/kg/day
    - **Initial glucose level at diagnosis unavailable**: start with 0.8 units/kg/day
  - Morning insulin should constitute ⅔ of the total daily dose
    - This amount should be divided further to ⅔ NPH and ⅓ regular insulin (Exhibit 30-1)
    - This dose should be given about 20 minutes before breakfast
  - The evening dose should constitute ⅓ of the total daily dose

Exhibit 30-1. Case Study: Insulin Dosing using Neutral Protamine Hagedorn and Regular Insulin

A 30-kg patient presents with an initial blood glucose of 558 mg/dL and serum bicarbonate of 20 mEq/L.
Administer 0.8 units/kg/day × 30 (24 units/day).

Morning:
⅔ of the total dose = 16 units total (10 units NPH and 6 units of regular insulin before breakfast)

Evening:
The remaining ⅓ total dose = 8 units total (4 units of NPH and 4 units of regular insulin before dinner)

NPH: Neutral Protamine Hagedorn

            - This amount should further be divided to ½ NPH and ½ regular insulin
        - This dosing plan places a child at risk for low blood sugar; the child should have small snacks in the midmorning, midafternoon, and at bedtime when this insulin plan is used
    - Children on insulin should have multiple blood sugar checks per day
    - A combination of rapid-acting insulin (lispro or aspart) and glargine is preferable to the regular and NPH insulin combination, if available, because it more closely approximates normal physiology (further pediatric endocrinology consultation is recommended)
    - In an austere environment, use a goal blood sugar of 150 mg/dL

Hypoglycemia

- Signs and symptoms
    - Nonspecific in infancy, but can include cyanotic episodes, apnea, respiratory distress, refusal to feed, myoclonic jerks, convulsions, somnolence, hypothermia, sweating, etc
    - For older children, symptoms include anxiety, weakness, hunger, shakiness, sweating, tachycardia, nausea, vomiting, headache, visual disturbances, lethargy/lassitude, restless-

ness, mental confusion, somnolence/stupor, convulsions, bizarre neurological signs, decreased intellectual ability, personality changes, bizarre behaviors, etc
    - Other suggestive physical findings include hepatomegaly, short stature, large size for gestational age (newborn), and hemihypertrophy of an extremity
- The definition of hypoglycemia is < 40 mg/dL in the first month of life (older infants, children, and teenagers should be able to maintain a blood sugar > 60 mg/dL)
- The differential diagnosis includes a host of congenital metabolic and hormonal disorders, systemic disease, and drug intoxications; the presence of urine ketones may be helpful in diagnosis
    - If urine ketones are positive, it is likely that a transient abnormality exists that can be treated with IV or oral glucose therapy
    - The absence of ketones in the face of profound hypoglycemia generally represents an excess of insulin secretion or the presence of a disorder of fatty acid metabolism
- Treatment varies by age
    - Neonates: 2–4 mL/kg 10% dextrose in water ($D_{10}W$) IV bolus
    - Children: 2–4 mL/kg 25% dextrose in water ($D_{25}W$) IV, administered slowly
        - Follow each immediately by continuous glucose infusion
        - If IV therapy is unavailable, oral or nasogastric therapy should be undertaken in a child that is awake and able to tolerate it
    - If a child is actively seizing or comatose due to low blood sugar, administer 1 mg of glucagon intramuscularly
        - Be aware that vomiting is common after glucagon administration; lay children on their sides after giving glucagon

Thyroid

- Hypothyroidism
    - Hypothyroidism can be congenital or acquired
        - Congenital hypothyroidism is almost impossible to recognize early on

- Signs and symptoms
  - Macroglossia
  - Open posterior fontanelle
  - Developmental delay
  - Constipation
  - Coarse facial features, including broad nasal bridges, eyelid edema, flat facies, and large heads
- Treatment is oral thyroid replacement
  - Starting dose is 12–15 μg/kg/day for neonates
  - Most children with congenital hypothyroidism are on 5 μg/kg/day of levothyroxine by 1 year of age
  - Most infants require 37.5 μg daily (given as 1½ 25-μg tablets)
  - Pills should be crushed and given directly to the patient mixed in formula or applesauce—**DO NOT** make elixirs for this therapy (stability may be affected)

- Acquired hypothyroidism
  - Signs and symptoms
    - Constipation
    - Fatigue
    - Cold intolerance
    - Enlarged thyroid gland
  - Most children with acquired hypothyroidism require an initial dose of 2–3 μg/kg/day of levothyroxine

- Hyperthyroidism
  - Symptoms in infants and children
    - Irritability
    - Flushing
    - Tachycardia
    - Hypertension
    - Poor weight gain
    - Goiter
    - Exophthalmos
    - Hepatosplenomegaly, jaundice, thrombocytopenia, and hypoprothrombinemia
  - Signs are typically subtle and slowly progressive; initial

signs of irritability and jitteriness should lead one to suspect sepsis or hypoglycemia first

- Treatment in infants and children is initiated with propanolol (1–2 mg/kg/day divided tid) and propylthiouracil (PTU) 5–10 mg/kg/day divided tid
- The female-to-male ratio of acquired hyperthyroidism in teenagers is 5:1
- Symptoms in teenagers
  - Tachycardia
  - Restlessness
  - Difficulty sleeping
  - Widened pulse pressure
  - Heat intolerance
  - Increased frequency of loose stools
  - Enlarged, nontender thyroid
- Etiology is generally autoimmune, but if a prominent thyroid nodule is palpable, it may be the cause
- Treatment in teenagers can be surgical resection of all or part of the thyroid gland, or medical or radioactive iodine ablation
  - Medical treatment consists of β-blocker therapy with atenolol (25–50 mg/day) until the marked symptoms have resolved, and with PTU at 5–10 mg/kg/day divided tid
    - If medical treatment is initiated, thyroid function tests should be obtained prior to therapy and sent to a referral lab (this should be possible in a deployment situation)
    - After the free thyroxine level has normalized or lowered, adding levothyroxine at 2 μg/kg/day allows maintenance of a euthyroid state
    - The thyroid can be adequately suppressed while treating with PTU

Adrenal Disorders

- Adrenal insufficiency is uncommon; however, an index of suspicion for adrenal disorders is critical because they can be fatal
- A patient with known autoimmune conditions, such as dia-

betes or thyroid disease, has the potential to develop adrenal insufficiency

- Tuberculosis, human immunodeficiency virus, adrenal hemorrhage, and traumatic adrenal resection may also lead to adrenal insufficiency
- Signs and symptoms
  - Unexplained hypotensive shock
  - Progressive weakness, fatigue, dehydration, and hypotension are most common
  - Anorexia, nausea, vomiting, myalgias, and personality changes are possible
  - Other suggestive physical findings include hyperpigmentation of the skin and mucous membranes (especially the creases and the nipples)
  - Vitiligo and alopecia may also be associated
  - Laboratory evidence suggestive of adrenal insufficiency includes hyponatremia, hyperkalemia, and hypoglycemia
- If adrenal insufficiency is suspected, obtain a blood specimen in a serum separator tube (red, tiger, yellow)
  - Separate the serum and freeze the specimen
- Treatment includes aggressive IV fluid therapy (20 cc/kg bolus of NS followed by reassessment)
  - Pressor agents are sometimes required
  - Hydrocortisone hemisuccinate should be given urgently by IV (50 mg/m^2)
    - Infants: 25 mg
    - Toddlers and young children (< 6 y): 50 mg
    - Older children and teenagers (> 6 y): 100 mg
  - Regular dosing (q6h) should be continued at a dose of 100 mg/m^2/day, divided in equal doses
  - If the adrenals have been removed or primary adrenal disorders are suspected, mineralocorticoid therapy (fludrocortisone) will be necessary when the hydrocortisone dose is dropped below 100 mg/m^2/day
    - Safe when the child stabilizes or the significant stressor (surgery, illness, etc) has resolved
    - Maintenance hydrocortisone dose is 12–15 mg/m^2/day (divided tid)
    - Fludrocortisone dose is 0.1 mg bid for infants, and 0.1 mg qid in patients ≥ 1 year old

Calcium and Vitamin D Disorders

- Hypocalcemia
  - Symptoms can range from nothing to severe (eg, tetany and seizures)
  - Long QT interval is apparent on electrocardiogram
  - Symptomatic hypocalcemia generally occurs when calcium levels in the blood are below 6 mg/dL
  - Managing acute hypocalcemia requires calcium and vitamin D
    - Administer 10% calcium gluconate at 1 mL/min, not to exceed 2 mL/kg
    - Give intravenously but with care; SQ infiltration of calcium can cause severe burns
    - Vitamin D is given as calcitriol at a dose of 20–60 ng/kg/day
    - Once acute symptoms have resolved, oral calcium should be given at 50–75 mg of elemental calcium per kilogram of body weight every 24 hours (oral calcium is much safer to give than IV calcium)
    - Vitamin D may be needed long term in some cases, such as in the presence of hypoparathyroidism
    - Hypocalcemia may not respond to therapy if the patient's magnesium level is also low (see Hypomagnesemia)
- Hypercalcemia
  - Severe hypercalcemia (> 13.5 mg/dL) requires treatment
  - Initiate treatment with IV NS to establish optimal fluid hydration
    - Once urine output is substantial (> 2 cc/kg/h), give furosemide at a dose of 1–2 mg/kg IV
    - If hypercalcemia persists, give hydrocortisone hemisuccinate 1 mg/kg IV every 6 hours
    - Bisphosphonates can also be used, but are not likely to be available in an austere environment
    - In the immobilized patient, it may be prudent to start a low-calcium diet and avoid vitamin D
    - Encourage copious fluid intake
- Hypomagnesemia
  - May cause hypocalcemia
  - Hypocalcemia will be resistant to treatment in the presence

of untreated hypomagnesemia
- Treat magnesium levels below 1.4 mg/dL
- Treatment consists of 50% magnesium sulfate 0.1–0.2 mL/kg
  - Repeat the dose in 12–24 hours if the magnesium level remains low

- Rickets
  - The most common cause of rickets is vitamin D deficiency
  - Infants and children at risk for vitamin D deficiency typically have a history of prolonged breast-feeding and live in a northern latitude
  - Signs and symptoms
    - Rachitic rosary
    - Bowed legs
    - Bowing forearms
    - Frontal bossing
    - Craniotabes
    - Short stature
    - Suboptimal weight
    - Systemic symptoms, including hypotonia, weakness, anorexia, and delay in walking
    - Vitamin D deficiency can present as seizures when severe hypocalcemia is present
  - Radiographic evidence of vitamin D deficiency consists of cupping, widening, and irregularity of the distal metaphyses; there is also evidence of osteopenia with cortical thinning
  - Treatment in an urgent situation includes administering IV calcium and providing vitamin D treatment
    - In an otherwise normal child, ergocalciferol should be administered in doses of 1,000–2,000 international units (IUs) per day
      - Start at the higher end of the dose and wean to 1,000 IU/day after 2–4 weeks
    - Supplemental vitamin D should be continued until there is radiographic evidence of healing
      - This usually takes 2–3 months, but can take longer in cases of severe vitamin deficiency
    - If symptoms of vitamin D deficiency persist despite

adequate replacement, changing vitamin D to 1,25-hydroxyvitamin D may alleviate the problem

  - ▹ Calcitriol should be used at a dose of 20–60 ng/kg/day
  - ▹ This form of medication has a long half-life and care should be taken not to overdose this medication

- ◦ To prevent rickets, breast-fed babies should receive a daily multivitamin containing 400 IU of vitamin D

Chapter 31

Common Neurological Problems

Pediatric Neurological Examination

- **Mental status**
  - Is the child alert? Is the child appropriately oriented (based on age)?
  - Is the child age-appropriately interactive? If upset, is the child consolable?
- **Cranial nerves** (modified for the young child)
  - Cranial nerve (CN) II: visual acuity. In a young child, it is unlikely that the optic nerve can be visualized; however, several methods can be used to determine a young child's visual acuity
    - Does the child track objects (eg, a name badge, face, or small toy)?
    - How small an object will the child reach for?
    - Visual fields: if there is a small toy in front of the child, does the child look when another one is brought out from behind the examiner's back?
  - CN III, IV, VI: extraocular muscles, pupils, and ptosis
    - Use an object to check tracking, or spin the patient around in different directions to see if the patient's eyes move appropriately
  - CN V: facial sensation, muscles of mastication, corneal reflex
    - Does the patient respond to touch on the face?
    - If concerned, test corneal reflexes
  - CN VII: facial muscle strength and symmetry
    - Observe the patient crying, smiling, etc; compare sides
  - CN VIII: hearing
    - For older children, whisper a question in each ear and determine if the child can answer
    - For infants, clap hands or ring a bell and watch for a blink or other response

   - CN IX, X, XII: palate elevation, straight tongue protrusion, strength with tongue deviation laterally
      - Observe swallowing and speech
      - Observe patient crying; observe palate elevation and tongue movements
   - CN XI: sternocleidomastoid and trapezius strength
      - Have patient rotate head against resistance in each direction
      - Have patient shrug shoulders against resistance
- Coordination
   - Have child perform finger and foot tap (rapid alternating movements); observe movements for accuracy and rhythm
   - Have child bring a finger to the nose and heel to the shin; observe for ataxia or inability to hit the mark
   - Note abnormal movements
   - Modifications
      - Watch patient reach for and manipulate objects
      - If the child is old enough, ask the child to touch different parts of a toy
- Motor
   - Strength
      - Infants are best examined when they are fighting the examination or crying; does the fighting infant move all extremities? If so, observe for any differences (eg, can the infant push the examiner away equally with bilateral upper and lower extremities?)
      - Examine older children in the same manner as adolescents and adults
   - Tone
      - Patient needs to be awake and calm
      - For infants: test with patient's head midline (reflexes can be induced and examination findings changed if the head is turned)
         - Hypotonia (see Evaluating for Hypotonia)
         - Hypertonia
            - Note resistance to passive motion
            - Vertical suspension: legs crossing or "scissoring" suggests hypertonia
      - For older children: passively move the patient at variable

rates; note increases or decreases in tone, "catches," or rigidity

- Reflexes
  - Crossed adductors can be normal in children up to 12 months old
  - Babinski reflex/extensor plantar response (the big toe turns upward and other toes fan out when foot is tickled): can be normal up to 2½ years old
  - Unsustained clonus can be common in a healthy neonate
  - Reflexes that should **disappear** with age (normal ranges listed below):
    - Birth to 3–6 months: Moro reflex (must resolve for the child to roll)
    - Birth to 4–9 months: asymmetric tonic neck reflex
      - With patient supine, rotate head
      - Examiner should see extension of limb on the chin side and flexion on occiput side
    - Birth to 9 months: palmar and plantar grasp
  - Reflexes that should **appear** with age (normal range of appearance listed below):
    - 4–5 months: anterior propping (child should extend arms when sitting)
    - 6–12 months: parachute (may not be complete until 11–12 mo)
      - Suspend child horizontally about the waist, face down, then project the infant suddenly toward the floor or table
      - The infant should extend arms and spread fingers
    - 6–7 months: lateral propping (child should extend arms to the side if falling from sitting)
- Sensory
  - Most subjective part of a neurological examination
  - Child should distinguish light touch, pinprick (eg, from a safety pin), temperature, and vibration
    - Anterior cord: pain, fine touch, and temperature can be distinguished when intact
    - Posterior cord: proprioception, vibration, and 2-point discrimination can be determined when intact
  - If concerned, check for levels on the torso and extremities

  - If a deficit is noted, complete a further examination to identify distribution and likely location
    - Check dermatomes, nerve roots, and peripheral nerve distribution
    - Cortical: all modalities; remember the sensory homunculus
    - Higher cortical testing: Rhomberg's test
      - Patient stands with feet together and arms fully extended, palms up, eyes closed
      - Observe the patient for swaying or falling to one side or another; note if patient always falls to the same side on repeated testing
- Gait
  - Native gait: should be appropriate for the patient's age
    - Note symmetry and amount of arm swing, stability, and toe walking (if any)
    - Note the patient's ability to walk in a straight line
    - Observe for ataxia, painful gait, and other abnormal gait patterns
  - Have patients walk on their toes, heels, in tandem (toe–heel), and run
    - Observe arm swing and gait abnormalities
    - These exercises are considered "stressed gaits"
    - Observe for upper-extremity posturing, including flexion at the elbow or wrist, cortical thumbing, fisting, internal rotation of the arm, or other abnormal posturing

Evaluating for Hypotonia in Infants

- Evaluation (Table 31-1)
  - Passively flap infant's hands and feet and note tone
  - Scarf sign
    - Place the infant in a semireclined position
    - Grasping the infant's hand, pull the infant's arm across the chest toward the opposite shoulder
    - If the elbow passes the midline, the patient is abnormally hypotonic
  - Vertical suspension
    - Support the patient in the axilla
    - Patient should not slip through the examiner's hand

Table 31-1. Distinguishing Examination Features of the Hypotonic Infant

Source	Tone	Strength	Sensation	Atrophy	Fasciculations	Deep Tendon Reflexes
Brain	Decreased truncal	Normal	Normal	Disuse	No	Normal or increased
Spinal cord	Above lesion: normal Below: decreased	Above lesion: normal Below: decreased	Above lesion: normal Below: decreased	Below	Occasionally below	Above lesion: normal Below: increased
Anterior horn cell	Decreased	Decreased	Normal	Occasionally	Marked	None
Nerve	Decreased	Decreased distal	Decreased distal	Present	Present	Decreased
Neuromuscular junction	Slight decrease	Fluctuates; worse with activity	Normal	None	None	Occasionally decreased
Muscle	Decreased	Decreased	Normal	None	None	Decreased over time
Ligament	Decreased	Normal	Normal	None	None	Normal

and should be able to maintain a sitting position

- Horizontal suspension
  - Suspend the prone infant above a table while supporting the abdomen
  - Infant should lift head and bottom, arching back
  - If hypotonic, the infant's head and legs will hang down
- Traction response
  - Place thumbs in the infant's palms and fingers around the infant's wrists
  - Gently pull the infant from the supine position
  - Infant should flex at the elbows, and head should rise and be maintained briefly in the axis of the trunk, even in full-term newborns
  - The time in which the head is aligned with the body should increase as the infant gets older

- History
  - Prenatal
    - Prenatal infections
    - Drugs
    - Fetal movement
  - Birth
    - Full-term or premature
    - Vaginal or cesarean-section birth
    - Breech or regular delivery
    - Complications
    - Newborn nursery or newborn intensive care unit
    - Time until discharged home
  - Feeding well or poorly
  - History of consuming honey or corn syrup
  - Consumption or construction in child's neighborhood
  - Static versus acute onset
  - Any developmental regression (or loss of milestones or abilities they previously could perform)
  - Family history
    - Muscular dystrophy
    - Myotonic dystrophy
    - Neuromuscular disorders
    - Sudden infant death syndrome
    - Consanguinity

    - Relatives requiring assistance to walk
- Localization
  - Brain
    - Causes include: hypoxic ischemic encephalopathy; stroke; prematurity; metabolic, chromosomal, and peroxisomal disorders; malformations; and delayed myelination
    - Head and trunk will be floppy; arms and legs may have increased tone
    - Sophisticated workup includes magnetic resonance imaging of the brain, chromosomal analysis, fluorescence in situ hybridization (FISH), positive or negative metabolic laboratory examinations, and specialist consultation, if available
  - Spinal cord
    - Lesions here are causes of hypotonia
    - Trauma, myelomeningocele, and tumor may be causes
    - Perform magnetic resonance imaging if possible
  - Anterior horn cell
    - Spinal muscular atrophy can cause hypotonia
      - Werdnig-Hoffmann disease (early)/type II
      - Kugelberg-Welander disease
    - Polio
    - Genetic disorders (sensory motor neuropathy) can also cause hypotonia
  - Nerve
    - Also a rare cause of hypotonia
    - Other causes include polyneuropathies, Guillain-Barré syndrome, and hereditary neuropathy
    - Test using electromyogram or nerve conduction, if available
  - Neuromuscular junction
    - Causes include botulism and myasthenia
    - Test a stool sample for botulinum toxin or myasthenia acetylcholine receptor antibodies, respectively, for confirmation (these tests are unlikely to be available outside large medical centers)
  - Muscle
    - Causes can include muscular dystrophy (progressive),

myopathy, human immunodeficiency virus, influenza, medications (eg, azidothymidine, steroids), inflammatory disorders (eg, dermatomyositis), Addison disease, Cushing disease, hypothyroidism, and hypophosphatemia
    - Metabolic causes include glycogen storage, Pompe's disease, and mitochondrial disease
    - Test using creatine kinase, biopsy, erythrocyte sedimentation rate, complete blood count, thyroid function test, lactate or pyruvate test, or blood chemistry test as directed by examination and other findings
  - Ligament
    - Causes may include Marfan syndrome, Ehlers-Danlos syndrome, hypermobility syndrome
    - Genetics can also cause ligament disorders that lead to hypotonia

Headaches in Children

- Acute headache
  - Defined as a single event without history of previous similar events
  - Can be generalized or localized
  - Can occur with or without neurological symptoms and signs
  - Types
    - Acute generalized: causes include fever, systemic infection, central nervous system (CNS) infection, toxins (eg, carbon monoxide, amphetamines), postictal state, hypertension, shunt malfunction, hypoxia, hypoglycemia, lumbar puncture, trauma, CNS hemorrhage, embolus, exertion, or electrolyte imbalance
    - Focal acute: causes include trauma, sinusitis, otitis, pharyngitis, Chiari malformation, glaucoma and other ocular disorders, temporomandibular joint disorder, dental disorder, or occipital neuralgia
- Acute recurrent
  - Periodic headaches that are separated by pain-free intervals
  - When associated with nausea, vomiting, and photophobia,

these headaches are usually migraines
  - Differential includes migraine; hypertension; vasculitis; substance abuse; shunt malfunction; atrioventricular malformation; mitochondrial myopathy, encephalopathy, lactic acidosis, and stroke-like episodes; postictal state; hypoglycemia; exertion; colloid cyst of the third ventricle; and dialysis
- Chronic progressive
  - Worsen in frequency and severity over time
  - May progress rapidly or slowly
  - May be accompanied by symptoms and signs of increased intracranial pressure (ICP) or progressive neurological disease
  - Neurological examination is frequently abnormal
  - Organic process/abnormality is usually present
  - Further investigation is usually warranted
  - Differential includes hydrocephalus, subdural hematoma, neoplasm, abscess, Dandy-Walker complex, Chiari malformation, subdural empyema, and pseudotumor cerebri
- Chronic nonprogressive
  - Chronic daily migraines (transformed migraines) begin with episodic migraines and a number of years later (depending on medication overuse and headache frequency) headaches evolve into daily vascular headaches
  - Chronic tension-type headaches may occur several times a week, more than 15 days a month, or may be constant
    - Usually not associated with symptoms of increased ICP or progressive neurological disease
    - Neurological examination is normal
    - Often related to school, stress, family dysfunction, or medication overuse

Evaluation of Children and Adolescents with Recurrent Headaches

- Diagnosed on a clinical basis rather than by testing
  - Diagnostic studies are not indicated when the clinical history shows no associated risk factors and the child's examination is normal
  - Lumbar puncture and electroencephalogram (EEG) are

not recommended unless history is concerning for CNS infection or seizure
  - EEG helps rule out benign occipital epilepsy, which presents with visual disturbances and can be associated with migraines
- Neuroimaging
  - Not recommended on a routine basis
  - Consider in children with abnormal neurological examinations
  - Concerning signs include focal findings, signs of increased ICP, significant alteration of consciousness, and coexistence of seizures
  - Consider in children with history of recent onset of severe headaches, change in type of headaches, or if associated features suggest neurological dysfunction
- Migraine presentation and management in children and adolescents are similar to adult presentation and management
  - Be cautious with drug dosing and aware that some medications are not approved for use in young children

Chapter 32

Hematology and Oncology

Anemia

- Normal red blood cell (RBC) values vary depending on the age of the child (Table 32-1)

Table 32-1. Normal Red Blood Cell Values

Age	HgB (g/dL) Mean (–2SD)	RBC Count ($x10^{12}$/L)	MCV (fL)	MCHC (g/%RBC)
0 days	16.5 (13.5)	3.9–5.5	108 (98)	33 (30)
1–3 days	18.5 (14.5)	4.0–6.6	108 (95)	33 (29)
2 wk	16.6 (13.4)	3.6–6.2	105 (88)	31.4 (28.1)
1 mo	13.9 (10.7)	3.0–5.4	101 (91)	31.8 (28.1)
6–8 wk	11.2 (9.4)	2.7–4.9	95 (84)	31.8 (28.3)
3–6 mo	12.6 (11.1)	3.1–4.5	76 (68)	35 (32.7)
6–24 mo	12.0 (10.5)	3.7–5.3	78 (70)	33 (30)
2–6 y	12.5 (11.5)	3.9–5.3	81 (75)	34 (31)
6–12 y	13.5 (11.5)	4.0–5.2	86 (77)	34 (31)
12–18 y				
female	14 (12)	4.1–5.1	90 (78)	34 (31)
male	14.5 (13)	4.5–5.3	88 (78)	34 (31)
18–49 y				
female	14 (12)	4.1–5.1	90 (80)	34 (31)
male	15.5 (13.5)	4.5–5.3	90 (80)	34 (31)

HgB: hemoglobin
MCHC: mean corpuscular hemoglobin concentration
MCV: mean corpuscular volume
RBC: red blood cell
SD: standard deviation
Data source: Nathan DG, Oski FA. *Nathan and Oski's Hematology of Infancy and Childhood.* 6th ed. Philadelphia, Pa: WB Saunders; 2003: 1841, App 11.

- Microcytic anemia
  - Iron deficiency
    - Reticulocyte count will be low; red cell distribution width (RDW) will be high; serum iron, high total iron binding capacity, and ferritin will be low
    - Treat with oral (PO) iron (4–6 mg elemental iron/kg daily divided bid or tid); recheck in 6 weeks

- Chronic lead poisoning
  - Lead prevents normal hemoglobin (HgB) synthesis
  - Reticulocyte count will be low, serum lead levels will be high
  - Treat levels greater than 45 μg/dL by removing lead exposure and administering DMSA (also called succimer or dimercaptosuccinic acid) tid for 5 days, then bid for 2 weeks or until lead levels are < 25 μg/dL
- Thalassemia
  - Inherited disorder of HgB synthesis (see below). May be either α-thalassemia or β-thalassemia, homozygous (severe) or heterozygous (mild)
  - Use Mentzer index to differentiate between iron deficiency anemia and β-thalassemia
    - If the result is < 12, thalassemia is likely
    - If > 13.5, iron deficiency is more likely

$$\frac{\text{mean corpuscular volume (MCV)}}{\text{RBC count}}$$

  - Laboratory results for thalassemia will show elevated reticulocyte count, normal RDW, and target cells on smear
  - Treat with folic acid (1 mg PO daily)
    - Patients with severe cases may need chronic blood transfusions with iron chelators, splenectomy, or both
    - Do not treat with iron unless iron is depleted
- Chronic inflammation
  - Inflammation causes iron to be trapped in the reticuloendothelial system
  - Low reticulocyte counts and mildly increased RDW may also be normocytic
  - Serum iron and total iron binding capacity will be low, ferritin will be elevated
  - Treat the underlying disease

- Normocytic anemia
  - Hemolytic
    - Characterized by premature RBC destruction and elevated reticulocyte count
    - Smear may show schistocytes, spherocytes, or bite cells
    - Bilirubin and lactate dehydrogenase levels will be high,

haptoglobin will be low
    - May need direct antibody testing, osmotic fragility testing, or glucose-6-phosphate dehydrogenase (G6PD) activity; however, G6PD may be normal immediately after an acute attack
  - Acute blood loss
  - Splenic sequestration
    - Occurs when RBCs become trapped in the spleen
    - Seen in sickle cell disease or hereditary spherocytosis
    - Characterized by elevated reticulocyte count and decreased platelet count
    - Pallor, shock, and enlarged spleen are diagnostic signs
    - **Treat the shock**; patients in splenic sequestration can rapidly decompensate
  - Transient erythroblastopenia of childhood
    - Typical age of onset is about 2–3 years
    - Child is usually pale and tachycardic, but otherwise appears well (may even have a HgB count of 5 g/dL)
    - Reticulocyte count is low, but MCV is normal before recovery
    - Observation is usually sufficient treatment
    - Transfuse only if there are signs of impending cardiovascular collapse
  - Chronic renal disease
    - Chronic renal disease can cause anemia through a variety of factors, including chronic inflammation, nutritional deficiency or uremia, and decreased erythropoietin
    - Reticulocyte count and erythropoietin levels will be low
    - Treat with erythropoietin (50–150 units/kg subcutaneous or intravenous [IV] three times weekly)
- Macrocytic anemia
  - Vitamin B_{12} deficiency
    - Vitamin B_{12} deficiency is seen in patients with poor diets, poor intestinal absorption, parasites, or bacterial overgrowth
    - The typical patient has anemia and peripheral neuropathy, though infants may present with tremors, micro-

cephaly, developmental regression, and/or failure to thrive

- Reticulocyte count will be low, neutropenia, and thrombocytopenia may be present, and RDW will be elevated
- Smear may show hypersegmented neutrophils (≥6 lobes)
- Serum B_{12} levels may be low
- Schilling test may be necessary to determine cause
- Treat with vitamin B_{12} alone or intrinsic factor

- Folic acid deficiency
  - Folic acid deficiency can be caused by a nutritional deficit (especially in children drinking goat's milk), poor intestinal absorption (celiac disease), increased body requirements (rapid growth or cell turnover), or metabolic disorders (inborn errors of metabolism or folate antagonistic drugs)
  - Reticulocyte count will be low, neutropenia, and thrombocytopenia may be present, and RDW will be elevated
  - Smear may show hypersegmented neutrophils (≥6 lobes)
  - Serum folate levels may be low
  - If the diagnosis between folic acid and B_{12} deficiency is unclear and laboratory tests for serum levels are unavailable, give low-dose folic acid (100–500 μg daily)
    - In folic acid deficiency, reticulocytosis will be seen in 2–4 days; no increase will be seen in B_{12} deficiency at that dose
    - Once B_{12} deficiency is ruled out, treat with folic acid (1 mg PO daily)
- Aplastic
  - In aplastic anemia, the bone marrow's ability for hematopoiesis is either reduced or completely lacking
  - Can be a result of acquired or congenital factors
  - Characterized by low reticulocyte count, pancytopenia, and normal RDW
  - Bone marrow biopsy and aspiration must be performed
  - Treatment is supportive with transfusions as needed until a definitive diagnosis is reached
- Bone marrow infiltration
  - Bone marrow spaces are occupied by tumor, fibrosis, or

storage disease
    - Low reticulocyte count, pancytopenia may be present
    - Bone marrow biopsy and aspiration must be performed
    - Treatment is supportive with transfusions as needed until a definitive diagnosis is reached
  - Liver disease
    - Shortened RBC survival
    - Smear will show burr cells or target cells
    - Prothrombin time (PT) / activated partial thromboplastin time (aPTT) may be prolonged in more severe liver disease
    - Treatment is supportive
  - Hypothyroidism
    - Low thyroid hormone down regulates precursor metabolism
    - MCV may also be normal
    - Spiculated RBCs are evident on smear
    - Thyroid function test is consistent with hypothyroidism
    - Treat the underlying disease
  - Dyserythropoiesis / myelodysplastic syndromes
    - Ineffective erythropoiesis
    - Presents with a decrease in one cell line that progresses to pancytopenia
    - Low reticulocyte count
    - Smear shows teardrop cells
    - Bone marrow has normal or increased cellularity
    - Treatment is supportive unless a bone marrow donor is available
- Sickle cell diseases
  - Sickle cell disease occurs frequently in people living in certain parts of Africa, India, and the Middle East; in the United States, it occurs in 0.2% of African Americans
  - It may be detected with a Sickledex (Strek, Inc, Omaha, Neb) or sickle prep solubility test, but the diagnosis is made with HgB electrophoresis
    - Severe: homozygous sickle HgB disease (HgBSS), HgBS-β^0-thalassemia
    - Less severe: a heterozygous sickle HgB disease (eg, HgB SC), HgBS-β^+-thalassemia

- Complications
  - 0–4 years old
    - **Dactylitis/pain crisis**: usually the first clinical manifestation of sickle cell disease
      - The child will present with swollen, tender hands or feet
      - Typically well tolerated and can often be treated with fluids and acetaminophen or nonsteroidal antiinflamatory drugs
    - **Splenic sequestration**: one of the leading causes of mortality
      - Often complicates sepsis
      - Usually occurs before 2 years of age
      - Patient presents with weakness, left-sided abdominal pain, and progressive shock; a large spleen will be palpated on physical examination
      - Hematocrit will fall to about 50% of the patient's baseline, with an associated drop in platelets; reticulocyte count will be higher than usual
      - **Volume resuscitate first, but patient may need simple or exchange transfusion**
      - HgB/hematocrit will increase more than is expected as RBCs are released from the spleen
      - Splenectomy will not help during sequestration, but is indicated for patients with recurrent episodes
    - **Pneumococcal sepsis**: risk is 400-fold in affected children and associated with a 30% mortality rate
      - Child is febrile and appears toxic
      - Admit and treat with appropriate antibiotics based on resistance patterns
      - Prevent with pneumococcal vaccination and penicillin prophylaxis (125 mg PO bid until 3 y, then 250 mg PO bid until at least 5 or 6 y) or erythromycin (10 mg/kg PO bid) for children allergic to penicillin
  - 4–10 years old
    - **Stroke**: occurs in about 7% of children; silent infarcts can be seen in up to almost 20%

- Children typically have ischemic strokes (in adults hemorrhagic strokes are more common)
- Diagnosis is made by a noncontrast computed tomography (CT) scan, though a CT scan may be negative in first 3–6 hours

▹ **Aplastic crisis**: most often caused by parvovirus B19

- Infection is more severe in all of the hemolytic anemias because of the shortened life span of the RBC
- HgB/hematocrit will be lower than baseline, with low or absent reticulocyte count
- Most cases will resolve on their own, but some patients may need transfusion if reticulocytosis is delayed

▸ 10–20 years

▹ **Acute chest syndrome**: second most common cause for hospitalization in sickle cell disease

- Usually occurs in older children
- Presents as fever with respiratory symptoms and a new infiltrate on radiography
- It is more common in the winter with increased upper respiratory infections
- Mortality rate is 5%
- More than half of patients with acute chest syndrome have pulmonary fat embolism or an associated infection
- Treat with: oxygen, incentive spirometry and bronchodilators, analgesics to prevent hypoventilation from pain, and antibiotics to cover atypicals (*Chlamydia* and *Mycoplasma* are common pathogens); hydration can decrease sickling, but overhydration will cause pulmonary edema and worsen the acute chest (typical rate is ⅔–1 × maintenance)
- Transfuse packed red blood cells (PRBCs) for partial pressure of oxygen (PO_2) < 70 mmHg or worsening pulmonary status; perform exchange transfusion if hematocrit is higher than patient's baseline

  - **Gallstones**: by age 15, more than 40% of children with sickle cell disease have developed cholelithiasis, though they are most often asymptomatic
  - **Priapism**: painful erection lasting for more than 30 minutes
    - Usually occurs in the early hours of the morning or following sexual activity
    - In most cases, it can be treated at home with frequent urination, vigorous exercise, increased fluid intake, and warm baths; if home treatment is unsuccessful after 3 hours, it is unlikely to be effective
    - Hydration, analgesia, and warm compresses may be helpful; if these methods fail within 6–8 hours, PRBC transfusion may be needed, though effect may not be seen for 24 hours
    - If the condition has not begun to resolve 24 hours after PRBC transfusion, surgical consultation is needed for possible shunting to prevent fibrosis and impotence
- All ages
  - **Fever**: considered an emergency in all age groups; infection is the most common cause of death in children with sickle cell disease
    - Most patients with sickle cell disease are functionally hyposplenic by 2 years old
    - A patient with a temperature ≥ 38.5°C should have a complete blood count (CBC), urinary analysis, and chest radiograph with cultures from the blood, urine, and throat, as well as a broad-spectrum antibiotic that penetrates the central nervous system and covers *Haemophilus influenzae* and *Streptococcus pneumoniae* (eg, ceftriaxone)
  - **Pain crisis**: the most common manifestation of acute vasoocclusive crisis
    - Most common locations are the lumbosacral spine, hip, femur, knee, shoulder, and elbow
    - Most episodes can be managed at home with increased fluid intake and analgesics, but treat-

ment with IV morphine (0.1–0.15 mg/kg loading dose) and hydration may be required
- Morphine doses of 5–10 mg are not uncommon, and a history of the patient's prior doses is often most helpful
- Fluids are typically run at 1½ × maintenance (D_5½NS + 20 mEq KCl/L)

- Hemolytic anemias
  - The normal RBC lives for about 120 days in circulation. Premature destruction can result in anemia. Patients generally present with anemia, elevated reticulocytosis, and hyperbilirubinemia. Once the diagnosis of hemolytic anemia is made, the cause needs to be determined
    - Autoimmune hemolytic anemia: group of disorders in which autoantibodies are formed that bind to RBCs and lead to premature destruction
    - G6PD deficiency: G6PD functions as a reducing enzyme and is found in all cells. The normal half-life of the protein is 60 days. Patients whose G6PD has a shorter half-life are susceptible to hemolysis when RBCs are exposed to oxidative stress
      - Presentation: G6PD deficiency is predominant in people of African and Mediterranean descent; in these geographical areas, males are more likely to be deficient, although females with G6PD deficiency are not uncommon
      - Diagnosis: G6PD levels will be normal in the acute phase because all the deficient RBCs will have lysed; once the patient has recovered from the oxidative insult, G6PD levels can be obtained
      - Treatment: patients should avoid agents that are known to cause hemolysis (most notable is primaquine treatment for malaria)
      - In the acute phase, patients may require RBC transfusions. Indications for transfusion are:
        - HgB < 7 g/dL
        - HgB < 9 g/dL with hemoglobinuria
    - Other causes: there are a host of other causes of hemolysis, including RBC membrane defects (spherocytosis,

elliptocytosis), immune and nonimmune drug-induced hemolysis, and microangiopathy

- Thrombocytopenia
  - Thrombocytopenia is defined as a platelet count < 150,000/mm^3. Isolated thrombocytopenia generally does not result in spontaneous bleeding unless the platelet count is less than 30,000/mm^3. Trauma or medical procedures may cause increased bleeding in a patient with a platelet count less than 100,000/m^3. Thrombocytopenia most commonly results in bleeding of the mucous membranes or the skin (petechiae or bruising)
    - Immune (idiopathic) thrombocytopenic purpura (ITP): ITP is a common cause of thrombocytopenia in kids
      - Results when autoantibodies attack platelets
      - Can be either acute or chronic
      - Acute ITP occurs most frequently in children between 2 and 8 years old
      - Presentation: bruising, petechiae, and mucous membrane involvement; splenomegaly is present in only about 10% of patients
      - Diagnosis: CBC shows a low platelet count, often less than 20,000/mm^3, but normal HgB and white blood cell (WBC) counts. Mean platelet volume is frequently elevated. PT/aPTT are normal. Bone marrow aspiration should be considered prior to treating with steroids if the history is not typical, the CBC shows abnormalities beyond thrombocytopenia, or hepatosplenomegaly is present. The aspirate will show increased megakaryocytes. Persistence of ITP for more than 6 months is considered chronic (chronic ITP occurs in 20% of patients with acute ITP)
      - Treatment of **acute** ITP: can often be treated with observation alone; treat if platelet count is less than 20,000/mm^3 with significant mucous membrane bleeding **or** less than 10,000/mm^3 with mild purpura
        - Prednisone (4–6 mg/kg/day divided bid, maximum dose of 60 mg/day) tapered in 5–7-day intervals for a total of 21–28 days
        - Methylprednisolone (30 mg/kg/day divided

bid, maximum dose of 1 g/day) for 3 days for more severe cases
- Anti-D immunoglobulin (50 μg/kg IV)
- IV immunoglobulin (0.4 g/kg IV daily) for 5 days, or (1 g/kg IV daily) for 2 days
- Platelet transfusions should be used only in emergency (eg, surgery, intracranial hemorrhage) because transfused platelets have a very short lifespan
- Splenectomy is indicated for severe, life-threatening bleeding that is not responsive to medical management
- Vaccination with meningococcal, pneumococcal, and *H influenzae* b vaccines should be performed, preferably 2 weeks prior to surgery

- Treatment of **chronic** ITP: evaluate patients for other autoimmune diseases, systemic lupus erythematosus, or human immunodeficiency virus infection; treatment for symptomatic patients is the same as that for acute ITP

- Hemolytic uremic syndrome (HUS)/thrombotic thrombocytopenic purpura (TTP): both conditions are forms of microangiopathic anemia associated with thrombosis. Thrombus formation consumes platelets and hemolyzes RBCs as they pass through the smaller vessels. HUS is often seen in association with *Shigella dysenteriae* or *Escherichia coli* O157:H7 infections. TTP can be seen following viral or bacterial infections, during pregnancy, or with certain drugs
  - Presentation: gastrointestinal infection, which can include bloody diarrhea; oliguria and hypertension develop early
    - In TTP, patients initially present with bleeding and neurological symptoms, then later develop fever
  - Differentiation
    - Patients with HUS or TTP will have thrombocytopenia and hemolytic anemia, though they are less severe in HUS than in TTP
    - The platelet count in HUS is greater than 100,000/mm^3 in half of patients

            - The age of onset for HUS is between 6 months old and 5 years old, whereas TTP is more commonly seen in adults
        - Treatment
            - HUS treatment should focus on the renal disease with fluid restriction and hypertension management; treat anemia with PRBC transfusions as needed; platelet transfusions are not indicated because life-threatening bleeding is rare and platelet transfusion can worsen thrombosis
            - Treat TTP with plasmapheresis
    - Disseminated intravascular coagulation: an acquired syndrome of intravascular activation of the coagulation cascade that occurs most commonly following sepsis
        - Presentation: depends upon the underlying disorder
            - Bleeding, petechiae or mucosal bleeding, or severe hemorrhage may not be present
            - Patients have prolonged PT / aPTT, decreased fibrinogen, and increased fibrin split products, including D-dimer
            - Thrombocytopenia is noted on CBC
        - Treatment: treat the underlying cause and provide replacement therapy
            - Transfuse platelets to maintain > 50,000 / mm^3
            - Administer fresh frozen plasma (10–15 mL / kg) to maintain prothrombin time < 2 × normal
            - Cryoprecipitate to maintain fibrinogen > 100 mg / dL

Coagulopathies

- Hemophilia A and B are X-linked deficiencies in either factor VIII or factor IX, respectively. The two factors work together to drive the coagulation cascade from the intrinsic pathway to the common pathway
    - Presentation
        - The two syndromes are clinically identical to each other
        - Both occur almost exclusively in males
        - Their first manifestation can be with bleeding at birth or prolonged bleeding after circumcision
        - Most cases are identified by the time the patient is 18 months old

- Joint bleeding is the hallmark of hemophilia, with the weight-bearing joints of the legs being most frequently affected

- Evaluation
  - PT will be normal, but aPTT will be prolonged
  - A mixing study will correct the defect if the patient has not developed inhibitors
  - Factor assays will show decreased activity in the factor that is deficient
- Treatment
  - Factor replacement (Table 32-2)
  - Patients with mild or moderate factor VIII deficiency can be treated with desmopressin acetate (0.3 μg/kg

Table 32-2. Factor Replacement*†

Type of Bleed	Desired Level (%)
Joint or simple hematoma	20–40
Simple dental extraction	50
Major soft tissue bleed	80–100
Head injury (prophylaxis)	100+
Major surgery (dental, orthopaedic, other)	100+

*For factor VIII, each unit/kg will increase level by 2% (eg, to increase from < 10% to 100%, use 50 units/kg).
†For factor IX, each unit/kg will increase level by 1% (eg, to increase from < 10% to 100%, use 100 units/kg).

IV over 15–30 min, or 1 puff [150 μg] intranasally for children < 50 kg, and 2 puffs [300 μg] intranasally for children > 50 kg) if they are known responders
    - **Note**: desmopressin acetate nasal spray for hemophilia is 15-fold the concentration of the spray for diabetes insipidus
    - If specific factors are unavailable, or if the type of hemophilia is not known, fresh frozen plasma can be used (40 mL/kg) because it contains all of the clotting factors
    - Volume overload can be a complication; for patients with hemophilia A, cryoprecipitate (50–100 units factor VII in 10 mL) can be used
    - Patients may develop inhibitors to factors
- Von Willebrand's disease: the most common inherited bleed-

ing diathesis, occurring in 1%–2% of the general population, though in most people, the disease is mild enough that they never seek medical attention
  - Presentation: history of easy bleeding or bruising
    - Bleeding is most often of the platelet type, with epistaxis and mucocutaneous bleeds
    - Oozing is seen after surgical procedures, especially after dental extractions
    - Females may have menorrhagia; there is often a family history of the same type of bleeding
  - Treatment
    - Prophylaxis for minor surgery or treatment of minor bleeding with desmopressin
    - Prophylaxis for major surgery or treatment of significant bleeding with cryoprecipitate, fresh frozen plasma, or platelets (see Chapter 5, Transfusion Medicine, for specifics on using blood products)

Oncology

- The most common malignancies in childhood include leukemia, brain tumors, lymphoma, and neuroblastoma
- Children with cancer are particularly susceptible to infection, which is the primary cause of death in oncology patients
  - This may be due to a deranged or suppressed immune system, poor nutritional status, mucous membrane damage, or indwelling central venous catheters
- In children with fever and neutropenia, initiate broad-spectrum antibiotic therapy with activity against both gram-positive and gram-negative bacteria
  - Carefully search for a source of infection, paying particular attention to mucous membranes, the perineum, and skin surrounding vascular access sites
  - The patient should be admitted until cultures are negative for 48–72 hours, the patient is afebrile for 24–48 hours, and bone marrow shows signs of recovery, with absolute neutrophil count > 200/mm^3 on at least two occasions and rising
  - Antibiotic therapy can be stopped at this time unless a bacterial source is identified

- For fevers that persist for 5 days, or fevers that recur after the patient has been treated for more than 5 days, start antifungal therapy

Chapter 33

Nephrology

Assessing Kidney Function in Children

- To estimate glomerular filtration rate (GFR), use the Schwartz formula
  - Two points are needed for this GFR calculation: patient height (in centimeters), and a stable serum creatinine measurement

$$\text{Estimated GFR (eGFR)} = \frac{(\text{height [cm]})\,(\text{k})}{(\text{serum creatinine mg/dL})}$$

  - Typical "k" values are as follows:
    - Preemies: 0.33
    - Infants (< 12 mo old): 0.45
    - Children and female adolescents: 0.55
    - Male adolescents: 0.7
  - If serum creatinine is rising, estimate GFR as 0 or < 20 mL/min/1.73 m^2
- When kidney function is questionable, dose all medications based on eGFR
- If GFR < 40 mL/min/1.73 m^2, especially in the presence of chronic kidney disease, associated findings include:
  - Anemia: due to erythropoietin deficiency, as well as the iron deficiency caused by the chronic disease; supplement with iron and epoetin alfa (if possible)
  - Secondary hyperparathyroidism: manifesting with high levels of intact parathyroid hormone (iPTH), phosphate, alkaline phosphatase, and low levels of calcium
    - Treat with calcium supplementation at meals to bind phosphate and raise calcium levels
    - Administer 1,25-dihydroxyvitamin D to suppress iPTH
  - Acidosis
    - Treat acidosis with citric acid/sodium citrate and calcium carbonate supplementation to neutralize hydrogen ion and promote growth

  - Elevated potassium causes severe acidosis and decreases GFR in children
    - Treat with sorbitol or osmolar potassium-binding resin to encourage rectal excretion of potassium
    - If urine output is present, consider a high-dose diuretic

Acute Kidney Injury

- Acute kidney injury is evident when GFR < 50 mL/min/1.73 m^2, or when creatinine rises by 0.5 mg/dL in children or 1.0 mg/dL in adolescents
- The most common cause in a field or combat environment is inadequate renal perfusion (inadequate intravascular volume)
  - Clinical examination of intravascular fluid status includes:
    - Checking blood pressure (BP) and heart rate to assess for evidence of shock
    - Examining mucous membranes, fontanelle, weight, etc
    - Checking urine sodium if possible; if the child is hypotensive, urine sodium is < 20 mmol/L, regardless of serum sodium
    - Urine osmolarity or urine-specific gravity
    - Assessing oncotic pressure with serum albumin as a cause of low renal perfusion
- Other causes of acute kidney injury in the field environment
  - Obstructive uropathy (eg, neurogenic bladder, posterior urethral valves, single kidney with renal stones, etc)
    - Look for lower extremity atrophy, sacral dimple, and hair tuft for spina bifida occulta, etc
    - Use kidney ultrasound to assess
    - Place Foley to drain
    - Watch serum creatinine after decompression
  - Acute glomerular injury
  - Hypertension
    - Cuff size should measure two-thirds the distance from the patient's olecranon to acromion; the bladder portion of the cuff should wrap completely around the arm
    - Hypertension criteria:

        - < 12 months old: 100/70
        - Quick formulas for children ages 1–10 years old
            - Systolic BP: age × 2 + 100 (95th percentile)
            - Diastolic BP: age × 1.5 + 70 (95th percentile)
        - > 10 years old: use adult measurement
    - Proteinuria with acute hematuria (gross or microscopic); red blood cell (RBC) casts and dysmorphic RBCs can be seen in a urine microscopic evaluation
    - Edema
    - Acute tubular necrosis (this is the same as acute glomerulonephritis above, except a granular cast is seen on urine microscopic evaluation)
- Treating acute kidney injury
    - Bolus initially with normal saline (NS; 20 mL/kg), or blood products or albumin 25% (1 g/kg); slowly (over 1–2 h) to establish intravascular volume and restore BP (some patients may be euvolemic or hypervolemic)
    - Place a urine Foley to drain and watch urine output
    - Place patient on ⅓ maintenance fluids (¼ NS without potassium)
    - Replace hourly urine output with an equal volume of ½ NS
    - Control or maintain BP with vasodilators or vasopressors based on the patient's BP
        - Low BP: use vasopressors
        - High BP: use diuretics or calcium-channel blockers
        - Titrate medications based on response
    - If the patient becomes oliguric or anuric, consider furosemide 3–5 mg/kg to establish urine output and help with volume status
    - Stabilize electrolytes, especially potassium, through established cellular shift and excretion methods
    - If access to Army Knowledge Online (AKO) is available, contact the nephrology consult service (nephrology.consult@us.army.mil)

Nephrotic Syndrome

- Hypoalbuminemia (< 2.5 g/dL)
- Hyperproteinuria

  - Spot urine protein-to-creatinine ratio > 2.0

OR

  - Urine dipstick or urinary analysis shows protein to be 2+ or more
- Hypercholesterolemia (total cholesterol > 200 mg/dL, low-density lipoprotein > 130 mg/dL)
- Edema presents with weight gain, tibial and eyelid swelling (usually first to show), and ascites
- Noted to be absent: hypertension, elevated serum creatinine or decreased GFR, active urine sediment (no RBC casts, etc)

Treating Edema and Nephrotic Syndrome

- Treat edema if the following are present:
  - Severe hyponatremia
  - Severe pleural effusion with respiratory distress
  - Severe anasarca with skin breakdown or severe swelling in the scrotum or labial areas
- Treat edema with albumin 25% (1 g/kg) over 4 hours
- Monitor on a cardiorespiratory monitor (if possible) to watch respiratory status
- Follow with furosemide (1 mg/kg intravenous [IV]), then albumin again in the same order over 4 hours ("albumin-furosemide-albumin sandwich"); this treats edema by increasing oncotic pressure and renal perfusion; diuretic therapy excretes free water
- Treatment of nephrotic syndrome: most cases will respond to prednisone at 2 mg/kg daily
- Contact nephrology consultation service on AKO if available

Renal Stones

- Renal stones are rare in children, but because of the climate and a lack of potable water, they are more common in current combat theaters
- Calcium oxalate kidney stones are the most common type found in children. Their clinical presentation is similar to that in adults and includes:
  - Gross hematuria (presents with pink or red urine)
  - Inguinal pain reproducible with palpation of the flank or abdomen
  - Fever, flank pain, and dysuria or a burning sensation, which

may present if the patient passes gravel or a stone (infection develops behind obstructing stones)

- Physical examination
  - Perform a urinary analysis; look for hematuria
  - Do a renal ultrasound or computed tomography scan, if available
  - If possible, send urine for a spot check for both calcium and creatinine levels, then calculate the calcium-to-creatinine ratio (a urine calcium-to-creatinine ratio > 0.2 is high)
- Treatment
  - Hydrate: 1.5 L/day of fluid in younger children (< 20 kg), or 2 L/day in older children
  - Consider citrate for increasing pH of urine, if possible, to decrease stone formation in the urinary tract
  - Maintain good urine output (5 voids per day)

Chapter 34

Dermatology

Introduction

Most pediatric dermatological conditions are not acute and may be managed through telemedicine specialty consultation if dermatological expertise is needed. This chapter includes guidelines for telemedicine and focuses on situations requiring expeditious treatment in which potential delays in consultation may be deleterious to the patient.

Teledermatology Consultation

Requesting a teledermatology consultation is relatively easy for members of the US military. The following components should be submitted via e-mail to the US Army consultation service (derm.consult@us.army.mil; be sure to remove any personal patient information):

- Multiple focused photographs of all lesions on the patient
  - Photographs are best taken in well-lit settings (natural sunlight is optimal) without use of the camera's flash
  - Use the camera's "macro" setting, usually indicated by a picture of a flower, for close-up photographs of individual skin lesions
- Basic dermatological history of a lesion or condition, including:
  - Onset
  - Evolution
  - Duration
  - Location
  - Symptoms such as itch or tenderness
  - Alleviating and exacerbating factors
  - Current skincare regimen, including hygiene and topical preparations
  - Associated systemic symptoms
- Past medical history, including:
  - Medications and allergies

  - Previous skin disease or cancer
  - Systemic disease
  - Evidence of atopic background (eg, eczema, asthma, allergies)
- Family/social history, including:
  - Skin diseases in other family members
  - Similar skin symptoms in close contacts
  - Pertinent environmental exposures, such as climate, pets, chemicals, harsh soaps, abrasive brushes, or radiation
- If basic laboratory facilities are accessible, a Gram stain, potassium hydroxide preparation, or Tzanck smear may immediately elucidate bacterial, fungal, or viral infections, respectively. If the facility is not equipped for these bedside tests, report laboratory test results that *have* been obtained, such as a complete blood count, and cultures or tissue specimens
- When describing the patient's physical examination, begin with vitals (especially fever) and general appearance
  - Remember that a thorough skin examination necessitates that the patient be fully disrobed and inspected from head to toe (eg, a common mistake to avoid is failing to examine the feet when a patient presents with hand dermatitis)
  - When describing the skin examination, use the following descriptive terms to aid communication with the dermatologist:
    - Primary skin lesions
      - Papule: an elevated, solid lesion up to 0.5 cm in diameter
      - Plaque: a circumscribed, elevated, superficial, solid lesion > 0.5 cm in diameter
      - Macule: a circumscribed, flat discoloration up to 0.5 cm in diameter
      - Patch: a circumscribed, flat discoloration > 0.5 cm in diameter
      - Nodule: a circumscribed, elevated, solid lesion > 0.5 cm in diameter; a larger, deeper papule
      - Pustule: a circumscribed collection of pus (cloudy, free fluid, and leukocytes)
      - Vesicle: a circumscribed collection of free, clear fluid

up to 0.5 cm in diameter
    - Bulla: a circumscribed collection of free fluid > 0.5 cm in diameter
    - Wheal (hive): a firm, edematous, transient plaque, which lasts hours at most
- Secondary changes
  - Crust (scab): collection of dried serum and cellular debris
  - Scale: excess dead epidermal cells, thickened stratum corneum
  - Erosion: a partial focal loss of epidermis
  - Ulcer: a full-thickness, focal loss of epidermis and dermis (deeper than erosion, heals with scarring)
  - Excoriation: an erosion caused by scratching, often linear
  - Atrophy: depression in the skin resulting from thinning of the epidermis or dermis
  - Lichenification: thickened epidermis induced by scratching (skin lines are accentuated)
- Special skin lesions and descriptors
  - Telangiectasia: dilated superficial blood vessels (blanchable—empty completely with compression)
  - Petechiae: circumscribed deposit of blood < 0.5 cm in diameter (not blanchable)
  - Purpura: circumscribed deposit of blood > 0.5 cm in diameter (not blanchable)
  - Erythema: an area of uniform redness that blanches with pressure
- Other important descriptors include:
  - Color (eg, erythematous, violaceous, hemorrhagic, dusky, skin-colored, blanchable / nonblanchable, beefy red, yellow, etc)
  - Size (eg, 4 mm, 2 cm, etc)
  - Shape (eg, ill-defined oval, well-defined linear streak)
  - Specific location (eg, generalized over arms and legs but spares the trunk, face, and palms or soles)
  - A complete description also includes some comment on the mucous membranes (mouth, eyes, genitals, etc) and skin appendages (hair, nails)

- A response should be sent from a dermatologist within 24

hours (often in as few as 6–8 h)

Febrile Child with Rash

Many inflammatory diseases and viral exanthems may give this type of clinical picture. The following diagnoses include the majority of diseases that need to be recognized and treated emergently:

- Rickettsial diseases
  - Rocky Mountain spotted fever, Mediterranean spotted fever, typhus, and others
  - Typically present with skin eruption, fever, headache, malaise, and prostration
  - Transmitted by ticks, fleas, or body lice
    - Original tick bite may be a clinical clue, and often morphs from inflamed papule to necrotic eschar (tache noir)
    - The skin eruption tends to become petechial as it progresses
  - Diagnosis is based on which diseases may be endemic, the clinical presentation, and indirect fluorescent antibody testing, which may be confirmed by Western blot
  - It is imperative, especially for the spotted fever group of rickettsial diseases, to treat preemptively with doxycycline (2.2 mg/kg/dose bid intravenous [IV]; maximum dose 200 mg/day) to prevent mortality (Figure 34-1)
- Meningococcemia
  - Typically presents acutely, with fever, chills, hypotension, and meningitic symptoms (eg, neck stiffness, photophobia)
  - Half to two thirds of patients develop a petechial or ecchymotic eruption, primarily on the trunk and lower extremities, as well as petechiae on the eyelids and acral surfaces (Figure 34-2)
  - The petechial eruption tends to progress to hemorrhagic bullae or frank necrosis
  - Diagnosis is made on clinical suspicion because treatment needs to be rapid
    - Blood cultures growing the gram-negative diplococci of *Neisseria meningitidis* confirm the diagnosis
    - Treat these patients emergently with aqueous penicillin G (100,000–400,000 units/kg/day divided every 4–6 h,

maximum dose of 24 million units / day) or ceftriaxone (100 mg / kg / day divided every 12 h IV, maximum dose 2g / day) for 7 days

    - Close contacts should receive prophylactic rifampin (children) or ciprofloxacin (adults)

- Measles (rubeola)
  - Extremely infectious and spread by respiratory droplets
  - A prodrome of high fever, malaise, conjunctivitis, cough, and coryza (head cold symptoms) is followed by a maculopapular eruption (ie, generalized erythematous macules and papules), which begins on the head and progresses down the body over 2–3 days (Figure 34-3)
  - Koplik spots (white papules on an erythematous background on the buccal mucosa) are pathognomonic and appear during the prodrome, lasting 3 days (Figure 34-4)
  - Complications of measles include pneumonia, encephalitis, lymphopenia, thrombocytopenic purpura (rarely also disseminated intravascular coagulation [DIC]), and fetal death in pregnant women
  - Diagnosis is clinical, and treatment is supportive (rest, antipyretics, analgesics)
  - Affected children should be given vitamin A (2 doses of 200,000 units 24 h apart) to reduce morbidity and mortality
    - Giving vitamin A supplements to the entire population at the start of an outbreak will significantly reduce mortality
- Scarlet fever
  - Caused by toxins of group A streptococcal infection
  - Primarily affects children < 10 years old and was often fatal before the era of antibiotics
  - Presents with sore throat (streptococcus pharyngitis or tonsillitis), malaise, headache, nausea, abdominal pain, and high fever; an erythematous, blanchable, sandpaper-like rash follows within 12–48 hours
    - The eruption looks like "a sunburn with goose pimples," and begins on the neck, groin, and axillae before spreading to the rest of the body (Figure 34-5)
    - Pastia sign, petechial linear streaks within flexural

    - creases, may also be seen
    - Palms, soles, and conjunctivae are typically unaffected
    - In addition to the pharyngitis, the child may have circumoral pallor, cervical lymphadenopathy, palatal petechiae, and white strawberry tongue, which later morphs into red strawberry tongue
  - Diagnosis is clinical, though a throat culture may be useful
  - Treatment with penicillin or amoxicillin should be initiated to prevent the development of rheumatic fever
  - Desquamation typically occurs 7–10 days after the eruption, and should not be cause for concern
  - Complications include otitis, peritonsillar abscess, pneumonia, myocarditis, meningitis, and arthritis, as well as the immune sequelae of glomerulonephritis and rheumatic fever
    - Consider measles, toxic shock syndrome, drug hypersensitivity, staphylococcal scalded skin, and Kawasaki disease in the differential
- Kawasaki disease (mucocutaneous lymph node syndrome; Figure 34-6) is typically seen in children > 5 years old and is diagnosed by the presence of fever for > 5 days plus four of the following criteria:
  - Polymorphous skin eruption
  - Stomatitis (injected pharynx, strawberry tongue, fissuring cheilitis)
  - Edema of the hands and feet
  - Conjunctival injection
  - Cervical lymphadenopathy
    - An erythematous, desquamating perianal rash is often an early sign
    - As the illness progresses over 10–20 days, fingers and toes may desquamate, starting around the nails
    - Diagnosis is clinical. Rapid treatment with IV immunoglobulin (IVIG), if available (2 g/kg given over 10–12 h, see package insert for specific administration guidance) and aspirin is imperative to prevent potentially fatal coronary artery aneurysm, which complicates up to 25% of untreated cases
- Toxic shock syndrome can be caused by either streptococcus

or staphylococcus

- Streptococcal toxic shock syndrome presents with fever, shock, multiorgan system failure, and usually soft-tissue infection, such as necrotizing fasciitis
    - Streptococcal toxins have direct effects on the major organs, leading to shock and ultimately a mortality rate of 30%
    - Do not wait for cultures; treat emergently with fluids and pressors (for hypotension), clindamycin (40 mg/kg/day divided every 6–8 h), and surgical debridement of any soft-tissue infection source
- Staphylococcal toxic shock syndrome, caused by an exotoxin of *Staphylococcus aureus,* is typically associated with staphylococcal wound or catheter infections, or surgical or nasal packing
    - Patients present with sudden onset of high fever, myalgias, vomiting, diarrhea, headache, and pharyngitis; progression to shock can be rapid and fatal
    - Patients typically develop a diffuse scarlatiniform exanthem, erythema, and edema of the palms and soles, strawberry tongue, hyperemia of the conjunctiva, and a nonpitting generalized edema
    - Treat with supportive care and penicillinase-resistant antibiotics; remove any nidus for infection, such as nasal packing, tampons, and catheters
    - When considering toxic shock syndrome, also include Kawasaki disease, scarlet fever, staphylococcal scalded skin, toxic epidermal necrolysis, systemic lupus, rickettsial spotted fevers, and leptospirosis in the differential diagnosis
    - Desquamation of the palms and soles typically follows toxic shock syndrome by 1–3 weeks

• Leptospirosis (Weil's disease, pretibial fever, Fort Bragg fever) presents with abrupt onset of chills, high fever, jaundice, renal disease (proteinuria, hematuria, azotemia), petechiae, and purpura on skin and mucous membranes
- Death occurs in 5%–10% of patients
- Anicteric leptospirosis may also occur, and is sometimes termed "pretibial fever" because of characteristic shin pain

associated with erythematous rash most marked on the shins
  - Conjunctival suffusion, hemorrhage, ocular pain, photophobia, and intense headache may be other clues to diagnosis
  - Acquired from contact with water or soil contaminated with urine or tissues of infected animals (often rats, dogs, and cats)
  - Diagnosis may be made by finding the spirochetes of Leptospira in the blood (using smear, culture)
  - Treatment with penicillin (IV if disease is severe) and/or doxycycline during the first week of illness will shorten the disease duration

Bullae, Erosions, and Desquamation in Neonates and Young Children

The differential diagnosis for bullae in the neonate is vast and may include a variety of incurable genetic disorders that must be managed with intensive supportive care. For this reason, in the deployed setting, it is best to determine if the bullae are related to something acute or treatable, such as bullous staphylococcal impetigo or acute burn injury

- Bullous staphylococcal impetigo
  - Can be life-threatening in neonates and often occurs between the fourth and tenth days of life
  - Bullae may appear on any part of the body, often starting on the face or hands
  - Weakness, fever, and diarrhea may follow; sepsis may occur without antistaphylococcal antibiotics
- Staphylococcal scalded skin syndrome (Figure 34-7)
  - Preferentially affects neonates and young children
  - Begins with abrupt fever, skin tenderness, and erythema involving the neck, groin, and axillae
  - Over the next few hours to days, erythema progresses to cover more surface area, before ultimately evolving into a very superficial, generalized desquamation (more superficial and less severe than in toxic epidermal necrolysis)
    - Large sheets of epidermis separate
    - Nikolsky's sign is positive (the upper layer of the skin

detaches with application of lateral fingertip pressure to intact skin adjacent to a lesion)
    - The affected skin extends far beyond areas of actual infection (usually the pharynx, nose, ear, conjunctiva, skin, or septicemia)
  - Cultures are best taken from the mucous membranes
  - Rapid diagnosis can be made by examining frozen sections of a skin biopsy from a blister
    - In Figure 34-8, the superficial blister (just beneath the stratum corneum) is caused by a staphylococcal toxin to desmoglein 1, a protein that helps link keratinocytes together
    - This helps differentiate staphylococcal scalded skin syndrome from pemphigus vulgaris or toxic epidermal necrolysis, both of which may also present with superficial (Nikolsky-positive) blistering or denudation, but would show a slightly deeper split in the epidermis, histologically
  - Treatment includes IV fluids and cefazolin (50–100 mg/kg/day IV divided every 8 h, maximum dose 6 g/day; adjust for methicillin-resistant *S aureus* as necessary according to cultures)
- Neonatal herpes simplex virus (HSV) can also be life-threatening
  - Presents with vesicles in the newborn (Figure 34-9)
  - The majority of transmission occurs during delivery, and almost all patients present at 4–21 days of life
  - May be localized to skin and/or eye, involve the central nervous system, or be disseminated (encephalitis, hepatitis, pneumonia, coagulopathy)
    - Encephalitis or disseminated HSV can be fatal in up to half of affected neonates
    - More than half of survivors suffer neurological disability
  - Classic HSV presentation involves painful clusters of vesicles on an erythematous base; however, in over a third of cases, vesicles may not be seen
    - Clusters of erosions tend to remain where vesicles were located

- When these clusters coalesce, they leave behind an erosion or shallow ulcer with scalloped borders
  - Confirm this diagnosis with direct fluorescent antibody staining or a Tzanck preparation of smears obtained from the base of an unroofed vesicle, and with viral culture
  - However, if neonatal HSV is suspected, begin IV acyclovir (60 mg/kg/day IV divided every 8 h × 21 days) immediately
    - Central nervous system involvement may be detected by polymerase chain reaction of cerebrospinal fluid
- Bullous drug reactions can vary dramatically in severity, and many dermatologists consider drug-induced erythema multiforme, drug-induced Stevens-Johnson syndrome (SJS), and toxic epidermal necrolysis (TEN) to represent variations of the same disease process but on a spectrum of severity (Figures 34-10 and 34-11)
  - The definitions of SJS and TEN are somewhat arbitrary and overlap exists; usually SJS affects < 10% body surface area and TEN affects > 30% body surface area
  - The more widespread and severe the epidermolysis, the worse the prognosis and the more likely the process is drug-induced
  - The separation of skin layers in TEN is deeper than that in staphylococcal scalded skin syndrome (see above), with resultant denudation comparable to widespread burns. Accordingly, patients with TEN require intensive supportive care in an intensive care unit or burn center
  - Patients with SJS have a better prognosis than those with TEN, but whether the mucocutaneous denudation is due to TEN or SJS, offending drugs should be discontinued immediately and the patient should be transferred to an intensive care unit for careful fluid management, wound care, nutritional support, and sepsis precautions
    - Early ophthalmologic intervention is needed to

avoid ocular scarring and blindness
        - The use of systemic corticosteroids and IVIG for either disease is controversial
    - Erythema multiforme (minor) typically occurs in the spring or fall, and is often associated with HSV or, less commonly, *Mycoplasma pneumoniae*
        - The lesions can have many different morphologies (hence "multiforme"), but are often targetoid in nature and can be acral in location (Figure 34-12)
        - Most cases are self-limited and do not require treatment
        - Daily suppressive anti-HSV therapy may be considered if the erythema multiforme recurs frequently
- Severe contact dermatitis can also present with widespread erythema and bullae
    - Even when severe and widespread, contact dermatitis typically displays a patterned distribution
    - Very pruritic
    - In severe cases, patients may require a 3–4 week taper of oral corticosteroids
    - Encourage good skin hygiene (at least twice daily gentle cleansing followed by bland emollient, such as petrolatum)
        - Antistaphylococcal antibiotics may also be necessary in cases of secondary infection (suggested by tenderness, expanding honey-colored crusts, and a positive bacterial culture)
- Atopic dermatitis (eczema)
    - A common inflammatory skin disease in childhood characterized by intense pruritus and cutaneous inflammation
    - In addition to affecting quality of life, atopic dermatitis can lead to disruption of the skin barrier and increase susceptibility to infection
    - Associated with asthma and seasonal allergies (the atopic triad)
    - Exacerbating factors may include irritants (soap, over-washing, drying chemicals) and allergens (skin contact

is far more detrimental than contact with foods or aeroallergens)
  - ▹ Presentation in infants and toddlers: erythematous papules and plaques often with overlying excoriation, crusting, and serous exudates; distribution is usually over the scalp, forehead, cheeks, trunk, and extensor surfaces of the extremities
  - ▹ Presentation in children and adults: dry, intensely pruritic papules and patches on flexor surfaces of the arms, neck, and legs. The dorsum of the hands and feet are often involved
    - ▪ Secondary changes, such as lichenification and postinflammatory hypopigmentation and hyperpigmentation are often seen
    - ▪ The differential diagnosis includes seborrheic dermatitis, psoriasis, pityriasis rosea, candidiasis, and keratosis pilaris
- ▸ Treatment
  - ▹ Avoid known allergens and irritants
  - ▹ Soak and smear: hydrate the skin by soaking in lukewarm water for 20 minutes; follow immediately (while the skin is still damp) by sealing in the moisture with emollient (ointment, cream, or thick lotion)
  - ▹ Moisturize frequently with less greasy lotions between soak-and-smear treatments
  - ▹ Use only mild soaps when necessary
  - ▹ Apply topical corticosteroids to localized plaques; taper off the steroids as the plaques clear
  - ▹ Use oral corticosteroids only in very severe cases (there is the potential for a rebound effect upon discontinuation)
  - ▹ Use topical or oral antibiotics directed against *S aureus* for superinfection

- ◦ Smallpox (variola major) has theoretically been eradicated since 1977, but is mentioned here due to its potential as a bioterrorism threat (smallpox was fatal in up to 40% of untreated patients)
  - ▸ Characterized by fever, severe headache and backache, and enanthem followed by exanthem

- Lesions progress simultaneously from erythematous macules to papules to vesicles, and finally pustules, which crust and collapse
  - This progression takes approximately 2 weeks
  - The lesions first appear on the palms and soles, then spread to the face and extremities (Figure 34-13)
  - By contrast, varicella (chickenpox) presents with lesions in varying stages of development (macules, papules, vesicles, crusts) and tends to involve the trunk and face preferentially
    - Varicella lesions evolve from vesicle to crust within 24 hours
    - Varicella can be identified at the bedside with a Tzanck smear, but a smear for direct fluorescent antibody staining and a viral culture confirm the diagnosis
  - Smallpox can be definitively diagnosed by viral culture, polymerase chain reaction, or electron microscopy; however, based on clinical suspicion, patients thought to have smallpox should be isolated, receive supportive care, and should be attended only by properly vaccinated healthcare workers
  - Smallpox is spread by respiratory route and patients are infectious from the onset of enanthem until about 10 days after the eruption begins (lesions are crusted)
  - Patients with varicella should also receive supportive care, but 20 mg/kg tid acyclovir over 5 days may speed recovery if initiated within 24 hours of the appearance of the eruption
    - Acyclovir should always be given to children > 13 years old and to any child with a history of atopic dermatitis
    - **Aspirin should never be given to varicella patients because of the risk of Reye's syndrome (fulminant hepatitis and encephalopathy)**

- Purpura in children
  - Henoch-Schönlein purpura (anaphylactoid purpura or allergic vasculitis; Figure 34-14) is the most common leukocytoclastic vasculitis in children ages 4–8 years old

(predominantly males)

- The trigger is often viral infection or streptococcal pharyngitis, as well as food, drugs, and lymphoma
- The rash is characterized by palpable purpura on the arms, legs, and buttocks
    - Patients can also have mild fever, abdominal colic, bloody stools, and arthralgias
    - Renal involvement with microscopic or gross hematuria is seen in half of patients, and a small percentage of patients go on to develop renal failure
    - Fatal pulmonary hemorrhage complicates rare cases
- Diagnosis is clinical
- Typically lasts 6–16 weeks
- Treatment is supportive, though oral corticosteroids can be given for abdominal pain
    - IVIG can be used in extreme cases
    - Nonsteroidal antiinflammatory drugs should be avoided (they may exacerbate renal or gastrointestinal problems)

- Purpura fulminans is a rapid, dramatic, and often fatal reaction seen in children (Figure 34-15)
    - The appearance of widespread ecchymoses on the extremities, followed by frank acral necrosis, is characteristic
    - DIC typically follows an infectious process, such as scarlet fever, meningitis, pneumonia, or superinfected varicella
    - Treatment is supportive and best managed in the intensive care unit
    - Many patients die from this complication and others require amputations

- **Necrosis in children**
    - Necrotizing fasciitis, or "flesh-eating bacteria," is most commonly caused by β-hemolytic streptococci, though other organisms, both aerobic and anaerobic, can be causative
    - Bacteria typically enter through a surgical or puncture wound, but necrotizing fasciitis may also occur de novo

  - Within 24–48 hours, as the bacteria spread along fascial planes and destroy tissue, the involved skin progresses from red, painful edema to dusky blue, anesthetic skin, with or without serosanguineous blisters
  - An early clue is tenderness outside the area of cellulitis
  - By the fourth or fifth day, the purple areas become gangrenous
  - Patients present in severe pain and are often hypotensive with leukocytosis
  - Mortality is around 20%
  - Prompt surgical intervention is necessary to conserve tissue and preserve the life of the patient
  - Neonatal necrotizing fasciitis most commonly affects the abdominal wall and incurs a higher mortality rate than fasciitis in adults
- **Disseminated intravascular coagulation**
  - Presents with widespread intravascular coagulation and, in two thirds of patients, skin eruption of petechiae and ecchymoses with or without hemorrhagic bullae
  - Purpura fulminans may supervene (see page 426)
  - Can be due to a number of disorders, including sepsis, arthropod venom, obstetric complications, and acidosis
  - Supportive care and replacement of appropriate coagulation factors (including vitamin K and IV heparin) are necessary for these patients
- **Anthrax**
  - May pose a bioterrorism threat, but otherwise typically occurs from the handling of animal hides or from contact with infected animals (alive or dead)
  - Patients present with a rapidly necrosing, painless eschar with suppurative regional adenitis (Figure 34-16)
  - Anthrax may be cutaneous (most common), inhalational, or gastrointestinal
  - Cutaneous anthrax begins as an inflamed papule at the inoculation site
    - The papule progresses to a bulla with surrounding edema
    - The bulla ruptures to leave behind a dark brown or black eschar, surrounded by vesicles over a red, hot, swollen base

- Although regional lymph nodes may be tender, the anthrax lesion itself is painless
- In about 20% of untreated cases, patients may develop high fever, prostration, and death over days to weeks
- Diagnosis is made by identifying the gram-positive bacillus in smears or culture (Figure 34-17)
- Treat early with ciprofloxacin or doxycycline for 60 days
  - If the child is < 2 years old, treat intravenously
  - Asymptomatic exposed individuals should be given 6 weeks of prophylactic doxycycline or ciprofloxacin

Further Reading

1. **www.learnderm.org**. Tutorial takes approximately 1½ hours and encompasses the essentials of the skin examination, including describing morphology and recognizing patterns of distribution and configuration.
2. **www.visualdx.com**. From any US military computer, click on the login tab (US military has purchased access). Comprehensive source of skin lesion photos. May enter diagnosis or key words to search to get a visual differential.

Figures 34-1 to 34-17 follow

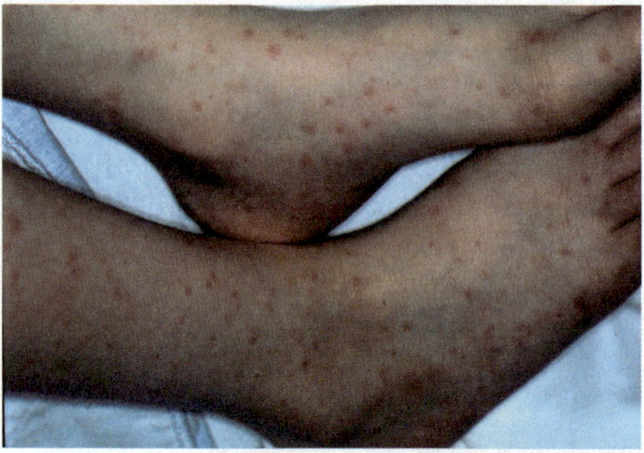

figure 34-1

figure 34-2

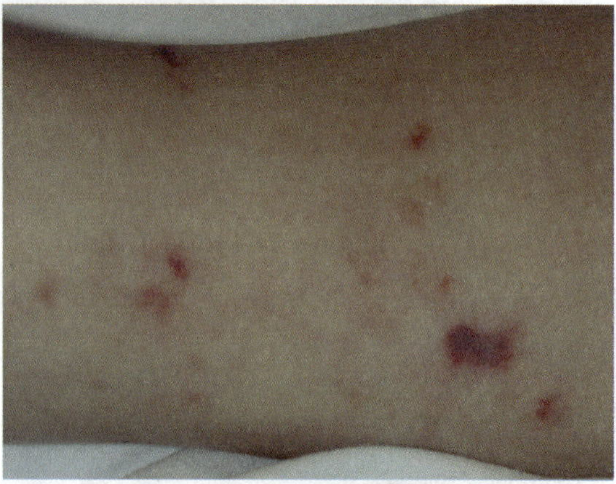

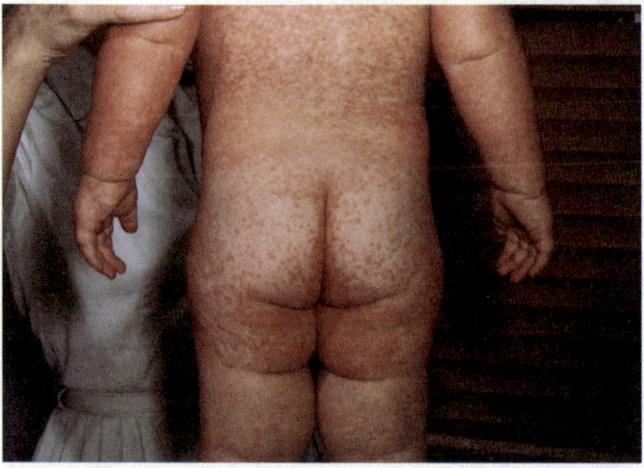

figure 34-3

Figure 34-1. This 9-year-old boy developed a red, partially blanching, papular eruption on his hands and feet, including his palms and soles, that progressed to the trunk over 3 days. He had a severe headache, high fever, arthralgias, and myalgias. His mother, who remembered removing a wood tick from her son's scalp 10 days earlier, also developed a rash, fever, and headache.
Reproduced with permission from: Dermatlas.org. http://www.dermatlas.org. Copyright Bernard Cohen, MD, 2001. Image rmsf_1_010907.

Figure 34-2. This 7-year-old boy developed a severe headache, fever, and a palpable purpuric rash on his arms and legs. He complained of nausea and severe episodic pain in his arms and legs. A blood culture grew *Neisseria meningitidis* within 24 hours, and broad-spectrum antibiotic coverage was switched to high-dose penicillin. He was afebrile and feeling much improved 2 days later. Note the irregularly shaped and angulated character of the purpuric papules, some of which showed central necrosis.
Reproduced with permission from: Dermatlas.org. http://www.dermatlas.org. Copyright Bernard Cohen, MD, 2002. Image meningococcemia_1_020403.

Figure 34-3. This child with measles is showing the characteristic red blotchy rash on his buttocks and back during the third day of the rash. Measles is an acute, highly communicable viral disease with prodromal fever, conjunctivitis, coryza, cough, and Koplik spots on the buccal mucosa. A red blotchy rash appears around day 3 of the illness, first on the face, then becoming generalized.
Reproduced from: Centers for Disease Control and Prevention Public Health Image Library Web site. http://phil.cdc.gov. Accessed November 12, 2009. Image 4497.

figure 34-4

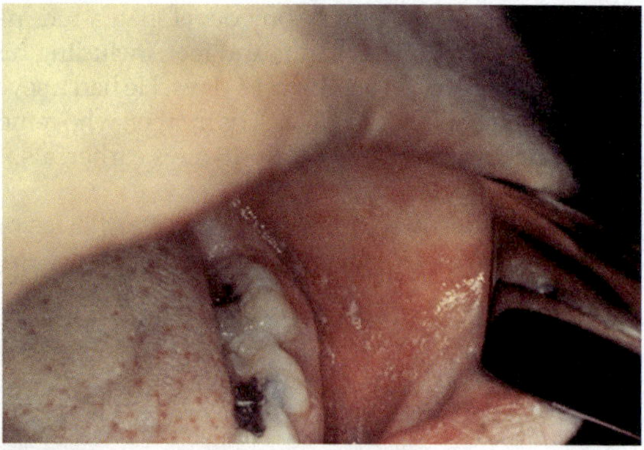

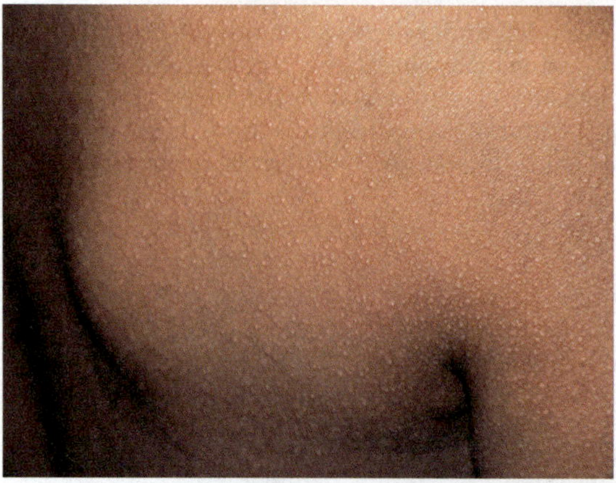

figure 34-5

figure 34-6

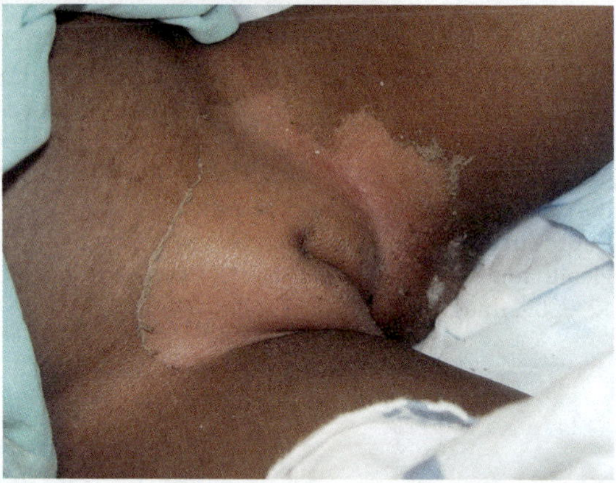

Figure 34-4. This individual with measles is displaying red Koplik spots on his buccal mucosa during the third day of the rash. Koplik spots occur 1–2 days before to 1–2 days after the cutaneous rash. Their presence is considered to be pathognomonic for measles, and they appear as punctate blue-white spots on the bright red background of the oral buccal (cheek) mucosa.
Reproduced from: Centers for Disease Control and Prevention Public Health Image Library Web site. http://phil.cdc.gov. Accessed November 12, 2009. Image 4500.

Figure 34-5. Scarlet fever. This 5-year-old boy had a 5-day history of sore throat and fever. He developed a generalized, fine, sandpaper-like rash on day 4 of illness. He also had red, swollen tonsils, and palatal petechiae. The case was prepared by University of Mississippi year 4 medical student, P Holland Alday.
Reproduced with permission from: Dermatlas.org. http://www.dermatlas.org. Copyright Will Sorey, MD, 2008. Image scarlatina_1_081007.

Figure 34-6. This previously healthy 4-year-old girl developed high fever for 6 days, widespread scarlatiniform eruption, tender right anterior cervical adenopathy, conjunctival injection, red swollen hands and feet, strawberry tongue, and a peeling, scaly, red diaper dermatitis. She began receiving intravenous immunoglobulin 4 hours before the images were taken, and her mother thought that her symptoms were already improving.
Reproduced with permission from: Dermatlas.org. http://www.dermatlas.org. Copyright Bernard Cohen, MD, 2004. Image kawasaki_2_040112.

figure 34-7

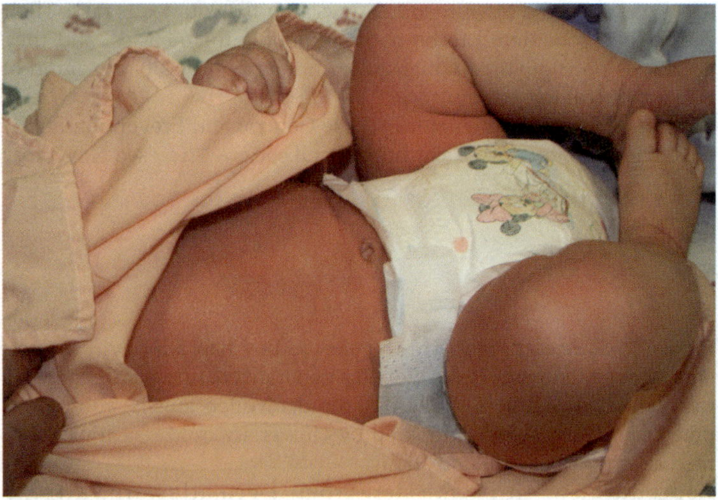

figure 34-8

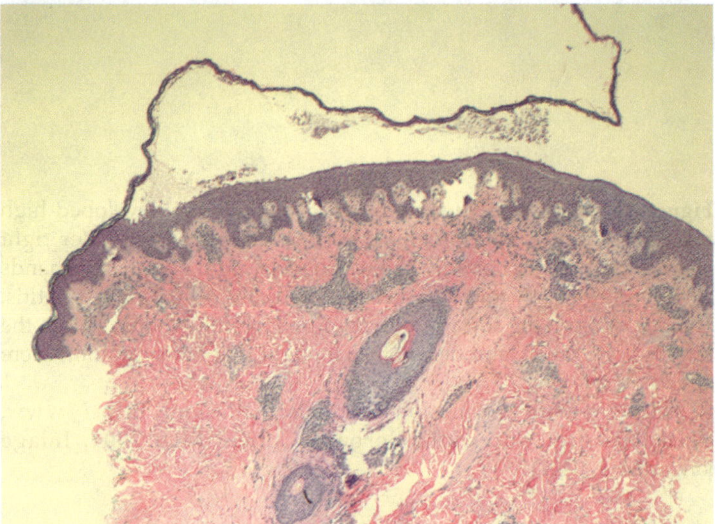

Figure 34-7. Staphylococcal scalded skin syndrome. This previously healthy 6-month-old girl developed a low-grade fever, increased fussiness, and generalized erythema with scaling, crusting, and fissuring accentuated around the mouth and skin creases. An erosion appeared after her mother placed her on the examining table, typical of a Nikolsky sign. Methicillin-sensitive *Staphylococcus aureus* grew from a skin culture taken from her nares. She did well on oral antibiotics, acetaminophen, and topical emollients, with drying of the crusts and clearing of the erythema in 2 days and diffuse desquamation 5 days later.
Reproduced with permission from: Dermatlas.org. http://www.dermatlas.org. Copyright Bernard Cohen, MD, 2009. Image staphylococcal_scalded_skin_syndrome_4_090120.

Figure 34-8. Staphylococcal scalded skin syndrome. This 15-year-old patient developed an erythematous eruption over her face, neck, and trunk, which spread to her extremities. Denudation followed. This patient is a little old for staphylococcal scalded skin syndrome, but it may occur in adults. The histology includes a superficial blister in a subcorneal location, caused by a toxin to desmoglein 1. Because of the pathophysiology, the histologic differential diagnosis includes pemphigus foliaceus and bullous impetigo. Staphylococcal scalded skin syndrome is usually paucicellular, more so than in this case, but inflammation may ramp up in older lesions. Few acantholytic cells are evident in the cleft, as are a few inflammatory cells and serum.
Reproduced with permission from: Dermatlas.org. http://www.dermatlas.org. Copyright Greg Hosler, MD, PhD, 2008. Image staph_scalded_skin_2_080801.

figure 34-9

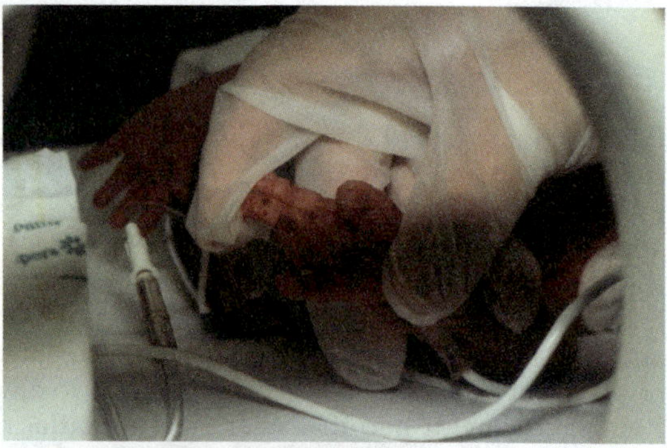

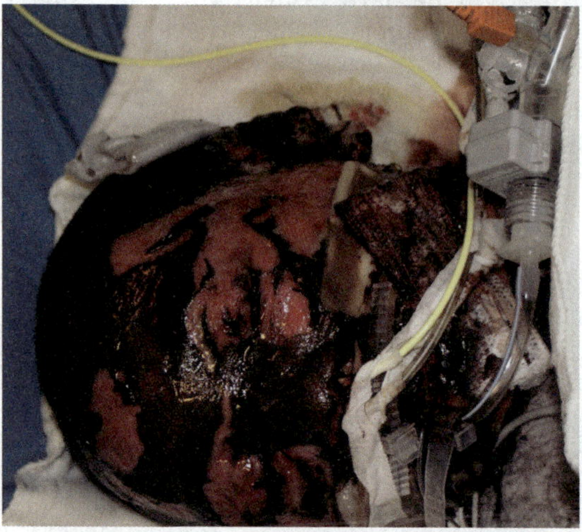

figure 34-10a

figure 34-10b

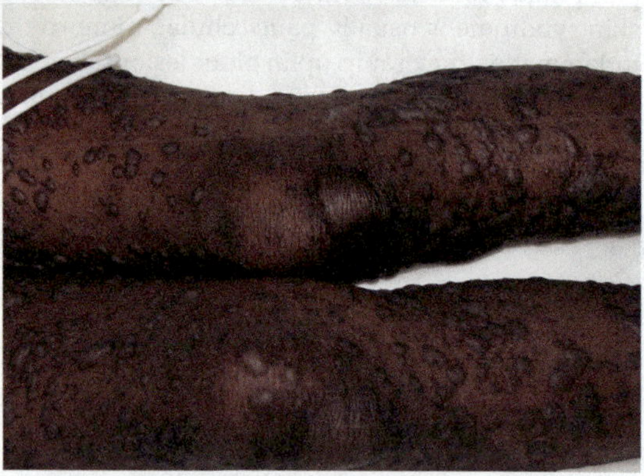

Figure 34-9. This premature infant had grouped vesicles on one hand and both feet at birth. A Tzanck smear was positive and a viral culture confirmed the diagnosis of neonatal herpes simplex virus infection. Reproduced with permission from: Dermatlas.org. http://www.dermatlas.org. Copyright Bernard Cohen, MD, 2005. Image newborn_herpes_simplex_2_050501.

Figure 34-10. (**a**) This previously healthy 10-year-old boy had a seizure and was started on oral phenytoin. Three weeks later, he developed conjunctivitis and oral mucositis. Note the Nikolsky sign with widespread erosions triggered by general skin care.
Reproduced with permission from: Dermatlas.org. http://www.dermatlas.org. Copyright Bernard Cohen, MD, 2006. Image ten_3_060424.

Figure 34-10. (**b**) Within 48 hours, he blossomed with confluent erosions above the waist and necrotic vesicles and bullae on the legs and feet.
Reproduced with permission from: Dermatlas.org. http://www.dermatlas.org. Copyright Bernard Cohen, MD, 2006. Image ten_1_060424.

figure 34-11

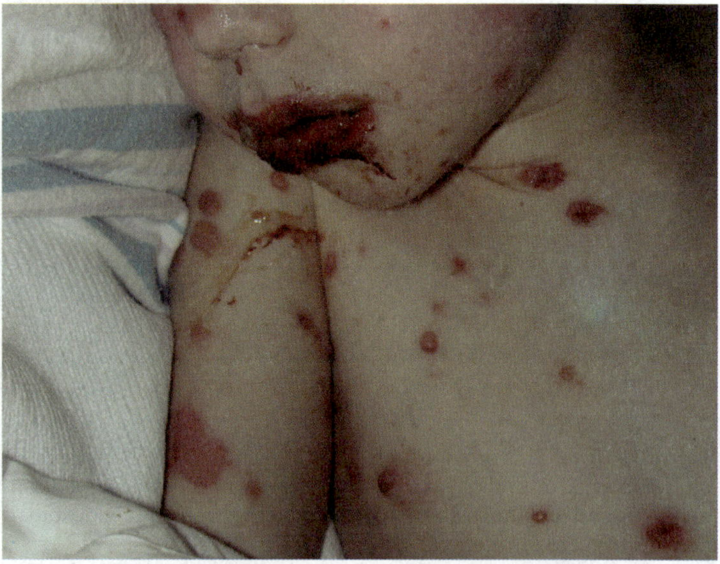

figure 34-12

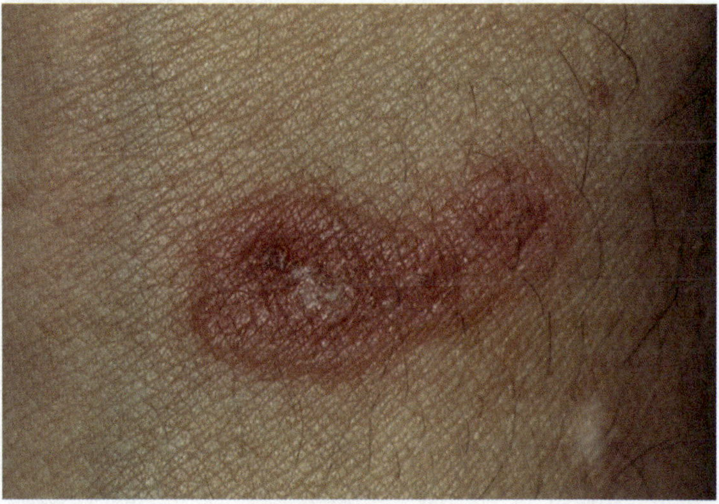

Figure 34-11. This 6-year-old boy developed a fever and pneumonitis with a left lingular infiltrate on chest x-ray. Ten days later, he complained of red itchy eyes, blisters in his mouth and red macules, some with central bullae, on the upper trunk, face, scalp, and extremities, including the palms and soles. Lesions progressed for 5 days before drying and healing with postinflammatory hyperpigmentation. He had no history of medication exposure before the illness, and mycoplasma titers were consistent with an acute infection.
Reproduced with permission from: Dermatlas.org. http://www.dermatlas.org. Copyright Bernard Cohen, MD, 2003. Image sjs_1_030223.

Figure 34-12. Erythema multiforme. A 16-year-old boy blossomed episodically with expanding red papules with central crust and bullous borders on his extremities, including palms and soles. Lesions appeared about twice a year and often involved the mouth as well. Skin biopsy of one of the arm lesions showed erythema multiforme, and culture of oral vesicles before one of the episodes yielded herpes simplex virus.
Reproduced with permission from: Dermatlas.org. http://www.dermatlas.org. Copyright Bernard Cohen, MD, 2001. Image em_2_010205.

figure 34-13

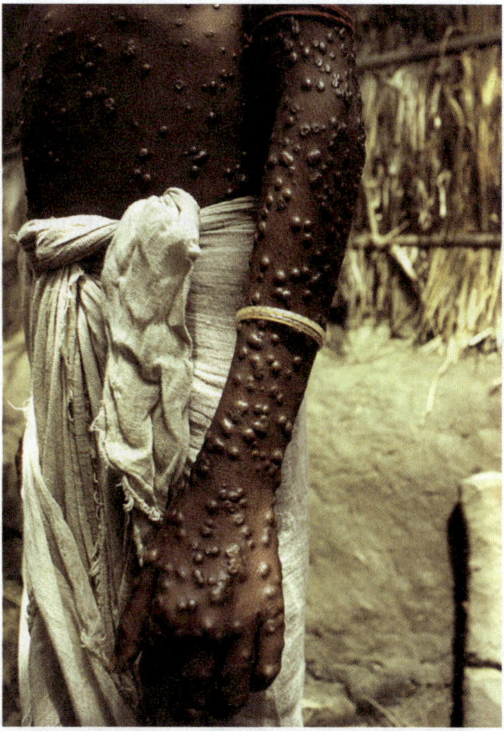

figure 34-14

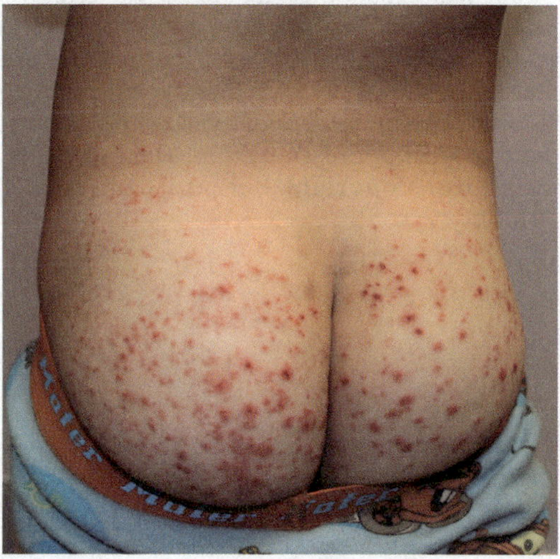

Figure 34-13. Smallpox. Depicted in this 1974 photograph is a Bengali boy who was an inhabitant of a Bangladesh village. As evidence from this image, he had sustained the ravages of smallpox, with the classic maculopapular rash evident on his torso and arm.
Reproduced from: Centers for Disease Control and Prevention Public Health Image Library Web site. Photograph courtesy of Jean Roy. http://phil.cdc.gov. Accessed November 12, 2009. Image 10661.

Figure 34-14. This previously healthy 4-year-old boy developed palpable purpuric lesions on his extremities, face, and buttocks 2 weeks after an upper respiratory infection. He subsequently experienced swelling of his ankles and wrists, colicky abdominal pain, and hematuria. His skin eruption and associated symptoms recurred for 3 weeks before resolving without complications.
Reproduced with permission from: Dermatlas.org. http://www.dermatlas.org. Copyright Bernard Cohen, MD, 2008. Image henoch_schonlein_purpura_10_080209.

figure 34-15

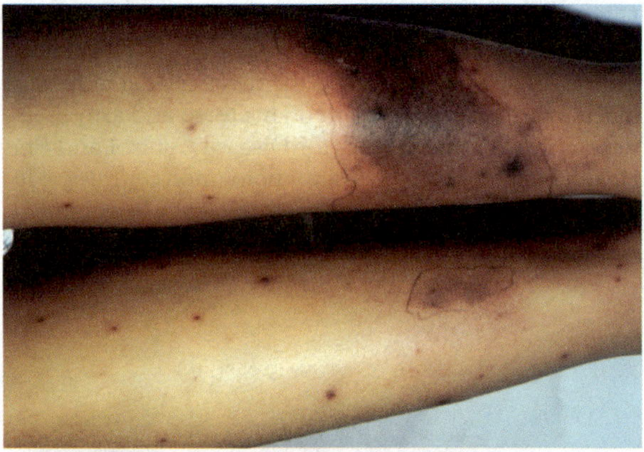

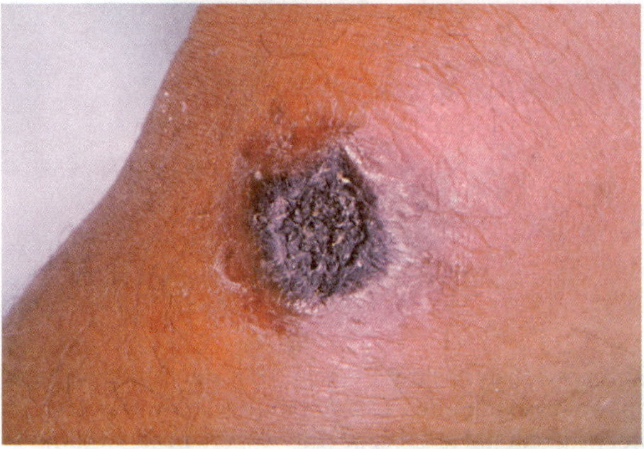

figure 34-16

figure 34-17

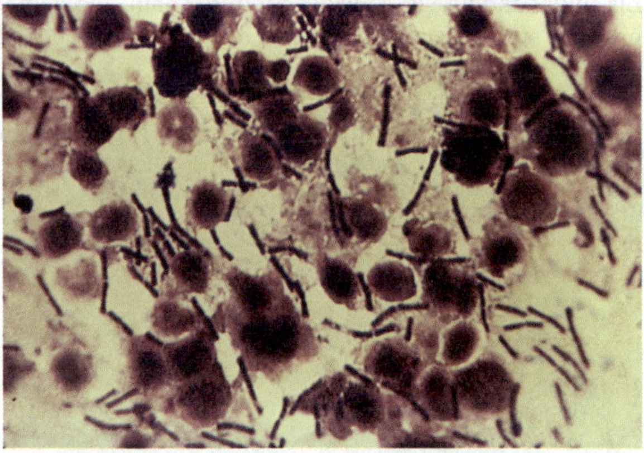

Figure 34-15. A healthy 10-year-old girl developed large expanding ecchymoses on her legs while she was recovering from varicella. She also bled into healing varicella crusts. Although she appeared well, she developed a high fever and laboratory signs of disseminated intravascular coagulation. A skin culture obtained from the crusted papules in the large ecchymoses grew Group A β-hemolytic streptococcus. She was treated with parenteral antibiotics and fluid resuscitation, and fortunately recovered without complications. The day after her admission to the hospital, a new systolic murmur was noted, and a subsequent echocardiogram showed a large clot in the ascending aorta. This also resolved uneventfully.
Reproduced with permission from: Dermatlas.org. http://www.dermatlas.org. Copyright Bernard Cohen, MD, 2001. Image purpurafulminans_1_010729.

Figure 34-16. Anthrax lesion on the skin of the forearm caused by the bacterium *Bacillus anthracis.* Here the disease has manifested itself as a cutaneous ulceration, which has begun to turn black, hence the origin of the name "anthrax," after the Greek name for coal.
Reproduced from: Centers for Disease Control and Prevention Public Health Image Library Web site. Photograph courtesy of James H Steele. http://phil.cdc.gov. Accessed November 12, 2009. Image 2033.

Figure 34-17. Photomicrograph of *Bacillus anthracis;* anthrax.
Reproduced from: Centers for Disease Control and Prevention Public Health Image Library Web site. http://phil.cdc.gov. Accessed November 12, 2009. Image 1811.

Chapter 35

Emergency Nutrition for Sick or Injured Infants and Children

Introduction

The goal of nutritional therapy in a critically ill infant or child is to provide sufficient calories and protein to spare mobilization of body reserves, prevent catabolism, promote wound healing, and protect from infection (Tables 35-1–35-3). In the initial phase of trauma or illness, metabolic rate decreases and the body becomes catabolic. As the patient becomes more stable, exogenous calories and protein can be used to promote anabolism. It is important to avoid both underfeeding, which can compromise healing, and overfeeding, which can lead to refeeding syndrome (see page 447).

Table 35-1. Average Weights and Heights for Age and Gender

	Males		Females	
Age	Length/Height (cm)	Weight (kg)	Length/Height (cm)	Weight (kg)
2–6 mo	62	6	62	6
7–12 mo	71	9	71	9
1–3 y	86	12	86	12
4–8 y	115	20	115	20
9–13 y	144	36	144	37
14–18 y	174	61	163	54
19–30 y	177	70	163	57

Table 35-2. Enteral and Oral Nutritional Needs (Nonspecific Range) in Infants and Children

Age (y)	Calories (per kg)	Protein (g/kg)	Distribution of kcals		
			Fat	Protein	Carbohydrate
0–1	80–120	2.5–3.5	35%–45%	8%–15%	45%–65%
1–10	60–90	2.0–2.5	30%–35%	10%–25%	45%–65%
11–18	30–75	1.5–2.0	25%–30%	12%–25%	45%–65%

Table 35-3. Parenteral Nutritional Needs (Nonspecific Range) of Infants and Children

Age (y)	Calories (per kg)	Protein (g/kg)	Distribution of kcals		
			Fat	Protein	Carbohydrate
0–1	80–120	2.0–2.5	35%–45%	8%–15%	45%–65%
1–10	60–90	1.7–2.0	30%–35%	10%–25%	45%–65%
11–18	30–75	1.0–1.5	25%–30%	12%–25%	45%–65%

Calories and Protein Needs

- Calorie needs are generally lower in extremely ill children than in healthy ones because of their lack of activity and catabolic state, which inhibits use of calories for growth; calorie needs will increase as the infant or child becomes stable
- Protein needs are elevated in sick infants and children, particularly those with open wounds, burns, or losses such as in diarrhea or ostomy output (Tables 35-4 and 35-5)

Table 35-4. World Health Organization's Equations for Estimating Resting Energy Expenditures*

Age (y)	Resting Energy Expenditure (kcal/day)	
	Males	Females
0–3	(60.9 × weight [kg]) – 54	(61.0 × weight [kg]) – 51
3–10	(22.7 × weight [kg]) + 495	(22.5 × weight [kg]) + 499
10–18	(17.5 × weight [kg]) + 651	(12.2 × weight [kg]) + 746

*Use in combination with an activity factor and stress factor to determine total energy expenditure.

Data source: World Health Organization. *Energy and Protein Requirements: Report of a Joint FAO/WHO/UNU Consultation*. Geneva, Switzerland: WHO; 1985. Technical Report 724.

- Calorie and protein needs are best calculated using the child's weight
  - If actual weight is not available, use the average weight for the child's age, or measure the patient's length and use the corresponding average weight (see Table 35-1)
    - **Note**: using average or ideal weights when calculating energy needs in severely malnourished patients can lead to serious metabolic intolerance (see Refeeding Syndrome and Overfeeding)

Table 35-5. Effects of Activity Factors and Stress Factors on Energy Requirements in Children

Type of Activity Factor	Multiply REE by
Nonambulatory, intubated, sedated	0.8–0.9
Bed rest	1.0–1.15
Mildly ambulatory	1.2–1.3
Type of Stress Factor	**Multiply REE by**
Starvation	0.70–0.9
Surgery	1.1–1.5
Sepsis	1.2–1.6
Closed head injury	1.3
Trauma	1.1–1.8
Growth failure	1.5–2.0
Burns	1.5–2.5
Cardiac failure	1.2–1.3

REE: resting energy expenditure

- Total Energy Expenditure (TEE) = Resting Energy Expenditure (REE) × Activity Factor (AF) × Stress Factor (SF) (see Tables 35-4 and 35-5)
  - **Example:** 4-year-old male who is paralyzed, has a closed head injury, and weighs 15.9 kg

$$\text{REE} = (22.7 \times 15.9) + 495 = 855 \text{ kcals}$$

$$\text{REE x } 0.8 \text{ AF} \times 1.3 \text{ SF} = 889 \text{ kcals}$$

Refeeding Syndrome

- Refeeding syndrome occurs when a malnourished patient is rapidly refed
  - Catabolism of fat and muscle leads to loss of lean muscle mass, water, and minerals, with total-body depletion of phosphorus (serum levels may remain normal)
  - When carbohydrates are given, insulin is released, enhancing uptake of glucose and phosphorus and increasing protein synthesis
  - This leads to a deficiency in phosphorus-containing compounds, which results in cardiac and neuromuscular dysfunction, anemia, and acute ventilatory failure
  - Potassium and magnesium stores may also become depleted; replace electrolytes as needed

- If laboratory data are not available, physical signs include muscle weakness, labored breathing, seizures, diarrhea, retching, and volume overload (Table 35-6)

Table 35-6. Metabolic Disturbances and Symptoms Associated With Refeeding Syndrome

Metabolic Disturbance	Symptoms
Hyperglycemia	Polyuria, polydypsia, polyphagia, weight loss, weakness, fatigue, blurred vision
Hypoglycemia	Decreased consciousness, sweating, anxiety, shakiness, palpitations, weakness, hunger, faintness, headaches, tremor, tachycardia
Hypophosphatemia	Respiratory failure, pyorrhea, fatigue, nervous disorders
Hypokalemia	Cardiac arrhythmia, muscle weakness, nocturia, elevated blood pressure or hypotension, atonia, paraesthesia, hyporeflexia
Hypomagnesemia	Seizure, muscle cramps, tetany, tremor, weakness, vertigo, dysphagia, confusion, hypocalcemia

- Treatment
  - Prevent by recognizing patients at risk
  - Slowly increase rate and concentration of carbohydrate delivery, maintain hydration, and measure electrolytes and blood glucose frequently; correct abnormalities
  - When beginning total parenteral nutrition (TPN) or tube feeding (TF), slowly increase the number of goal calories given per day
    - Give 50% of the patient's goal calories on day 1 of TPN or TF
    - Give 75% of goal calories on day 2 of TPN or TF
    - Give 100% of goal calories on day 3 of TPN or TF
  - With TPN patients, maintain a favorable distribution of calories from protein, carbohydrates, and fats

Overfeeding

Overfeeding can occur in any patient who is being fed more calories than needed. Overfeeding can cause metabolic and respiratory stress leading to hyperglycemia, diarrhea, tachypnea, carbon dioxide retention, and failure to wean off ventilation.

Because calculations for estimating energy needs are not exact, signs of overfeeding should always be considered whenever a patient is on nutrition support.

Tube Feedings

- Use an age-appropriate TF product, if available
  - Standard adult formulas are acceptable in children > 1 year old and can be used if they are the only type available
    - Protein content will be 1½–2-fold that of pediatric products
    - Avoid exceeding 4 g of protein per kilogram (higher protein concentrations will stress the kidneys; be sure fluid intake is adequate)
  - Minimum calories can usually be met, even while giving the maximum amount of protein
  - Additional calories can be given using vegetable oil (100 kcal/15 mL) and sugar (48 calories per 15 mL) or intravenous (IV) dextrose
- Goal rate for enteral feedings depends on caloric and fluid needs (Table 35-7)
  - If the patient is on IV fluids, adjust volume
  - Enteral feeds are advanced so calculated fluid requirements are not exceeded

Table 35-7. Guidelines for Initiating and Advancing Continuous Enteral Feeding

Age (y)	Initial Infusion	Incremental Advances
0–1	1–2 mL/kg/h	10–20 mL/kg/day
1–6	1 mL/kg/h	1 mL/kg q 2–8 h
>7	10–25 mL/h	20–25 mL q 2–8 h

*Hourly infusion increases incrementally until goal calories are achieved.

Breast-Feeding

- Whenever possible, give breast milk (orally or enterally) rather than commercial formulas, particularly if powdered formulas need to be reconstituted with potentially contaminated water
- Breast milk can routinely be given to children up to age 2 or older and occasionally to children as old as 5 or 6
- If clean equipment is available to obtain pumped breast milk,

additional calories and protein can be added to expressed milk if the volume of the milk or the child's volume tolerance is limited

- If formula is necessary, the standard powdered infant type is recommended
  - One scoop (8–9 g) of infant formula powder added to 8 ounces of pumped breast milk will yield 24 calories per ounce
  - If necessary, add a carbohydrate from a clean source, such as granulated sugar (2 teaspoons per 8 oz breast milk will yield 24 calories per ounce)

Nutrient Needs in Specific Conditions

- Burns, open wounds, gunshot wounds, and fragment injuries
  - Give the mid- to upper range of calories (see Table 35-5)
  - Give the high value of protein
  - Supplement with vitamin C and zinc if available (otherwise use a standard multivitamin-mineral supplement)
- Ventilated, sedated, or paralyzed patients
  - Use lower-end calorie values (see Table 35-5)
  - Give goal protein value
- Sepsis
  - Give the midrange calorie value and goal protein
  - If the patient is febrile, use the upper-range calorie value and goal protein (see Table 35-5)
- Amputation

Table 35-8. Parenteral Electrolyte Needs

Electrolyte	Infants/Toddlers (Birth–2 y)	Children (2–11 y)	Adolescents (≥ 12 y)
Sodium	2–5 mEq/kg/day	3–5 mEq/kg/day	60–150 mEq/day
Potassium	1–4 mEq/kg/day	2–4 mEq/kg/day	70–180 mEq/day
Chloride	2–3 mEq/kg/day	3–5 mEq/kg/day	60–150 mEq/day
Calcium	0.5–4.0 mEq/kg/day	0.5–3.0 mEq/kg/day	10–40 mEq/day
Magnesium	0.15–1.0 mEq/kg/day	0.25–1.0 mEq/kg/day	8–32 mEq/day
Phosphorus	0.5–2.0 mmol/kg/day	0.5–2.0 mmol/kg/day	9–30 mmol/day

Table 35-9. Signs of Specific Nutrient Deficiencies

Nutrient	Deficiency Symptoms
Protein	Kwashiorkor, weakness, lethargy, edema, ascites, fatty liver, dermatitis, depigmented hair, alopecia, decubitus ulcers, moon face, muscle wasting, growth failure, hypotension, cheilosis, stomatitis, delayed wound healing
Protein/ energy	Marasmus; dry, dull hair; drawn-in cheeks; carious teeth; ascites; diarrhea; weakness; irritability; increased appetite; muscle wasting; growth failure; other vitamin deficiencies
Fat/EFAs	Xerosis; flaking; scaly skin; dermatitis; follicular hyperkeratosis; dry, dull hair
Vitamin A	Eggshell nails, night blindness, dermatitis, taste changes, xerosis, keratomalacia
Vitamin C	Decubitus ulcers, perifolliculitis, petechiae, bleeding gums, swollen gums, stomatitis, bone pain, dry or rough pigmented skin, poor wound healing, anemia
Vitamin D	Rickets, bowed legs, prone to fractures, restlessness, frequent crying, sweating, muscular atony, weakness, scoliosis, back pain, bone pain, spinal changes
Calcium	Weight loss, muscle weakness, bone pain, skeletal deformities
Vitamin B_{12}	Megaloblastic anemia, scarlet tongue, fatigue, weight loss, jaundice, oral mucosa ulcerations, dementia, sensory loss, yellow skin pallor, hypertrophy, gait sensory ataxia
Iron	Fatigue, weight loss, glossitis, stomatitis, tachycardia, tachypnea, thin or spoon-shaped nails
Zinc	Delayed wound healing, alopecia, night blindness, taste changes, decubitus ulcers, delayed wound healing, dermatitis, erythema, xerosis
Iodine	Goiter, outer third of eyebrow missing
Thiamine	Edema, weakness, irritability, burning feet, pruritus, nausea, vomiting, anorexia, muscle wasting, muscle tenderness and cramps, beriberi, photophobia, confusion
Niacin	Pellagra, dermatitis, diarrhea, dementia, red/scarlet tongue, erythema, depression, irritability, stomatitis, glossitis, cheilosis, hyperpigmentation
Folic acid	Megaloblastic anemia, skin pallor, stomatitis, scarlet tongue, glossitis, sensory loss, oral mucosa ulcerations
Riboflavin	Flaking, scaly dermatitis, conjunctivitis, magenta tongue, stomatitis, glossitis, cheilosis, hypertrophy

EFAs: essential fatty acids

  - If no actual weight is available, estimate needs and ideal body weight based on metabolically active tissue

Total Parenteral Nutrition

- Premixed adult TPN solutions are higher in protein and some electrolytes, such as potassium (Table 35-8)
- Calculate the maximum volume of premixed adult TPN solution to avoid excessive intakes in a pediatric patient, then titrate in additional dextrose 50% to meet estimated calorie needs
- Maintain a balanced distribution of calories from protein, carbohydrate, and fat (see Table 35-3) to maintain nutrient efficiency and to minimize hepatic damage from TPN
- Watch for signs of specific nutrient deficiencies (Table 35-9)

Chapter 36

Bites and Stings

Arthropod, insect, and snake envenomation are sources of great concern and anxiety in transient populations, but in reality are not highly life threatening. Mortality rates in humans from most venom exposures are low. In animals, venom has three purposes: (1) defense, (2) prey immobilization, and (3) digestion.

There are specific problems with envenomation in children. Smaller children do worse with envenomation than adults because the snake or arthropod injects the same amount of venom into a much smaller host. Children are also poor historians, so a reliable story of the incident may be difficult to obtain. Unnecessary procedures, such as incision and suction over wounds and tourniquets, increase morbidity.

- History
  - Focus on the following when taking a history after envenomation:
    - Timing of the event
    - Location of the bite or sting
    - Nature of what happened
    - Whether or not spiders, snakes, or scorpions have been seen in the area or home
- Physical examination

  When performing the physical examination, look at all areas of the body, paying special attention to the hands, feet, legs, buttocks, and genitalia. Look for tiny marks, erythema, and edema. Local tenderness is a sign of envenomation
- Specific sources of envenomation
  - Black widow spider
    - Found in every state except Alaska
    - Females are considerably larger than males and are responsible for all human envenomations because their teeth can penetrate human skin; they have a characteristic red hourglass on their abdomens and make irregular webs in fields

- There have been no deaths from black widow spiders in the United States in decades
- Signs and symptoms
  - The initial presentation can vary greatly; the bite can range from painless to excruciating. Pain, which will be worst in first 8–12 hours, may linger
  - Muscle fasciculations, weakness, and ptosis
  - Vomiting, salivation, hypertension, and priapism (rarely)
  - Fasciculations may be so severe that, when the abdominal muscles are involved, condition may mimic acute abdomen
- Treatment
  - Clean the bite area, ice the wound, and provide tetanus prophylaxis
  - Look for serious pain and neurological symptoms
  - Administer adjuncts for symptomatic treatment, such as the following:
    - Calcium gluconate (50–100 mg/kg for fasciculations; maximum dose of 2 g)
    - Muscle relaxants and benzodiazepines for severe muscle spasms
  - There is an antivenin available in the United States; however, it has been associated with serum sickness

- Brown recluse spider
  - From genus *Loxasceles*; body measures 1 cm, leg length is 2–3 cm
  - Brown with a dark violin shape on the anterior head and neck area (nicknamed "fiddle back")
  - Hides in wood piles and closets and will bite when threatened (eg, when trapped in clothes or bed linens)
  - Signs and symptoms
    - Classic lesion has an area of central necrosis within an erythematous ring
    - Venom contains hemolysin and cytotoxin
    - Bite can result in dramatic hemolysis and renal injury; envenomation can lead to renal failure or herald coagulopathy
  - Treatment

    - Check for hemoglobinuria and proteinuria in children
    - Use blood urea nitrogen, creatinine, and liver function tests as well as urinary analysis and coagulation studies for seriously ill patients
    - Provide supportive care
- Tarantula
  - Large, hairy, slow spiders
  - Will bite when threatened; depending on the size and strength of the spider, the bite can be painful, but most are only as painful as a bee sting
  - Far less dangerous than the black widow or the brown recluse
  - Some Latin American varieties have urticating hairs that they flick at prey by the thousands
  - Arabian Peninsula and Iran/Afghanistan varieties
    - Common variety is called "Camel Spider," but is actually the Near Eastern Solpugid, a nonspider arachnid
    - Maximum body size is 5 cm
    - They are nonvenomous
    - They are fast, moving at speeds up to 10 mph (if they run toward a person, they are likely trying to escape the hot sun)
    - Contrary to common belief, they do not eat the flesh of large animals
    - Bite may become secondarily infected
- Scorpion
  - Scorpions are common around the world; most bites are only as dangerous and painful as a bee sting
  - In the United States, only one indigenous scorpion, the bark scorpion (*Centruoides*), is life threatening
    - The bark scorpion is a nocturnal hunter
    - Found from southwest Texas to Arizona (there have not been any deaths related to bark scorpion stings in Arizona in over 30 y)
    - Venom contains at least five different neurotoxins
    - Signs and symptoms
      - The sting can affect the parasympathetic and sympathetic nervous systems and may also result in neuromotor effects

    - Young children are more likely to have severe cardiorespiratory symptoms
    - Up to 80% of children < 2 years old manifest with severe symptoms (as opposed to 5% of adults)
  - Treatment
    - Because children can be poor historians, it may be helpful to use a diagnostic "tap test"; tapping over the inoculation site will elicit significant pain
    - Routine wound care includes cleaning the area and administering ice and acetaminophen (for pain) as needed; the inoculation site can be injected with 1% lidocaine
    - Treat any serious respiratory or neuromuscular symptoms with supportive measures
    - A sheep-derived antivenin is available through the University of Arizona
- In the Arabian Peninsula / Iraq, there are 14 indigenous scorpion species
  - *Androctonus crassicauda*: black or dark brown
  - *Leiurus quinquestriatus*: yellow; stings more people than *Androctonus*
  - *Hemiscorpius lepturus*: caused all winter stings in an Iranian study (10%–15% of all stings overall)
  - *Mesobuthus eupeus*: venom contains a neurotoxin; caused approximately 45% of stings in Iran
  - Up to 4% of all children hospitalized in Saudi Arabia from May through August have sustained scorpion stings
  - Most envenomations occur at night, mainly in barefooted children or shepherds
  - Males are at least twice as likely as females to be stung
  - Mortality rate is 2%–5%
  - Signs and symptoms
    - Stings cause hypertension and central nervous system manifestations and are very painful
    - Generalized erythema occurs in 20%–25% of children under age 5 (unclear mechanism)
    - Cholinergic signs include exocrine gland hypersecretion, urinary frequency and incontinence, and

increased gastrointestinal motility

        - Neurological symptoms include delirium, confusion, coma, restlessness, seizures, localized muscle spasm near sting site, opisthotonus, and paralysis
    - Treatment
        - There is a polyvalent antivenin, but an Iranian case series failed to show effectiveness in humans
        - There is no antivenin available for cytotoxic venom
- Bees and wasps
    - Bees, wasps, and other stinging insects account for roughly one third of all envenomations
    - Bees are apids and sting defensively with a barbed stinger that stays in the victim; the bee dies after the sting
    - Wasps, hornets, and yellow jackets are vespids and have a smooth stinger used for hunting and protection; they can sting multiple times
    - Killer bees were imported to Brazil from Africa in 1956; they escaped captivity and have slowly been spreading north. They are aggressive and attack in swarms
    - Treatment
        - Most reactions are local and can be treated with acetaminophen and antihistamines
        - Consider steroid burst with antihistamine for large reactions
        - For anaphylaxis or anaphylactic reactions, treat with:
            - Epinephrine: 0.01 mg/kg of a 1:1,000 preparation, intramuscular; maximum pediatric dose is 0.3 mg
            - Steroids: 2 mg/kg intravenous (IV) methylprednisolone sodium succinate

              AND
            - Antihistamines: diphenhydramine 1 mg/kg IV
            - Observe for several hours for the late effects of anaphylaxis
- Fire ants
    - Venom is similar to that of bees and can be treated in much the same way
    - Found in southern United States to mid-Atlantic states

- Snakes
  - There are five families of poisonous snakes; only *Crotalidae* are common in North America (eg, rattlesnakes, water moccasins, copperheads)
  - There are 8,000 poisonous snake bites annually in the United States; only 10–15 are fatal
  - The higher venom-to-size ratio in young children means greater morbidity per bite
  - Young children tend to get bit on the lower extremities when they wander into a snake's area
  - Older children and teenagers tend to get bit on the upper extremities, presumably after trying to catch the snake
  - Treatment
    - Clean the wound
    - Remove all jewelry on affected limb
    - Treat pain, bleeding, and respiratory weakness
    - Apparent hypovolemia is due to distributive shock
    - Sheep-derived monoclonal antibody can also be used; it is associated with less serum sickness than horse-derived antibody
    - Crotalidae polyvalent immune fragment antigen binding (ovine), marketed as "CroFab" (Protherics, Inc, Nashville, Tenn), is currently the only licensed treatment for severe envenomations in the United States
      - To treat with CroFab, first mix 4–6 vials with 250 mL normal saline
      - Give 1 mL/min for the first 10 minutes
      - If the patient tolerates initial infusion, give the whole amount at 250 mL/h
      - Observe for 1 hour. If the patient's condition worsens, repeat the procedure; if not, give 2 vials IV every 6 hours for 18 hours
      - The dose does not vary based on the child's weight because the antibody is directed at the venom

Chapter 37

Heat and Cold Injuries

Cold Weather Injuries

Hypothermia is when a person's core temperature drops below 35°C. Smaller children have larger surface-area-to-mass ratios and are more susceptible to hypothermia than adults (ie, the smaller the body, the greater the susceptibility to hypothermia). Heat is lost through four mechanisms: (1) radiation, which accounts for approximately 60% of heat loss; (2) conduction, which is more of a concern with cold-water immersion or in the presence of wet clothing (clothes should be removed and the patient dried quickly); (3) convection, which increases with exposure to wind chill (eg, in the desert at night); and (4) evaporation, which accounts for 20%–25% of heat loss, usually from sweating and respiration.

- Effects on the body
  - Cardiovascular: tachycardia is the initial heat-generating protective measure, but heart rate and mean arterial pressure decrease as core temperature decreases. Atrial, then ventricular, dysrhythmias occur as the temperature decreases below 32°C
  - Neurological: neuronal enzyme activity declines with hypothermia, but cerebral perfusion pressure is maintained until temperature reaches 25°C
  - Respiratory: initial tachypnea diminishes with a steady decline in minute ventilation and eventual cold bronchorrhea, which mimics pulmonary edema
  - Renal: as peripheral vasoconstriction creates total body fluid overload, there is rapid diuresis of dilute fluid; effects are enhanced by alcohol and cold-water immersion
  - Gastrointestinal: motility is decreased, leading to constipation and ileus
- Treatment
  - Check airway, breathing, and circulation (ABCs); treat aggressively

  - Hypothermia associated with icy water immersion can lead to the diving reflex, with good neurological outcomes even after prolonged cardiopulmonary resuscitation (CPR) and rewarming
  - The cold myocardium is resistant to defibrillation; continue CPR
  - Some patients convert spontaneously when their temperature reaches above 32°C
  - Actively rewarm
    - Remove all wet clothing, dry the patient, and wrap with warm blankets (warming lights work best on exposed skin)
    - Administer warmed IV fluids and consider warm nasogastric fluids and warm rectal lavage
- Frostbite: cold damage to the skin that causes vasoconstriction and eventual tissue freezing
  - Use the same degree system as burns for classification
  - Treat by immediate immersion in warm water; however, rewarmed tissue is more susceptible to refreezing. If refreezing is likely, consider not rewarming until the patient has reached a warmer environment

Warm Weather Injuries

Heat injuries are common in soldiers deployed to Iraq and Afghanistan. Infants are predisposed to these injuries because of their high body-surface-area-to-mass ratio. Adolescents who compete in summer sporting events are also at risk. There are three types of heat illness (same as adults):

- Heat cramps
  - Muscle cramps from dilutional hyponatremia
  - No central nervous system signs
  - Treat by repleting fluids and sodium
- Heat exhaustion
  - Manifests with dizziness, nausea, vomiting, and weakness without significant change to mental status
  - Skin is moist from excessive sweating
  - Occurs with mild elevation to 39°C–40°C
  - Treat by replacing fluids and sodium
- Heatstroke

- This is a true medical emergency with a high rate of mortality; it needs to be recognized and treated promptly
- Presents as a combination of altered mental status, dry skin, and hyperpyrexia
- Complications include rhabdomyolysis, renal insufficiency, and hepatic failure
- Treatment: immediate active cooling (eg, ice to the neck and groin, fanning the skin after spraying with water, etc), administering IV fluids and diazepam to prevent shivering (which raises body heat)
- Look for and treat complications

Chapter 38

Chemical, Biological, Radiological, Nuclear, and Explosive Injuries

Background

Pediatric casualties are unavoidable in every conflict. Children are virtually certain to be among the victims of future terrorist attacks, including those potentially involving chemical, biological, radiological, nuclear, and explosive (CBRNE) agents.

Unique Considerations in the Pediatric CBRNE Victim

The saying that "children are not just small adults" is a mantra familiar to all pediatric caregivers. Perhaps nowhere is this more relevant than in the case of pediatric CBRNE victims, who differ from adults in myriad ways that make their care more problematic

- Anatomical and physiological differences
  - Children have a higher surface-area-to-volume ratio than adults, making them more susceptible to transdermal absorption and the effects of volume loss
  - Children have increased minute ventilation, a thinner and less-well-keratinized epidermis, and a less mature blood–brain barrier than adults
- Differences in disease manifestation and severity
  - In some cases, children may be more prone than adults to developing severe disease from a given agent
  - In other cases, children may simply present with different signs and symptoms
    - Venezuelan equine encephalitis, an incapacitating agent in adults, can be lethal in young children
    - Melioidosis sometimes causes a parotitis in children, but not in adults
    - Few, if any, children are immune to smallpox, but many adults may have some degree of residual immunity from long-distant vaccination

    - ▸ Radiation injury disproportionately affects rapidly growing tissues, posing a special problem for young children
- Treatment difficulties
    - Many agents routinely used to treat adults are relatively unfamiliar to those who typically care for children (eg, fluoroquinolone and tetracycline antibiotics are rarely used in young children because of possible toxicities and side effects)
    - Many of the drugs recommended for use in infants and children in this chapter are not specifically approved by the US Food and Drug Administration for those indications; in some cases the dosing is extrapolated from adult dosing
- Prophylactic difficulties
    - Certain immunizations approved for adults are not licensed for use in children (eg, anthrax vaccine adsorbed [AVA] is approved only for those 18–65 y old)
    - Some vaccines (eg, vaccinia and yellow fever) have a higher incidence of complications in children
- Developmental considerations
    - Children, who "live closer to the ground," are less able to flee in an emergency, follow the instructions of public safety personnel, and distinguish reality from fantasy (eg, repeated media broadcasts of an event may be interpreted by young children as multiple events)
    - Children may be more prone to developing posttraumatic stress disorder than adults
- Other considerations
    - Drugs and antidotes are often unavailable in pediatric (liquid) dosing forms, and medical equipment is often unavailable in sizes suitable for children
    - Hospitals may not be equipped to care for large numbers of children

Pediatric Chemical Casualties

- Background. There are hundreds of chemical agents that may be used by terrorists; this chapter deals with those "military-grade" agents that have gained widespread acceptance as potent and viable terrorist threats

- Military-grade agents
  - Nerve agents
    - Organophosphates that inhibit anticholinesterase
    - Nerve agents cause acetylcholine to accumulate at the neuromuscular junction, resulting in cholinergic crisis
    - This category can be divided into persistent nerve agents (eg, VX) and nonpersistent agents (eg, tabun, soman, and sarin)
    - Signs and symptoms
      - Symptoms can be summed up by the mnemonic **SLUDGE** (salivation, lacrimation, urination, defecation, gastrointestinal upset, and emesis)
      - Central effects include ataxia, seizures, coma, and respiratory depression
    - Laboratory findings: none are available rapidly enough to be of use in the setting of warfare or terrorism
    - Treatment: the same for children as for adults
      - Give atropine and pralidoxime chloride (2-PAM Cl) 25 mg/kg (intravenous [IV] or intramuscular [IM]) initially
      - There is no maximum dose for atropine, although experts recommend an initial dose of 0.05 mg/kg IV or IM, titrating to effect (ie, secretions are dry and the patient no longer shows signs of respiratory distress)
      - Many experts also feel that adult autoinjectors may be safely used in young children
      - Seizures should be managed with benzodiazepines (either diazepam [0.3 mg/kg] or lorazepam [0.1 mg/kg] initially, titrating to effect)
  - Blister agents (vesicants)
    - Cellular poisons widely used in World War I, as well as by the Iraqi Army during the Iran–Iraq war
    - Mustard and lewisite are the most notable
    - Signs and symptoms
      - Burning eyes, skin, and respiratory tract, with higher exposures leading to systemic effects and eventual bone marrow suppression
      - Mustard gas has a delayed onset of symptoms;

lewisite exposure manifests more rapidly

- Laboratory findings: none are available rapidly enough to be of use in the setting of warfare or terrorism
- Treatment includes rapid decontamination
  - Soap and water are fine for most casualties; diluted bleach from a standard military decontamination kit is equally effective
  - Supportive care is the hallmark of therapy, although patients with blister agent burns require less fluid than those with conventional burns

- Pulmonary agents: those intended to prevent or inhibit breathing; used extensively during World War I
  - Chlorine and phosgene are the two primary examples of pulmonary agents in use today; an additional pulmonary agent that can be inadvertently released from burning military vehicles is perfluoroisobutylene
  - Signs and symptoms: the chemical generates hydrochloric acid in the exposed victim and leads to an oxygen free-radical cascade
    - Upper-airway and conjunctival irritation develops first, followed by wheezing and pulmonary edema
    - The onset of symptoms within a few hours is an ominous finding
    - Phosgene smells of newly mown hay
  - Laboratory findings: none are specific, although monitoring blood gases or transcutaneous oxygen saturation may help guide supportive therapy
  - Treatment begins with removing the victim from the area and providing supportive care (oxygen, albuterol, and ipratropium are the mainstays of treatment)
    - Enforce bed rest for phosgene victims to prevent or help ameliorate pulmonary edema, which usually occurs 4–6 hours postexposure, but may be delayed for up to 24 hours
    - Because children are shorter than adults and these chemicals are denser than air, pediatric victims will have a proportionately higher exposure than adults in the same attack
    - Children frequently need higher doses of albuterol than adults; they are much less likely to have adverse

cardiac reactions to it
    - Corticosteroids may be required for severe bronchospasm
- Blood agents
  - Chemicals distributed through the body via blood
  - Cyanide, a volatile chemical that disperses easily in the air, is the prototypical blood agent
  - Signs and symptoms: cyanide inhibits cytochrome A3 and halts normal oxidative metabolism, leading to cellular hypoxia and acidosis; it strikes metabolically active tissues hardest, specifically the heart and brain
    - Toxicity is dose dependent, with mild exposures causing tachypnea, tachycardia, and dizziness
    - More substantial exposures lead to severe toxicity, which causes seizure, coma, apnea, cardiac arrest, and, eventually, death
  - Laboratory findings: anion gap metabolic acidosis and elevated mixed venous oxygen saturation
  - Treatment includes moving the patient to fresh air and administering a cyanide antidote kit
    - Start by administering 0.33 mL/kg (9 mg/kg) of 3% sodium or amyl nitrite (300 mg/10 mL) IV over 5 minutes (assuming a normal hemoglobin of 12 g/dL), which causes the formation of methemoglobin (which, in turn, binds cyanide ion); dosage can be adjusted based on hemoglobin levels
    - Follow by administering 1.65 mL/kg (400 mg/kg) of 25% sodium thiosulfate (12.5 g in 50 mL) IV over 10–20 minutes (12.5 g maximum dose; used by the liver to convert cyanide to thiocyanate, which is renally excreted)
    - Nitrate-induced hypotension, as well as excessive methemoglobin formation, can be hazardous to pediatric patients; **weight-based dosing of antidotes is especially important**
- Riot control agents
  - Designed to incapacitate victims rather than permanently injure them
  - Examples include *O*-chlorobenzylidene malononitrile (CS; military-grade tear gas), 1-chloroacetophenone (CN

gas; eg, mace), and capsaicin (pepper spray)

- Signs and symptoms
  - Mild exposure causes eye burning and tearing with eventual blepharospasm
  - The nose, throat, and upper airway become irritated
  - In high-dose exposures, victims' skin may blister and they may develop tracheobronchitis (eventually resulting in pulmonary edema)
- Laboratory findings are nonspecific
- Treatment for riot control agents is supportive
  - Begin by moving the victim from the contaminated area and removing potentially saturated clothing
  - For patients with pulmonary symptoms, provide supplemental oxygen as needed
  - In patients experiencing airway reactivity or wheezing, use albuterol, ipratropium bromide, and steroids as indicated

Pediatric Biological Casualties

- Background. In 1999, the Centers for Disease Control and Prevention developed a list of infectious and toxic agents that, if employed by terrorists, would pose the greatest threats to public health. "Category A" agents are those deemed to present the greatest risk. All six of these agents also routinely appear at the top of state-sponsored biological weapons threat lists
- Category A agents
  - Inhalational anthrax
    - Etiologic agent is *Bacillus anthracis*, a gram-positive, spore-forming rod
    - Signs and symptoms
      - Inhalational anthrax typically has an incubation period of 1–6 days
      - A flu-like illness ensues, with fever, myalgia, headache, and cough
      - A brief intervening period of improvement sometimes follows 1–2 days of these symptoms
      - The patient rapidly deteriorates; high fever, dyspnea, cyanosis, and shock mark this second phase
      - Hemorrhagic meningitis occurs in up to 50% of cases

    - Laboratory findings
        - Sporulating gram-positive bacilli in skin biopsy material (in the case of cutaneous disease) or in blood smears
        - Chest radiographs demonstrating a widened mediastinum in the context of fever and constitutional signs, and in the absence of another obvious explanation (such as blunt trauma or postsurgical infection)
        - Confirmation is obtained by blood culture on standard media
    - Treatment and prophylaxis: see Table 38-1
    - Infection control: standard precautions, including use of gloves, gowns, masks, and protective eyewear when contact with blood, body secretions containing blood, or other moist body substances is anticipated
- Plague
    - Etiologic agent is *Yersinia pestis*, a small safety-pin-appearing, gram-negative bacillus
    - Signs and symptoms
        - Symptoms of pneumonic plague include fever, chills, malaise, headache, and cough
        - Chest radiographs may reveal a patchy consolidation; classic clinical finding is one of blood-streaked sputum
        - Disseminated intravascular coagulation (DIC) and overwhelming sepsis typically develop as the disease progresses
        - Meningitis occurs in 6% of cases
        - Untreated pneumonic plague has a fatality rate approaching 100%
    - Laboratory findings
        - Bipolar safety-pin–staining bacilli in Gram or Wayson stains of sputum or aspirated lymph node material
        - Confirmation is obtained by culturing *Y pestis* from blood, sputum, or lymph-node aspirate
        - The organism grows on standard blood or MacConkey agar, but is often misidentified by automated systems
    - Treatment and prophylaxis: see Table 38-1

Table 38-1. Recommended Therapy and Prophylaxis for Diseases Caused by Category A Biothreat Agents

Condition	Therapy	Prophylaxis
Anthrax, inhalational*	Ciprofloxacin† 10–15 mg/kg IV q12h **OR** Doxycycline 2.2 mg/kg IV q12h **AND** Clindamycin‡ 10–15 mg/kg IV q8h **AND** Penicillin G§ 400–600k units/kg/d IV ÷ q4h	Postexposure (60-day course) Ciprofloxacin 10–15 mg/kg PO q12h **OR** Doxycycline 2.2 mg/kg PO q12h
Anthrax, cutaneous, in terrorism setting¥	Ciprofloxacin 10–15 mg/kg PO q12h **OR** Doxycycline 2.2 mg/kg PO q12h	NA
Plague	Gentamicin 2.5 mg/kg IV q8h **OR** Doxycycline 2.2 mg/kg IV q12h **OR** Ciprofloxacin 15 mg/kg IV q12h	Doxycycline 2.2 mg/kg PO q12h **OR** Ciprofloxacin 20 mg/kg PO q12h
Tularemia	Same as for plague	Same as for plague
Smallpox	Supportive care	Vaccination may be effective if given within the first several days after exposure
Botulism	Supportive care; antitoxin may halt the progression of symptoms but is unlikely to reverse them	NA
Viral hemorrhagic fevers	Supportive care; ribavirin may be beneficial in select cases	NA

IV: intravenous
NA: not applicable
PO: per os (oral)
*In a mass casualty setting where resources are severely constrained, oral therapy may need to be substituted for the preferred parenteral option. Patients who are clinically stable after 14 days can be switched to a single oral agent (ciprofloxacin or doxycycline) to complete a 60-day course. Assuming the organism is sensitive, children may be switched

(**Table 38-1** notes *continue*)

Table 38-1 notes, *continued*

to oral amoxicillin (80 mg/kg/day q8h) to complete the course. However, the first 14 days of therapy or postexposure prophylaxis should include ciprofloxacin and/or doxycycline, regardless of age. A 3-dose series of anthrax vaccine absorbed may permit shortening of the antibiotic course to 30 days.
†Levofloxacin or ofloxacin may be acceptable alternatives to ciprofloxacin.
‡Rifampin or clarithromycin may be acceptable alternatives to clindamycin as drugs that target bacterial protein synthesis. If ciprofloxacin or another quinolone is employed, doxycycline may be used as a second agent (it also targets protein synthesis).
§Ampicillin, imipenem, meropenem, or chloramphenicol may be acceptable alternatives to penicillin; they are also effective at penetrating the central nervous system.
¥10 days of therapy may be adequate for endemic cutaneous disease. However, a full 60-day course should be used in the setting of terrorism because of the possibility of a concomitant inhalational exposure.

    - Infection control: droplet precautions
- Tularemia
    - Etiologic agent is *Francisella tularensis*, a gram-negative coccobacillus
    - Signs and symptoms
        - Multiple clinical forms of endemic tularemia are known
        - Inhalational exposure in a terrorist attack would likely lead to pneumonia or typhoidal tularemia, manifest as a variety of nonspecific symptoms (eg, fever, malaise, and abdominal pain)
    - Laboratory findings
        - Most findings (pneumonia, leukocytosis) are nonspecific
        - Confirmation can be obtained by *F tularensis* culture from blood using standard media
    - Treatment and prophylaxis: see Table 38-1
    - Infection control: standard precautions (see Category A agents, Infection control)
- Botulism
    - The etiologic agent is any of seven toxins produced by *Clostridium botulinum*, a gram-positive anaerobic bacterium
    - Signs and symptoms
        - A latent period, ranging from 24 hours to several days, is required before clinical manifestations develop
        - Initial clinical manifestations include cranial nerve dysfunction, manifested as bulbar palsies, ptosis,

  - photophobia, and blurred vision owing to difficulty in accommodation
  - Symptoms progress to include dysarthria, dysphonia, and dysphagia
  - Finally, a descending symmetric paralysis develops and death may result from respiratory muscle failure
- No specific laboratory findings
- Treatment and prophylaxis: see Table 38-1
- Infection control: standard precautions (see Category A agents, Infection control, page 469)

- Smallpox
  - Etiologic agent is the Variola virus, a member of the orthopoxvirus family
  - Signs and symptoms
    - During the incubation period (7–17 days), the virus replicates in the upper respiratory tract, ultimately giving rise to a primary viremia
    - Amplification of virus occurs following seeding of the liver and spleen; a secondary viremia then develops
    - The skin is seeded during secondary viremia, and the classic exanthem of smallpox appears
    - Clinical illness begins abruptly and is characterized by fever, rigors, vomiting, headache, backache, and extreme malaise; the classical exanthem begins 2–4 days later
    - Macules are initially seen on the face and extremities
      - They progress in synchronous fashion to papules, then to pustules, and finally to scabs
      - As the scabs separate, survivors can be left with disfiguring, depigmented scars
      - The synchronous nature of the rash and its centrifugal distribution distinguish smallpox from chickenpox, which has a centripetal distribution
    - Death occurs in 30% of variola major patients
  - Laboratory findings: classic orthopoxvirus appearance can be seen on electron microscopic examination of material obtained from lesions
  - Treatment and prophylaxis: see Table 38-1
  - Infection control: strict airborne and contact precautions

- Viral hemorrhagic fevers
  - Etiologic agents include a number of ribonucleic acid (RNA) viruses belonging to one of four taxonomic families: the *Arenaviridae, Filoviridae, Flaviviridae*, and *Bunyaviridae*
  - Signs and symptoms: the diseases produced by these agents differ considerably in their clinical manifestations, severity, and modes of transmission; however, they share a propensity to cause a bleeding diathesis
  - No laboratory finding is specific; however, many patients with a viral hemorrhagic fever show evidence of DIC
  - Treatment and prophylaxis: see Table 38-1
  - Infection control: contact precautions

Pediatric Nuclear and Radiological Casualties

- Background. Pediatric nuclear and radiological casualties present a divergent scope. Nuclear casualties are those that result from the immediate effects of a nuclear detonation. A so-called "dirty bomb" scatters a radioactive source across an area in a manner similar to local fallout. Because this material is usually from an industrial source, it is "preformed," and the radiation output decays at a steady half-life rate. Nuclear fission products from detonation decay extremely rapidly. Thus, by 48 hours after the detonation, the dose rate is < 1% of the initial fallout output.

  Radiological casualties result from exposure to ionizing radiation and contamination with radioactive material. Ionizing radiation exposure, as a total body injury, may be more hazardous to a pediatric population because of children's rapid cell turnover rate. Children are also at risk because of their increased metabolism, higher caloric requirements, and baseline respiratory rates. Children have thinner skin and a larger surface-to-mass ratio, increased fluid losses secondary to burns, and are more sensitive to the volume and electrolyte deficits induced by diarrhea, nausea, and vomiting. Small physical mass makes children less tolerant of total-body radiation injury. In industrial accidents, large adults have had better survival rates than smaller adults

- Medical effects of nuclear detonation
  - Blast
    - Overpressure results in pulmonary, solid organ, and ear damage
    - The instantaneous pressure change does not allow for internal stabilization, so pressure gradients that would not ordinarily cause damage result in structural injury
      - 5 psi is sufficient to rupture eardrums
      - 15 psi can cause alveolar hemorrhage
    - Blast winds cause debris entrapment, crush injuries, translocation injury, and missile wounds
      - Nuclear detonation results in sudden hurricane-force winds sufficient to lift children and displace them into solid structures
      - Collapsed buildings and other structures can trap children
      - Disorientation because of sudden destruction of the normal environment, loss of family members, and trauma will diminish normal survival instincts
        - Children will be particularly unable to distinguish potential escape routes
        - Hiding in close quarters may offer immediate comfort, but may result in fatal entrapment
  - Thermal
    - Partial and full-thickness burns will occur from secondary fires and the direct thermal pulse
    - After the detonation of a weapon of 10 kilotons or less, most casualties who receive direct infrared burns from the thermal pulse will also receive lethal-dose irradiation
    - Infrared burns will "mature" like a sunburn and may not be immediately evident
    - Fires caused by the blast will ignite rubble and cause traditional thermal injuries, which must be treated aggressively (any concomitant irradiation injury will worsen the total prognosis for a patient with combined injuries)
    - Retinal burns will occur if a child looks directly at the

detonation (these burns result when the lens on the retina focuses on the infrared pulse)

  - Total foveal destruction may occur, resulting in permanent loss of usable vision
    - Flash blindness is a temporary condition lasting several minutes and is due to massive overstimulation of the retinal cells
    - The brilliance of the detonation, reflected in the atmosphere and off structures, can cause temporary "flash-bulb" effects at distances of tens of miles at night (during daylight, the effect still occurs but at a shorter range)

- Ionizing radiation exposure
  - Signs and symptoms
    - Deterministic effects are directly dose-related—the higher the total radiation dose, the more severe the physical effects, the sooner they are expressed, and the more severe the damage
    - Early nausea and vomiting (within 4–12 h) indicates immune system failure may occur at 5–10 weeks following exposure
    - Acute local skin erythema in the first hours after the infrared pulse indicates a high probability of lethal injury
    - Radiation dermatitis is related to effective dose
      - Erythema occurs at 6–20 Sv (600–1,200 rem)
      - Exposure to 20–40 Sv will cause the skin to ulcerate in approximately 14 days, starting in the region that received the highest dose and progressing to lower dose areas
      - Above 3,000 Sv, the skin will blister immediately; this local dose will probably be associated with a lethal radiation injury
  - Laboratory findings
    - Leukopenia may be seen within 2–4 days of radiation exposure
    - Anemia and thrombocytopenia are later findings
  - Treatment
    - The basic clinical management for children is the same

as for adults: relieve nausea and vomiting, manage pain, and control infection

- The need for acute management is generally limited to patients experiencing dose rates > 1 cGy/h
- Treat and prevent neutropenia with cytokines such as filgrastim (5 μg/kg/day subcutaneous) or sargramostim (250 mg/m²/day subcutaneous) until neutrophil recovery may prevent death from sepsis and lessen the duration of prophylactic antibiotics
- Use of broad-spectrum antibiotics is appropriate during the period of absolute neutropenia; specific infections should be treated in accordance with standard practice

- Radiological contamination
  - Contamination evaluation and therapy must never take precedence over treatment of acute injury
    - Caregivers are not at risk of irradiation from contaminated patients
    - Normal barrier clothing will significantly limit cross-contamination
  - External contamination usually occurs in the form of dust, which can be washed off the skin and clothing
    - Signs and symptoms
      - Most radioactive materials emit β particles, which, when emitted on or near the skin, cause direct cell damage; this becomes evident as the cells migrate to the surface via normal desquamation (ie, "β burns")
      - Normally there is no initial visible effect because the stratum corneum consists of dead tissue
    - Laboratory findings: standard radiac instruments (eg, Geiger counter) detect and measure γ radiation
    - Treatment and prophylaxis: thorough decontamination will prevent further injury and should be undertaken as soon as is practical
  - Internal contamination occurs when children ingest, inhale, or are wounded by radioactive material
    - Signs and symptoms: normal metabolism of the nonradioactive isotope of the same element determines the metabolic pathway of a radionuclide
      - Once a radionuclide is absorbed, it crosses capillary

membranes through passive and active diffusion mechanisms and is distributed throughout the body

- The rate of distribution to each organ is related to organ metabolism, the ease of chemical transport, and the affinity of the radionuclide for chemicals within the organ
- The liver, kidney, adipose tissue, and bone have higher capacities for binding radionuclides due to their high protein and lipid makeup
- Nursing mothers should discontinue breast-feeding when internal contamination is suspected
- Inhaled particles < 5 μm in diameter may be deposited in the alveoli and microbronchioles
  - Larger particles will be cleared to the oropharynx by the mucociliary apparatus, where they will be swallowed and processed through the digestive tract
  - Soluble particles will either be absorbed into the bloodstream directly or will pass through the lymphatic system
  - Insoluble particles, until cleared from the alveoli, will continue to irradiate surrounding tissue
- Most radioisotopes in nuclear weapons, such as plutonium, uranium, radium, and strontium, are insoluble and, when ingested, pass through the gastrointestinal tract unabsorbed
- Certain radioactive elements, such as cesium (a potassium analogue) and iodine, are readily absorbed
- Avoiding contaminated food by eating only packaged foods significantly decreases internal contamination by this route; infants, with their predilection for placing items in their mouths, must be removed from contaminated areas
- Skin is impermeable to most radionuclides, but any element that is in a water-soluble form may pass through; skin is particularly vulnerable to water containing tritium as the hydrogen moiety
- Open wounds provide a direct route for absorption
  - Wounds should be carefully examined with an appropriate radiation detector after the surrounding

skin is cleaned

- Wounds and burns create a portal for any particulate contamination to bypass the epithelial barrier
- Thorough irrigation and cleansing is mandatory to diminish uptake by this route

- Laboratory findings
  - Standard radiac instruments (eg, Geiger counter) detect and measure γ radiation; many also detect and measure α and β activity
  - These instruments are hand held and have a range of several feet
- Treatment and prophylaxis: mobilizing or chelating agents should be initiated as soon as practical when the probable exposure is judged to be significant
  - Gastric lavage and emetics can be used to empty the stomach promptly and completely after the ingestion of poisonous materials
  - Purgatives, laxatives, and enemas can reduce the residence time of radioactive materials in the colon
  - Ion exchange resins may limit gastrointestinal uptake of ingested or inhaled radionuclides (like Prussian blue)
  - Ferric ferrocyanide (Prussian blue) and alginates have been used in humans to accelerate fecal excretion of cesium-137
    - The recommended dose of Prussian blue for children is 1 g orally (PO) tid
    - Treatment should continue for a minimum of 30 days
  - Blocking agents, such as potassium iodide, must be given as soon as possible after radioiodine exposure
    - Neonates: administer 16 mg (¼ of a 65-mg tablet OR ¼ mL of the solution; **use caution**, concentrations of potassium iodide solutions vary by manufacturer)
    - 1 month–3 years old: administer 32 mg (½ tablet OR ½ mL of solution)

        - Older children: administer 65 mg (1 mL of solution)
    - Mobilizing agents are more effective the sooner they are given after the exposure to the isotope (see below)
    - Propylthiouracil (PO, 5–7 mg/kg/day divided tid) or methimazole (0.5–0.7 mg/kg/day divided tid) may reduce the thyroid's retention of radioiodine
    - Chelation agents may be used to remove many metals from the body
    - Edetate CALCIUM disodium (CaEDTA), diethylenetriaminepentaacetic acid (DTPA), dimercaprol, and penicillamine can all be used to chelate various heavy metal radioisotopes (seek formal consultation before initiating any of these complex therapies)

Toxicology Consultation

- Available by e-mail at: toxicology.consult@us.army.mil
- Other links to the teleconsultation pages within Army Knowledge Online (www.us.army.mil)
    - Deployed providers briefing (https://www.us.army.mil/suite/files/19174202)
    - Case studies (https://www.us.army.mil/suite/files/19174257)
    - Reference materials (https://www.us.army.mil/suite/files/19174300)

Chapter 39

Pharmacotherapeutics

Factors Affecting Pharmacokinetics

Many nonpediatric providers think of children as small adults, but this is not the case. As children grow, their bodies undergo changes in absorption, distribution, metabolism, and excretion; all of which affect the pharmacokinetics of drugs in this population. Many of the drugs and dosages used in infants and children are not specifically approved by the US Food and Drug Administration (FDA) for those indications of patient populations. Some of the drugs and dosages recommended in this text are not FDA approved, but are widely accepted as appropriate

- Absorption
  - Influenced by:
    - Age
    - Physiological condition
    - Drug dosage, form, and physical properties
    - Interactions with concurrent medications and foods
  - Absorption of oral drugs
    - Absorption mostly takes place in the small intestine, where pH range is 4–8
    - The pH of neonatal gastric fluid is neutral to slightly acidic, but becomes more acidic as the infant matures. It usually reaches adult values by 2 years of age, but may take as long as 6 years of age; this higher gastric pH affects the absorption of some drugs (eg, phenytoin, phenobarbital, ampicillin, nafcillin, and penicillin G)
    - Neonates have erratic, prolonged gastric emptying times and intestinal transit times, which leads to increased absorption; gastric emptying time reaches adult values by 6–8 months of age
    - Older children have faster gastric emptying and transit time, which leads to decreased absorption
    - During the first few months of life, neonates have

immature biliary function that results in a decreased amount of bile salts and decreased absorption of lipid-soluble drugs (eg, vitamin E)

        - Concurrent administration of infant formulas or milk products temporarily increases pH and may impede absorption of acidic drugs
        - Critical illness often shunts blood from the gut to the heart and brain, effectively decreasing the gut's ability to absorb medication
        - Neonates, infants, and young children should receive oral medications on an empty stomach unless the pharmacokinetics for the specific medication will be affected by the presence of food and change in pH
    - Absorption of parenteral drugs
        - Because neonates and young infants have small skeletal muscle mass and variable blood flow, the absorption of drugs administered via the intramuscular (IM) and subcutaneous (SQ) routes may be unpredictable
        - Properties of some medications influence IM absorption (eg, phenobarbital [rapid], diazepam [slow])
    - Absorption of topical drugs
        - Neonates and infants have enhanced absorption of topical drugs due to the relative thinness and the high water concentration of their skin
        - Neonates and infants possess a high proportion of body surface area (BSA) to total body mass, which can lead to systemic, toxic, and/or adverse reactions to topical agents (eg, isopropyl alcohol, steroid ointments, and hexachlorophene soaps)
- Distribution
    - Developmental changes in body composition affect drug distribution
        - Term neonate: body fluid equals 55%–70% of total body weight
        - Premature infant: body fluid equals up to 85% of total body weight
        - Adult: body fluid equals 50%–55% of total body weight
        - During the first 12 months after birth, total body fluid decreases dramatically, then gradually decreases to

adult proportions by 12 years of age
- Extracellular fluid is 40% of a neonate's weight (as opposed to 20% of adult's weight)

- Solubility in lipids versus water affects distribution of drugs and dosages
  - A higher proportion of fluid to body weight greatly enhances the distribution of water-soluble drugs
  - The low ratio of fat to muscle in children limits the distribution of fat-soluble drugs
- Plasma protein binding affects distribution; only free (unbound) drug can exert a pharmacological effect
  - Children < 3 months old have significantly less albumin and α_1-acid glycoprotein than adults; drugs that bind primarily to these proteins must be administered in reduced doses
  - Drug binding to plasma protein reaches adult levels by approximately 12 months of age
  - The affinity of plasma proteins to bind with drugs is reduced in the neonate
  - Bilirubin and free fatty acids compete with drugs for binding sites on plasma proteins and further reduce the protein-binding abilities of drugs in neonates; sulfonamides, salicylates, penicillins, and furosemide displace bilirubin from plasma proteins
- Immaturity of the blood–brain barrier in neonates results in greater drug penetration of cerebrospinal fluid (eg, aminoglycosides)

- Metabolism
  - Most drugs are metabolized in the liver
    - Neonates have a large liver (40% of body mass vs 2% in adults); therefore, they have a relatively larger surface area for metabolism
    - A neonate's immature liver and enzyme system may impede metabolism
      - Some enzymes reach adult levels at a few months of age, while others may take years
      - The ability of a child to metabolize many drugs may not be developed fully until 12–15 months of age
    - Older infants and children metabolize some drugs more

rapidly than adults (eg, carbamazepine, quinidine, phenytoin)
- Enzymatic functions mature at different ages
  - Glucuronidation (mechanism to assist the liver in eliminating toxins) is not sufficiently developed until 1 month of age
  - Standard pediatric dosages of some drugs may produce adverse or toxic reactions in neonates (eg, chloramphenicol)
  - Older infants and children can metabolize some drugs more rapidly than adults and may require larger doses to achieve a therapeutic effect
  - Intrauterine exposure to drugs may induce early development of hepatic enzymes, which will result in increased capacity to metabolize drugs
- Concurrent drug use can produce interactions that may stimulate or reduce liver enzyme activity (eg, phenobarbital can increase metabolism of phenytoin, requiring an increased dose of phenytoin)

- Excretion
  - Most drugs and metabolites are excreted in the urine
  - Renal excretion involves glomerular filtration and tubular secretion, the former being more developed at birth
  - Glomerular filtration rate reaches adult levels by 12 months of age in most full-term infants; premature infants will take longer to reach adult levels
  - Renal tubular secretion mechanisms become fully functional after glomerular filtration rate has reached adult levels
  - Maturity of the renal system and presence of renal disease can affect drug dosage requirements; renal function is much more developed in full-term neonates than in premature infants
  - Inadequate renal excretion results in drug accumulation and possible toxicity unless doses are reduced, dosing interval is increased, or both, depending on the medication

Administering Drugs to Children

- General rules
  - Pediatric medication doses should not be extrapolated from

adult doses

- There are no standardized units for pediatric drug dosing
  - Most drug dosages are expressed in mg/kg/*dose* or mg/kg/*day*; some references list the units in "mg/kg/d." The "d" may stand for dose or day. Confirm with source
- Some dosages are calculated using body surface area (BSA) in units expressed as mg/m²/dose or mg/m²/day
  - The BSA for children and adults (in m²) may be calculated using the following:

$$\sqrt{\frac{\text{Ht (cm)} \times \text{Wt (kg)}}{3{,}600}}$$

- Many drug regimens require modification because of renal insufficiency or failure; usually the dose is decreased, the dosing interval is changed, or both
- The standard method to determine renal status in children is to calculate the creatinine clearance (Cl_{Cr}) as described below (**this formula may not provide an accurate estimation of Cl_{Cr} for infants < 6 m of age or for patients with severe starvation or muscle wasting**)

$$Cl_{Cr} = (K) \times (L/S_{Cr})$$

Cl_{Cr} = creatinine clearance in mL/min/1.733 m^2
L = length in centimeters
S_{Cr} = serum creatinine concentration in mg/dL
K = constant of proportionality that is age specific (Table 39-1)

Table 39-1. Age-Specific Constant of Proportionality to Determine Creatinine Clearance

Age (y)	K
Low birth weight < 1	0.33
Full term < 1	0.45
2–12	0.55
13–21 (female)	0.55
13–21 (male)	0.70

- The change in medication regimen depends on the drug
  - Common cut-off points for regimen modification are $Cl_{Cr} \leq 70$, ≤ 50, ≤ 25, and ≤ 10 mL/minute/1.73^2
  - The lower the Cl_{Cr}, the more severe the renal insufficiency
  - Consult a pharmacist or pediatric drug reference for specific regimen changes
- Reevaluate dosages at regular intervals to ensure proper adjustment as the child develops
- Ensure that the BSA or body weight dosage is age-appropriate
- When calculating amounts per kilogram, **do not exceed the maximum adult dosage**
- **Always** double-check all computations

- Tips for administering drugs to children
  - Take a confident, positive approach; be kind but assertive
  - Allow the child some control by offering appropriate choices, such as which arm to use for an injection or the flavor of an oral drug chaser (never give the child a choice when none exists)
  - Be truthful about the pain and discomfort associated with the procedure; compare expected sensation with something the child has likely experienced before (eg, a pinch or a pinprick)
  - When explaining how long a procedure will take, remember that children generally do not fully understand the concept of time until approximately age 7–8 years of age; use terms the child can understand (eg, "by the time you count to 3, it will be over")
  - Children tend to take language literally; avoid using imprecise and potentially frightening jargon, such as, "I'll have to shoot you again," "dye" (may be confused with "die"), "put to sleep" (may be confused with euthanizing an animal), "ICU" ("I see you"), and "stool" (confused with something to sit on)
  - Because needles and syringes can produce anxiety, keep them out of the child's view until ready to administer the medication
- Oral administration
  - Check gag reflex and ability to maintain airway in the

presence of fluids; assess for nausea and vomiting
- Liquid dosage form ensures more accurate dose for children; use whenever it is available (exceptions include phenytoin, carbamazepine)
  - If only tablets are available, crush and mix with compatible syrup or food
    - Crushing may reduce the effectiveness of some drugs
    - Check with a pharmacist or consult a drug manual before crushing and mixing medications
- To administer oral drugs to infants,
  - Raise the infant's head to prevent aspiration
  - Gently press down on the infant's chin with thumb to open the infant's mouth
  - Administer the dose
    - Syringe:
      - Place the tip of the syringe in the pocket between the patient's cheek mucosa and gum
      - Administer slowly and steadily to prevent aspiration
    - Nipple: place medication in rubber nipple and allow infant to suck the contents. **Never** mix medications into a baby's bottle (if the child does not finish the entire bottle, the correct dosage will not be ingested; also, some formulas interfere with drug absorption)
    - For safety, never refer to a drug as "candy" or a "treat," even if it has a pleasant taste
  - See Table 39-2 for examples of common oral antibiotic dosing regimens

- Nasogastric route: check nasogastric residuals if giving enteral feedings that interfere with drug absorption
- Rectal
  - Be aware of the special significance of this part of the body to children
  - Toddlers in toilet training will resist the rectal route
  - Older children perceive this as an invasion of privacy and may react with embarrassment, anger, or hostility
  - To reduce a child's anxiety, explain the procedure and reassure that it will not hurt

Table 39–2. Common Oral Liquid Antimicrobial Medications Used in Children

Generic Name	Strength (mg/mL)	Average Dose (mg/kg/day)	Interval (h)	Maximum Dose
Amoxicillin	25, 40, 50, 80	Infants < 3 mo old: 20–30	12	2–3 g/day
		> 3 mo old: 25–50	8–12	
		Acute OM due to resistant *Streptococcus pneumoniae*: 80–90	12	
Amoxicillin + clavulanic acid	25, 40, 50, 80 AMX	Infants < 3 mo old: 30 AMX component	12	Use 25 mg/mL (AMX component) formulation for infants < 3 mo old
		Children < 40 kg: 25–45 AMX component	8–12	Use 4:1 (AMX:CA) formulation (25 or 50 mg AMX/mL) with tid dosing regimen
	120 AMX	> 3 mo old **and** > 40 kg with multidrug–resistant pneumococcal OM 80–90 AMX component	12	Use 7:1 (AMX:CA) or ES formulation for bid dosing regimen to avoid higher dose of CA
Azithromycin	20, 40	**URI and OM** in children > 6 mo old: 10 on day 1, followed by 5 on days 2–5	24	500 mg/day for day 1; 250 mg/day for days 2–5
		OM: 10 for 3 days	24	500 mg/day
		or 30 × 1 single dose		1,500 mg/day
		Pharyngitis in children > 2 y old: 12 for 5 days	24	500 mg/day

(**Table 39-1** *continues*)

Table 39-2 *continued*

Cephalexin	25, 50	25–100	6	4 g/day
Clarithromycin	25, 50	15	12	1 g/day
Clindamycin	15	10–30	6–8	1.8 g/day
Nitrofurantoin	5	Children > 1 mo old: 5–7	6	400 mg/day
		UTI prophylaxis: 1–2	24	100 mg/day
Penicillin V potassium	25, 50	25–50	6–8	3 g/day
Sulfamethoxazole + trimethoprim	8 TMP + 40 SMX	Children > 2 mo old: 6–12 TMP component	12	160 mg TMP component/dose
		Serious infection in children > 2 mo old: 15–20 TMP component	6–8	
Sulfasoxazole	100	Children > 2 mo old: 75 for initial dose then 120–150	4–6	6 g/day

AMX: amoxicillin
CA: clavulanic acid
ES: extra strength
OM: otitis media
SMX: sulfamethoxazole
TMP: trimethoprim
URI: upper respiratory infection
UTI: urinary tract infection

- Use the fifth finger for administration in children under 3 years old
- After administering the suppository, hold the child's buttocks together for a few minutes to prevent expulsion
- Concurrent critical illness may impair absorption

- Intravenous (IV) infusion
  - To reduce pain at the injection site, offer to use topical anesthetic preparations (eg, lidocaine/prilocaine) with occlusive dressing 30–60 minutes prior to IV access attempt
  - IV access may be more difficult to obtain in young children because they have small veins covered by SQ fat
  - It is difficult to secure IV access in small children
  - There is a greater incidence of infiltration and phlebitis in children than adults; however, this is the most effective route used to deliver medications during critical illness; when properly administered, IV infusion will lead to complete absorption and rapid attainment of drug levels
  - Check compatibility of the solution
    - Ensure IV medications, flushes, and parenteral nutritional fluids infused in the same IV line are physically and chemically compatible
    - In infants, hyperosmolar drugs must be diluted to prevent radical fluid shifts that may cause intracerebral hemorrhage
  - Use an arm board when necessary
  - Use soft restraints to minimize movement and risk of kinking or dislodgment
- IM injection
  - Skeletal muscle mass is decreased in newborns and critically ill children
  - Do not use lidocaine as a diluent for drugs needing reconstitution; doing so places the patient at risk for local anesthetic toxicity
  - Reconstitute medication in the highest concentration possible to avoid having to administer two separate injections to give the entire dose
  - The optimum site for IM injection depends on the child's age
    - < 3 years old: vastus lateralus (lateral thigh) muscle
    - > 3 years old: gluteus muscle or ventrogluteal area

- Appropriate needle size depends on the child's age and muscle mass
  - ⅝-inch needle is usually used in young infants
  - Children or thin, debilitated adolescents may require a 1-inch or smaller (⅝-in.) needle
  - For most children and adolescents, use a 1-inch or 1½-inch needle, respectively
- Needle gauge is determined by the viscosity of the drug formulation
  - A 19-gauge needle is used for viscous drugs (eg, penicillin G procaine)
  - A 21-gauge needle is used for aqueous formulations (eg, penicillin G)
- To avoid unnecessary tissue damage, use the shortest length and highest gauge needle
- The optimum amount of drug to administer via an IM site varies with the child's age, size, and health; volume is generally ≤ 2 mL
- Before IM injection
  - Explain that the injection will hurt, but that the medicine will help
  - If necessary, restrain the child
  - Always offer comfort after injection
  - Rotate sites
- See Table 39-3 for examples of antibiotics that can be given intramuscularly

• SQ injection
- Infants and children have less SQ fat than adults
- The SQ injection procedure is similar to IM injection, but uses shorter needles, and volume should be limited to ≤ 1.5 mL
- Use a 25-gauge to 27.5-gauge
  - For infants and small children ≤ 3 years old, use a ⅜-inch or ½-inch needle
  - For larger children, use a ⅝-inch needle
  - Obese children and adolescents may require a 1-inch needle

• Inhalants
- Correct administration depends on child's cooperation
- Inhalants can be used in children as young as 3 months

Table 39-3. Common Intramuscular Antimicrobial Medications Used in Children

Drug Name	Concentration (mg/mL)	Dosage Range (mg/kg/day)	Interval (h)	Maximum Dose	Change Dose/ Interval Due to Renal Dysfunction	Comments
Ampicillin	250	50–400	6	12 g/day	Yes	3 mEq Na^+/1 g ampicillin; use within 1 h of reconstitution
Cefazolin	225 or 330*	40–100	6–8	6 g/day	Yes	2 mEq Na^+/1 g cefazolin
Cefepime	280	50–150	8	2 g/dose, 6 g/day	Yes	No dosage adjustment for burn patients
Ceftriaxone	350	50–100	12	2 g/dose, 4 g/day	No	3.6 mEq Na^+/1 g ceftriaxone May cause primary cholelithiasis, nephrolithiasis, and hemolytic anemia; gallstones resolve after discontinuation Not recommended for neonates with hyperbilirubinemia
Gentamicin	40	2.0–3.5 or 5.0–7.5	8 or 24	According to serum levels	Yes	Peak concentration 4–12 µg/mL (2–3 times higher with once-daily dosing regimen) Trough concentration 0.5–2 µg/mL Contains sulfites, which may exacerbate asthma symptoms May cause cochlear and/or vestibular ototoxicity

*This concentration is only approved for use with the 1-g vial.

old if an appropriate spacer (valved-holding chamber with mask) is available
  - New spacers should be primed with 16 puffs of an albuterol metered-dose inhaler if they are not already static free
  - Clean spacer with warm water and mild soap every week to minimize bacterial contamination; do not rinse soap from the inside of holding chamber; the soap film acts as a surfactant and reduces static charge so that medication particles do not adhere to the sides of the chamber
  - Use a different spacer for each child (do not share spacers)
  - If a nebulizer is to be used to deliver medication, the child needs to wear the mask at all times during drug delivery
    - Nebulized medicines with a blow-by technique lose 90% of drug delivery
  - Common spacer instructions (spacer instructions may vary; read package insert for specific instructions):
    - Shake canister well before each puff
    - Properly assemble canister-spacer
    - Inhale and exhale slowly (if possible)
    - Place spacer mouthpiece between lips (or mask on face)
    - Press canister down one time
    - Inhale slowly (if a whistle sound is heard, patient is inhaling too fast)
    - Take spacer out of mouth and close mouth
    - Hold breath for 10 seconds (if unable to hold for 10 sec, exhale and inhale into spacer up to 3 times)
    - Exhale slowly

Emergency Pediatric Drug Therapy

- Requires quick, accurate dosage calculations and proper administration techniques (Table 39-4)
- Many drugs used for pediatric resuscitation are the same as those used for adults, but with different dosages or concentrations based on weight or BSA
- Emergency drug sheets must be filled out individually and kept at the child's bedside
- Medication administered via peripheral vascular access (followed by a flush), a central line, or IO access is equally efficacious

Table 39-4. Drugs Used During Pediatric Cardiopulmonary Arrests

Drug (Generic)	Class	Indications	Dose	Comments
Epinephrine	Catecholamine with α and β effects	Cardiac arrest; symptomatic bradycardia; PEA, VF, VT Use infusion postarrest if intermittent boluses failed to restore perfusing cardiac rhythm	Initial: 0.01 mg/kg IV/IO; 0.10 mg/kg via ET Repeat every 3–5 min during resuscitation	The volume given is always 0.10 mL/kg (ie, 0.10 mL of 1:10,000 solution = 0.01 mg/kg) For ET delivery (0.10 mL of 1:1,000 solution = 0.10 mg/kg) Follow with 5-cc NS flush Can cause local tissue necrosis
Atropine	Parasympatholytic agent	Symptomatic bradycardia refractory to optimal airway management	0.02 mg/kg IV, IO, ETT Min dose: 0.1 mg Max dose: child = 0.5 mg adolescent = 1 mg	CO is HR-dependent Symptomatic bradycardia MUST be treated Doses < minimum recommend may cause bradycardia in infants
Adenosine	Antiarrhythmic agent	Reentrant SVT	Initial: 0.1 mg/kg rapid IV /IO bolus Repeat dose: 0.2 mg/kg Max single dose: 12 mg	Short half-life; bolus rapidly and as centrally as possible Follow immediately with 5–10-cc NS flush via 3-way stopcock Be alert for possible asthma exacerbation
Sodium bicarbonate	Alkalinizing agent	Documented severe metabolic acidosis due to prolonged arrest; hyperkalemia; TCA overdose	1 mEq/kg IV or IO May empirically dose 0.5 mEq/kg every 10 min over 1–2 min if ABG results not available	Infuse slowly and only if ventilation is adequate May decrease ionized Ca^{2+} levels May cause Na^+ and H_2O overload

(**Table 39-4** *continues*)

Table 39-4 *continued*

Glucose	Carbohydrate	Hypoglycemia	0.5–1 g/kg IV (1–2 mL/kg 50%; 2–4 mL/kg 25%; 5–10 mL/kg 10%) Max concentration: $D_{25}W$	Hypertonic glucose ($D_{25}W$ or $D_{50}W$) may harden peripheral veins if it extravasates Do not exceed 12.5% glucose in neonates
Calcium chloride	Calcium salt	Hypocalcemia, hyperkalemia	0.2 mL/kg of elemental calcium (20 mg/kg) Repeat after 10 min prn if ionized calcium deficiency persists	Infuse no faster than 100 mg/min. May induce bradycardia or asystole, especially if patient is also on digoxin Extravasation can cause chemical burn or sclerosis of peripheral veins
Naloxone	Narcotic agonist	Narcotic poisoning	**Birth–5 y (≤ 20 lb)**: 0.1 mg/kg IV/ETT > 5 y (≥ 20 lb): 0.4–2 mg/dose IV/ETT **Continuous infusion**: 0.04–0.16 mg/kg/h, titrated to effect	Rare side effects usually related to abrupt narcotic reversal Administer with caution immediately after birth to infants of addicted mothers to avoid abrupt withdrawal and seizures in infant
Magnesium sulfate	Antiarrhythmic agent; electrolyte	Hypomagnesemia; torsades de pointes	25–50 mg/kg IV/IO (max dose: 2 g/dose)	Monitor serum Mg^{2+} level Use with caution in patients also on digoxin (can lead to heart block)
Lidocaine	Antiarrhythmic agent	Ventricular dysrhythmias	**Loading**: 1 mg/kg **Infusion**: 20–50 μg/kg/min (concentration: 120 mg lidocaine/100 mL D_5W)	Toxic levels can cause myocardial, circulatory, and/or CNS depression Metabolized by the liver

Table 39-4 notes:

ABG: arterial blood gas
CNS: central nervous system
CO: cardiac output
D_5W: 5% dextrose in water
$D_{25}W$: 25% dextrose in water
$D_{50}W$: 50% dextrose in water
ET: endotracheal
ETT: endotracheal tube
HR: heart rate
IO: intraosseous
IV: intravenous
NS: normal saline
PEA: pulseless electrical activity
prn: pro re nata (as needed)
SVT: supraventricular tachycardia
TCA: tricyclic antidepressant
VF: ventricular fibrillation
VT: ventricular tachycardia

- The endotracheal route may be used to administer epinephrine, atropine, and lidocaine
  - Usually the dose is 1½–10-fold that for the IV route
  - Follow drug administration with a 5-cc flush of normal saline to aid in drug delivery to the peripheral airways
  - Endotracheal administration of drugs is no longer recommended by the Neonatal Resuscitation Program
- Usual maximum volume for IM administration:
  - Neonate: 0.5 mL
  - Children: 1–2 mL
  - Adult: 2–3 mL

Further Reading

1. Phelps SJ, HakEB, Crill CM. *Pediatric Injectable Drugs: The Teddy Bear Book*. 8th ed. Bethesda, Md: American Society of Health-System Pharmacists; 2007.

2. Taketomo CT, Hodding JH, Kraus DM. *Pediatric Dosage Handbook: Including Neonatal Dosing, Drug Administration, & Extemporaneous Preparations*. 16th ed. Hudson, Ohio: American Pharmaceutical Association-Lexicomp; 2009.

3. Custer JW, Rau RE, Lee CK. *The Harriet Lane Handbook: Mobile Medicine Series, Expert Consult: Online and Print*. 18th ed. Philadelphia, Pa: Mosby; 2008.

4. Mosteller RD. Simplified calculation of body surface area. *N Engl J Med*. 1987;317(17):1098 (Letter).

5. Lam TK, Leung DT. Moreon simplified calculation of body surface area. *N Engl J Med*. 1998;318(17):1098 (Letter).

6. Pagliaro LA, Pagliaro AM. *Problems in Pediatric Drug Therapy*. 4th ed. Washington, DC: American Pharmaceutical Association; 2002.

ABBREVIATIONS AND ACRONYMS

A

ABC: airway, breathing, circulation
ABCDE: airway, breathing, circulation, disability, exposure/environmental control
ABG: arterial blood gas
ACLS: Advanced Cardiac Life Support
ADH: antidiuretic hormone
ADR: adverse drug reaction
AE: aeromedical evacuation
AF: activity factor
AKO: Army Knowledge Online
AMP: ampicillin
AMPLE: allergies, medications, past illnesses, last meal, events/environment
AMX: amoxicillin
aPTT: activated partial thromboplastin time
ARDS: acute respiratory distress syndrome
ATLS: Advanced Trauma Life Support
AV: arteriovenous
AVA: anthrax vaccine adsorbed
AVM: arteriovenous malformations

B

b-hCG: β-human chorionic gonadotrophin
BP: blood pressure
BPM: beats per minute or breaths per minute
BSA: body surface area
BUN: blood urea nitrogen

C

CA: clavulanic acid
CaEDTA: edetate calcium disodium
cAMP: cyclic adenosine monophosphate
CaO_2: changes in arterial oxygen concentration
CAR: cabin altitude restriction

CBC: complete blood count
CBRNE: chemical, biological, radiological, nuclear, and explosive
CCATTs: Critical Care Air Transport Teams
CHF: congestive heart failure
CI: cardiac index
Cl_{Cr}: creatinine clearance
CN: cranial nerve
CNS: central nervous system
CO: cardiac output
COMM: commercial
CONUS: continental United States
CPAP: continuous positive airway pressure
CPK-MB: creatine phosphokinase, muscle band
CPP: cerebral perfusion pressure
CPR: cardiopulmonary resuscitation
CRP: C-reactive protein
CRT: capillary refill time
CSF: cerebrospinal fluid
CSH: combat support hospital
CSW: cerebral salt wasting
CT: computed tomography
CTG: childhood traumatic grief
CVP: central venous pressure

D

D_5W: 5% dextrose in water
$D_{25}W$: 25% dextrose in water
$D_{50}W$: 50% dextrose in water
DIC: disseminated intravascular coagulation
DKA: diabetic ketoacidosis
DM1: diabetes mellitus type 1
DM2: diabetes mellitus type 2
DNA: deoxyribonucleic acid
DSN: Defense Switched Network
DTPA: diethylenetriaminepentaacetic acid

E

EA: esophageal atresia
EBV: estimated blood volume

ECG: electrocardiogram
EEG: electroencephalogram
EFA: essential fatty acid
eGFR: estimated glomerular filtration rate
ERCP: endoscopic retrograde cholangiopancreatography
ES: extra strength
ESR: erythrocyte sedimentation rate
ET: endotracheal
ETT: endotracheal tube

F

FAST: focused assessment with sonography for trauma
FDA: Food and Drug Administration
FFP: fresh frozen plasma
FiO_2: fraction of inspired oxygen
FISH: fluorescence in situ hybridization
FWWB: fresh warm whole blood

G

G6PD: glucose-6-phosphate dehydrogenase
GABHS: group A β-hemolytic streptococci
GCS: Glasgow Coma Scale
GE: gastroesophageal
GFR: glomerular filtration rate
GI: gastrointestinal
GPMRC: Global Patient Movement Requirements Center

H

HCT: hematocrit
HgB: hemoglobin
Hib: *Haemophilus influenzae* type B
HIV: human immunodeficiency virus
HPS: hypertrophic pyloric stenosis
HR: heart rate
HSV: herpes simplex virus
HUS: hemolytic uremic syndrome
Hx: history

I

ICP: intracranial pressure
ICU: intensive care unit

IDA: information-decision-action
IgM: immunoglobulin M
IM: intramuscular
IMV: intermittent mandatory ventilation
IO: intraosseous
iPTH: intact parathyroid hormone
IRM: intermediate restorative material
ITP: idiopathic thrombocytopenic purpura
IU: international unit
IV: intravenous
IVF: intravenous fluid
IVIG: intravenous immunoglobulin

K
KUB: kidney, ureter, and bladder

L
LFT: liver function test

M
MCHC: mean corpuscular hemoglobin concentration
MCV: mean corpuscular volume
MDI: metered-dose inhaler
$MgSO_4$: magnesium sulfate
MRCP: magnetic resonance cholangiopancreatography
MRI: magnetic resonance imaging
MSL: mean sea level

N
NE: norepinephrine
neb: nebulized
NG: nasogastric
nl: normal
NO: nitric oxide
NPH: Neutral Protamine Hagedorn
NPO: nil per os (nothing by mouth)
NRP: Neonatal Resuscitation Program
NS: normal saline

O
OEF: Operation Enduring Freedom

OIF: Operation Iraqi Freedom
OM: otitis media
ORS: oral rehydration solution

P
$PaCO_2$: partial pressure of carbon dioxide in arterial blood
PALS: pediatric advanced life support
2-PAM Cl: pralidoxime chloride
PaO_2: partial pressure of oxygen in arterial blood
PC: pressure control
PCA: patient-controlled analgesia
PCO_2: partial pressure of carbon dioxide
PE: physical examination
PEA: pulseless electrical activity
PEEP: positive end-expiratory pressure
PEFR: peak expiratory flow rate
PFA: psychological first aid
PICU: pediatric intensive care unit
PIP: peak inspiratory pressure
PMR: patient movement request
PMRC: patient movement requirements center
PO: per os (by mouth)
PRBC: packed red blood cell
prn: pro re nata (as needed)
PS: pressure support
PT: prothrombin time
PTU: propylthiouracil
PVC: premature ventricular contraction
PVR: pulmonary vascular resistance

R
RBC: red blood cell
RDW: red cell distribution width
REE: resting energy expenditure
RNA: ribonucleic acid
RSV: respiratory syncytial virus

S
SAM: structural aluminum malleable
SaO_2: arterial oxygen saturation

sat: saturation
SD: standard deviation
SF: stress factor
SIADH: syndrome of inappropriate antidiuretic hormone
SIPRNet: Secure Internet Protocol Router Network
SJS: Stevens-Johnson syndrome
SMX: sulfamethoxazole
SPT: suprapubic tube
SQ: subcutaneous
SVR: systemic vascular resistance
SVT: supraventricular tachycardia

T

TB: tuberculosis
TBSA: total body surface area
TBW: total body water
TCA: tricyclic antidepressant
TEE: total energy expenditure
TEF: tracheoesophageal fistula
TEN: toxic epidermal necrolysis
TF: tube feeding
TMP: trimethoprim
TPMRC-E: Theater Patient Movement Requirements Center–Europe
TPMRC-P: Theater Patient Movement Requirements Center–Pacific
TPN: total parenteral nutrition
TRAC2ES: TRANSCOM Regulating and Command and Control Evacuation System
TRANSCOM: US Transportation Command
TTP: thrombotic thrombocytopenic purpura

U

UA: urinary analysis
UDT: undescended testes
UGI: upper gastrointestinal
UPJ: ureteropelvic junction
URI: upper respiratory infection
USAF: US Air Force
UTI: urinary tract infection

V

VACTERRL: vertebral, anorectal, cardiac, tracheoesophageal fistula, renal, and radial limb
VATS: video-assisted thoracoscopic surgery
VBG: venous blood gas
VF: ventricular fibrillation
Vt: tidal volume
VT: ventricular tachycardia

W

WBC: white blood cell
WHO: World Health Organization

INDEX

D